Diagnosis and Therapies in Chinese Medicine

Diagnosis and Therapies in Chinese Medicine

Edited by **Patrick Lampard**

Callisto Reference
New York

Published by Callisto Reference,
106 Park Avenue, Suite 200,
New York, NY 10016, USA
www.callistoreference.com

Diagnosis and Therapies in Chinese Medicine
Edited by Patrick Lampard

International Standard Book Number: 978-1-63239-725-6 (Hardback)

Printed in China.

Contents

Preface

Chinese Medicine is an ancient science and is still used as a common way of treating disorders. The techniques used in chinese medicine such as acupuncture, massage and exercise and the use of herbal antidotes as opposed to modern medicine, are regarded as efficient ways of treating disorders. It uses the concept of yin and yang to divide the human body and then heal them with respective techniques. This book will discuss in detail the diverse concepts of chinese medicine, its diagnostics and theoretical applications and their efficiency. For readers who are interested in this field, the case studies and analysis included in the book will serve as an excellent guide to develop a comprehensive understanding of this field.

This book is the end result of constructive efforts and intensive research done by experts in this field. The aim of this book is to enlighten the readers with recent information in this area of research. The information provided in this profound book would serve as a valuable reference to students and researchers in this field.

At the end, I would like to thank all the authors for devoting their precious time and providing their valuable contributions to this book. I would also like to express my gratitude to my fellow colleagues who encouraged me throughout the process.

Editor

1

The Antidepressant-Like Effects of *Punica granatum* (Pomegranate) Extract in Mice

Mahsa Hadipour Jahromy[1*], Shahrzad Khakpour[2], Zhinoos Khorgami[3]

[1]Department of Pharmacology, Tehran Medical Sciences Branch, Islamic Azad University, Tehran, Iran
[2]Department of Physiology, Tehran Medical Sciences Branch, Islamic Azad University, Tehran, Iran
[3]Iranian Tissue Bank and Research Center, Tehran University of Medical Sciences, Tehran, Iran
Email: [*]Jahromymh@yahoo.com

Abstract

The aim of the present work is to evaluate the putative antidepressant-like effects of pomegranate fruit extract including seeds (PFE) on the performance of male mice in the forced swimming test (FST), after acute administration, after short-term treatment (7 days) and, after repeated administration in a 24-h period (24, 12 and 1 h before swimming test). A single dose (20 ml/kg p.o.) of PFE, in male mice provoked a significant reduction of the immobility time. Such effect was also observed with short-term treatment (7 days) with doses of 1 and 10 ml/kg/day of PFE. Moreover, it was noted that there were important differences in the onset of the antidepressant-like effect in the FST, depending on the modality of treatment with PFE. Both efficacy and potency were higher when repeated administration of PFE was used, and surprisingly the dose of 10 ml/kg (24, 12 and 1 h before swimming test) was as effective as Fluoxetine. In the same way, the short term administration (7 days) improved significantly efficacy and potency of the PFE in comparison to a single dose treatment. These results indicate an antidepressant-like profile of action for PFE which deserves further research.

Keywords

Pomegranate; Antidepressant Effect; Forced Swimming Test

1. Introduction

Depression is a major disease affecting nearly 13% - 20% of the population [1]. Roughly, 90% of patients with depressive symptoms suffer from mild to moderate depression, while only 10% are severely depressed. In mild

[*]Corresponding author.

to moderate depression, in particular, some practitioners and patients are reluctant to use standard antidepressants like tricyclic antidepressants or specific serotonin reuptake inhibitors (SSRIs), because of their side effects. Therefore, additional treatment strategies with fewer side effect profile, credible benefits and moderate costs are of particular interest [2] [3]. In the search for new molecules useful for the treatment of neurological disorders, medicinal plant research, worldwide, has progressed constantly, demonstrating the pharmacological effectiveness of different plant species in a variety of animal models [4]. At the present time, forced swimming test (FST) is the most widely used model for assessing potential antidepressant activity in rodents, following acute and short-term treatment [5].

Pomegranate (*Punica granatum*), a small tree originating in the Orient, belongs to the Punicaceae family [6]. It is grown mainly in Iran, India and in most Near and Far East countries. The main use of pomegranate is as table fruit, but large amounts are used in the beverage and liquor industries [7]. In folk medicine, pomegranate preparations have a number of therapeutic actions [8].

The edible part of pomegranate is rich in anthocyanins thus; the major class of phytochemical present in pomegranate is the polyphenols and includes flavonoids, condensed tannins and hydrolysable tannins. Hydrolysable tannins are predominant polyphenols found in pomegranate juice and account for 92% of its antioxidant activity [9] [10].

The present research was undertaken to study the duration of immobility in mice in the FST, after acute administration, after short-term treatment (7 days) and, after repeated administration in a 24-h period (24, 12 and 1 h before swimming test) following oral ingestion of a standardized preparation of pomegranate fruit extract (PFE).

2. Materials and Methods

2.1. Pomegranate Extract

Pomegranates (*Punica granatum* L.), was collected by one of the colleagues from the agriculture garden (under supervision of Agricultural Research Organization in Fars Province) in Shiraz, a city where known to have one of the best pomegranate native in Iran. Then washed, chilled to 4˚C, and stored. The seeds of the fruit containing the intact juice sacs were manually separated from the pericarp, and the whole juice extracted by the aid of electric juicer so that seeds break. Then filtered and stored in clean jars in fridge.

2.2. Animals

Male BALB/c mice, weighing 25 - 30 g were used in these experiments. They were group housed under the following laboratory conditions: temperature 23˚C ± 1˚C, humidity 40% - 60%, 12 h:12 h L/D cycle, lights on at 07:00 h. Food and water were available *ad libitum*. All the experiments were carried out between 10:00 and 15:00 h in testing rooms adjacent to the animal rooms. Each experimental group consisted of ten mice. Mice were treated in accordance with the current law and the NIH Guide for the Care and Use of Laboratory.

2.3. Drugs

Fluoxetine (Sigma) were suspended in normal saline (0.9% NaCl).

2.4. Behavioral Tests

This test was performed according to the procedure described by Porsolt *et al.* [11]-[13], with slight modifications [14]. Briefly, 1 h after dosing, the animals were individually forced to swim in a transparent glass vessel (25 cm high, 15 cm in diameter) filled with (12.5 cm high) water at 21˚C - 24˚C. The total duration of immobility (in seconds) was measured during the last 4 min of a single 6 min test session. Five groups of 10 mice were treated acutely with single dose of vehicle, PFE (1, 10 and 20 ml/kg) p.o. (Gavage), Fluoxetine i.p. (10 mg/kg) and 1 h later mice were individually forced to swim in the glass vessel. Other five groups of mice were short-term treated (7 days) with a single daily dose of vehicle, PFE (1, 10 and 20 ml/kg) p.o., or Fluoxetine i.p. (10 mg/kg), and 1 h after the last administration they were individually forced to swim in same conditions. In a different set of experiments, five groups of 10 animals were subjected to repeated administration of three doses of vehicle, PFE using 1, 10 and 20 ml/kg p.o., Fluoxetine i.p. (10 mg/kg), 24, 12 and 1 h prior to the swimming test. Behaviour was monitored from the frontal side by a video camera for subsequent analysis. Mice were considered immobile when they made no further attempts to escape except the movements necessary to keep their heads above the water.

2.5. Statistical Analysis

The results are expressed as mean ± S.D, and statistical analysis of the data was performed by Origin VI. $^{***}p < 0.001$; $^{**}p < 0.01$ were considered significantly different from vehicle, after non-parametric ANOVA.

3. Results

Effects of PFE on the Immobility Time

A significant shortening of the immobility time was observed when an acute dose of either 20 ml/kg p.o., of PFE ($p < 0.01$) or fluoxetine (10 mg/kg i.p.) ($p < 0.001$) was administered to mice compared to vehicle treated animals. The reduction of immobility time, between these two mentioned groups was at the same level, statistically (**Figure 1**). Short-term treatment (7 days) induced a decrease of the immobility time when the animals were exposed to the FST after dosing orally, once a day, with 1 ($p < 0.001$) and 10 ($p < 0.001$) ml/kg of PFE (**Figure 1**). In addition, repeated administration in a 24 h period showed a significant reduction of the immobility time with 1 ($p < 0.01$) and 10 ml/kg ($p < 0.001$) of PFE in different groups of mice submitted to FST in comparison to control group (**Figure 2**).

4. Discussion

The present study characterized the effects of the administration of PFE on mice performance in FST following acute, short-term and repeated treatment. In many previous papers the antioxidant and anti-inflammatory properties of pomegranate fruit juice in animal labs has been emphasized [15]-[18]. Also, it has been reported that Pomegranate extract improves a depressive state and bone properties in menopausal syndrome model ovariectomized mice [19]. Besides that, it was demonstrated that PFE exhibits low toxicity, no lethality, was well tolerated, did not induce significant changes in several behavioural and physiological parameters and is devoid of any hypnosedative activity, when administered to mice [15]. Recently, the antidepressant action of some herbal medicines has been reported focusing on polyphenols as their major component [3] [4] [14]. The edible part of pomegranate is rich in anthocyanins thus; the major class of phytochemical present in pomegranate is the polyphenols.

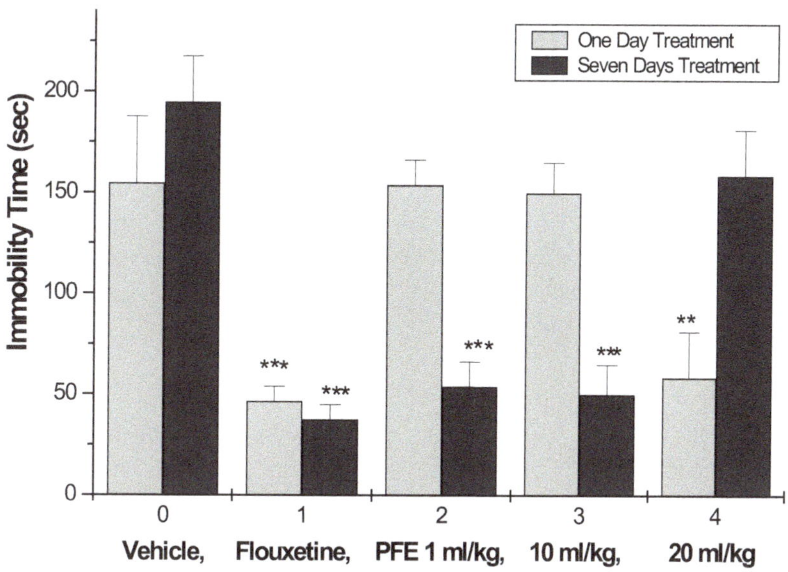

Figure 1. Effect of the vehicle, fluoxetine (10 mg/kg, i.p.) and increasing single doses of PFE (1, 10 and 20 ml/kg p.o) on the forced swimming test (FTS) in mice. Each bar represents the mean ± SD of 10 animals. $^{***}p < 0.001$; $^{**}p < 0.01$, significantly different from vehicle, after non-parametric ANOVA.

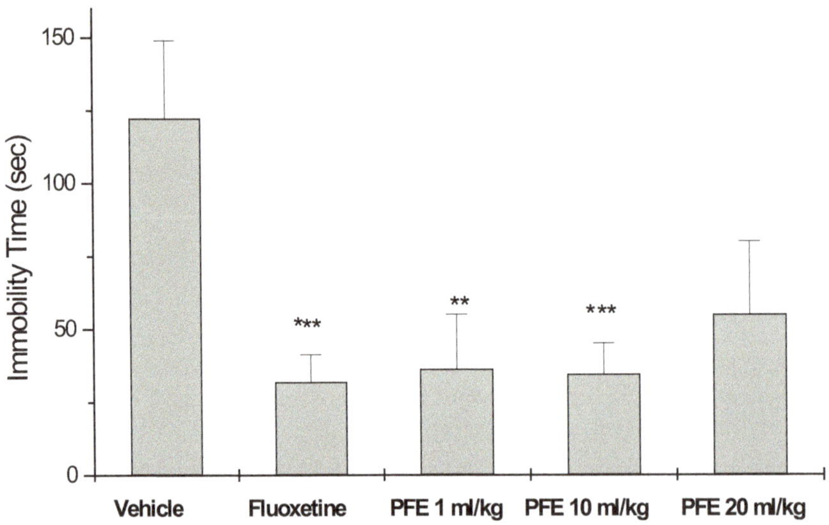

Figure 2. Effect of repeated administration of three doses in 24 h of vehicle, fluoxetine (10 mg/kg i.p) and increasing doses of PFE (1, 10, and 20 ml/kg p.o) on the forced swimming test (FTS) in mice. Each bar represents the mean ± SD of 10 animals. $^{***}p < 0.001$; $^{**}p < 0.01$, significantly different from vehicle, after non-parametric ANOVA.

Because the pharmacotherapy of depression typically requires chronic drug treatment to obtain a full response in terms of antidepressant effect, it is critical to perform, not only acute, but also short-term, chronic and repeated treatments in the FST mice model. Certainly, the administration of PFE produced a diminution of immobility time of mice exposed to the FST under acute, short-term or repeated modalities. Indeed, single dose of 20 ml/kg p.o., of PFE provoked a highly significant reduction of immobility time ($p < 0.01$). Similar results were also observed with short-term treatment (7 days) with single dose of 1 ($p < 0.001$), and 10 ($p < 0.001$) ml/kg/day of PFE, but not with higher dose. Additionally, in a different set of experiments, repeated administration in a 24-h period (24, 12 and 1 h before swimming) doses of 1 ($p < 0.01$) and 10 ($p < 0.001$) ml/kg p.o., of PFE provoke significant reduction of the immobility time of male mice subjected to the FST, when compared to control group (vehicle) but not with higher dose. It is important to note that although single acute high dose, showed antidepressant effect as fluoxetine, no significant effects observed in high dose of 20 mg/kg of PFE in repeated administration. This can be interpreted as acute tolerance or tacyfilaxy that might have happened in receptor responses. Moreover, depending on the modality of treatment with PFE (acute, short-term or repeated) in the FST, it was observed important differences in the onset of the antidepressant-like effect. In fact, both efficacy and potency of PFE as antidepressant were higher when repeated administration was used, and interestingly 10 mg/kg (24, 12 and 1 h before swimming) was as effective as fluoxetine (10 mg kg i.p.) used as positive control. In the same way, the short term administration (7 days), improves significantly the efficacy and potency of the PFE, in comparison to single dose treatments. These behavioural effects were similar to those seen in mice treated with conventional antidepressant drugs, such as tricyclic, monoamine oxidase inhibitors and selective serotonine reuptake inhibitors agents [5] [11] [20].

5. Conclusion

In conclusion, the results of this preclinical study provide evidence about the antidepressant effects of the pomegranate fruit extract administered either acute or repeatedly in mice. These results contribute to the scientific validation of the indications of this plant in Iranian folk medicine. However, further experiments are needed to identify its active compounds and the corresponding mechanisms of action. Our results encourage us to pursue the identification of the molecules associated to the effect observed in PFE.

Acknowledgements

The authors would like to thank M. Aghakhani, for his help during experiments. The experimental work has been done at physiology and pharmacology laboratory of medical sciences research center, Tehran Medical Sciences Branch, Islamic Azad University.

References

[1] Licinio, J. and Wong, M.L. (1999) The Role of Inflammatory Mediators in the Biology of Major Depression: Central Nervous System Cytokines Modulate the Biological Substrate of Depressive Symptoms, Regulate Stress-Responsive Systems, and Contribute to Neurotoxicity and Neuroprotection. *Molecular Psychiatry*, **4**, 317-327.

[2] Ernst, E. (1995) St. John's Wort, an Antidepressant? A Systematic, Criteria-Based Review. *Phytomedicine*, **2**, 67-71. http://dx.doi.org/10.1016/S0944-7113(11)80051-6

[3] Laakmann, G., Dienel, A. and Kieser, M. (1998) Clinical Significance of Hyperforin for the Efficacy of Hypericum Extracts on Depressive Disorders of Different Severities. *Phytomedicine*, **5**, 435-442. http://dx.doi.org/10.1016/S0944-7113(98)80039-1

[4] Zhang, Z.J. (2004) Therapeutic Effects of Herbal Extracts and Constituents in Animal Models of Psychiatric Disorders. *Life Sciences*, **75**, 1659-1699. http://dx.doi.org/10.1016/j.lfs.2004.04.014

[5] Cryan, J.F., Page, M.E. and Lucki, I. (2005) Differential Behavioural Effects of the Antidepressant Reboxetine, Fluoxetine, and Moclobemide in a Modified Forced Swim Test Following Chronic Treatment. *Psychopharmacology*, **182**, 335-344. http://dx.doi.org/10.1007/s00213-005-0093-5

[6] Harde, H., Schumacher, W., Firbas, F. and Denffer, D. (1970) Strasburg's Textbook of Botany.

[7] Nagy, P., Shaw, P.E. and Wardowski, W.F. (1990) Fruits of Tropical and Subtropical Origin.

[8] Bianchini, F. and Corbetta, F. (1979) Health Plants of the World.

[9] Longtin, R. (2003) The Pomegranate: Nature's Power Fruit? *Journal of the National Cancer Institute*, **95**, 346-348. http://dx.doi.org/10.1093/jnci/95.5.346

[10] Gil, M.I., Tomas-Barberan, F.A., Hess-Pierce, B., Holcraft, D.M. and Kedar, A.A. (2000) Antioxidant Activity of Pomegranate Juice and Its Relationship with Phenolic Composition and Processing. *Journal of Agricultural and Food Chemistry*, **10**, 4581-4589. http://dx.doi.org/10.1021/jf000404a

[11] Porsolt, R.D., Le Pichon, M. and Jalfre, M. (1977) Depression: A New Animal Model Sensitive to Antidepressant Treatments. *Nature*, **266**, 730-732. http://dx.doi.org/10.1038/266730a0

[12] Porsolt, R.D., Brossard, G., Hautbois, C. and Roux, S. (2001) Rodent Models of Depression: Forced Swimming and Tail Suspension Behavioural Despair Tests in Rats and Mice. In: Crawley, J.N., Ed., *Current Protocols in Neuroscience*, John Wiley & Sons, Inc., Hoboken, pp. 8.10A.1-8.10A.10.

[13] Petit-Demouliere, B., Chenu, F. and Bourin, M. (2005) Forced Swimming Test in Mice: A Review of Antidepressant Activity. *Psychopharmacology*, **177**, 245-255. http://dx.doi.org/10.1007/s00213-004-2048-7

[14] Hellión-Ibarrola, M.C., Ibarrola, D.A., Montalbetti, Y., Kennedy, M.L., Heinichen, O., Campuzano, M., Ferro, E.A., Alvarenga, N., Tortoriello, J., De Lima, T.C. and Mora, S. (2008) The Antidepressant-Like Effects of *Aloysia polystachya* (Griseb.) Moldenke (Verbenaceae) in Mice. *Phytomedicine*, **15**, 478-483.

[15] Lansky, E.P. and Newmana, R.A. (2007) *Punica granatum* (Pomegranate) and Its Potential for Prevention and Treatment of Inflammation and Cancer. *Journal of Ethnopharmacology*, **109**, 177-206. http://dx.doi.org/10.1016/j.jep.2006.09.006

[16] Schubert, S.Y., Lansky, E.Ph. and Neeman, I. (1999) Antioxidant and Eicosanoid Enzyme Inhibition Properties of Pomegranate Seed Oil and Fermented Juice Flavonoids. *Journal of Ethnopharmacology*, **66**, 11-17. http://dx.doi.org/10.1016/S0378-8741(98)00222-0

[17] N.P. Seeram, L.S. Adams, S.M. Henning, Y.T. Niu, Y.J. Zhang, M.G. Nair and D. Heber (2005) *In Vitro* Antiproliferative, Apoptotic and Antioxidant Activities of Punicalagin, Ellagic acid and a Total Pomegranate Tannin Extract Are Enhanced in Combination with Other Polyphenols as Found in Pomegranate Juice. *The Journal of Nutritional Biochemistry*, **16**, 360-367. http://dx.doi.org/10.1016/j.jnutbio.2005.01.006

[18] Aslama, M.N., Lansky, E.Ph. and Varani, J. (2006) Pomegranate as a Cosmeceutical Source: Pomegranate Fractions Promote Proliferation and Procollagen Synthesis and Inhibit Matrix Metalloproteinase-1 Production in Human Skin Cells. *Journal of Ethnopharmacology*, **103**, 311-318. http://dx.doi.org/10.1016/j.jep.2005.07.027

[19] Mori-Okamoto, J., Otawara-Hamamoto, Y., Yamato, H. and Yoshimur, H. (2004) Pomegranate Extract Improves a Depressive State and Bone Properties in Menopausal Syndrome Model Ovariectomized Mice. *Journal of Ethnopharmacology*, **92**, 93-101. http://dx.doi.org/10.1016/j.jep.2004.02.006

[20] Borsini, F. and Meli, A. (1988) Is the Forced Swimming Test a Suitable Model for Revealing Antidepressant Activity? *Psychopharmacology* (*Berlin*), **94**, 147-160.

Note List of Abbreviations

Pomegranate fruit extract (PFE)
Forced swimming test (FST)
Specific serotonin reuptake inhibitors (SSRIs)

2

Enhanced Satellite Cell Activity in Aging Skeletal Muscle after Manual Acupuncture-Induced Injury

Sonya K. Sobrian[1*], Eric Walters[2]

[1]Department of Pharmacology, Howard University College of Medicine, Washington, USA
[2]Department of Biochemistry and Molecular Biology, Howard University College of Medicine, Washington, USA
Email: *ssobrian@howard.edu

Abstract

Skeletal muscle injury stimulates normally quiescent resident satellite (stem) cells to re-enter the cell cycle and execute the myogenic program to restore muscle structure and function. Previously, we reported that manual acupuncture needling of the tibialis anterior (TA) (ST36 = Zusanli) muscle of young male rats produced focal injury and morphological changes that accompanied the presence of activated satellite cells (SC) 72 hours post-needling. To investigate whether aging TA muscle responds in a similar fashion to acupuncture needling, 17-month-old female rats were subjected to a single insertion and manual manipulation of an acupuncture needle. At 72 hours' post-needling, hematoxylin staining of the TA revealed increased mononuclear cell infiltration that was indicative of localized injury. Moreover, this was accompanied by a four-fold increase in the expression of proliferating cell nuclear antigen within cells of needled tissues. Heightened immunofluorescence for MyoD was found within SC in the needled muscle, which correlated with a 6- and 10-fold increase in two MyoD isoforms (~38 and 42 kDa, respectively), when analyzed by Western blotting. An additional 56 kDa MyoD immunoreactive species was observed in both needled and control muscle of the aging rats. The present study in pre-senile female rats, in conjunction with our previous study in young male rats, suggests that muscle remodeling and restructuring after injury may constitute the initial cellular and molecular mechanisms that underlie the benefits associated with acupuncture throughout the life-span.

Keywords

Aging Rat; Manual Acupuncture; Muscle Injury; Regeneration; ST 36 = Zusanli; Stem Cells

*Corresponding author.

1. Introduction

Skeletal muscle contains specialized somatic stem cells that are termed satellite cells (SC) because of their location on the periphery of myofibers under the surrounding basal lamina [1] [2]. These resident satellite cells are responsible for muscle growth and repair after injury throughout the life span [3]. In normal undisturbed muscle, these cells remain in a quiescent stage [4]. After muscle injury, satellite cells become mitotically active. The transcription factor MyoD is essential for promoting gene expression that regulates proliferation, differentiation and the regeneration of new muscle fiber [3]-[6]. The activated phenotype is defined by the presence of MyoD [7].

Satellite cell activation, which is necessary for muscle regeneration, has been analyzed using experimental models that induce injury by crushing [4], or injection of notexin [8] [9]. These methods are, however, invasive and/or prohibited in therapeutic settings, and may produce extensive damage to elements within muscle that are crucial for regeneration [10]. In contrast, muscle injury as a consequence of exercise can also activate satellite cell proliferation in both humans and laboratory animals [11] [12]. There is an increasing acceptance of acupuncture as a treatment modality for a variety of muscle-related illnesses [13], and acupuncture needling has been shown to provide clinically relevant short- and long-term benefits for low back pain, osteoarthritis, rheumatoid arthritis, chronic neck pain, myofacial pain syndrome, and headache [14] [15]. In Chinese medicine, disease is understood as a consequence of an imbalance in energy flow within 12 channels, or meridians, throughout the body [16], and acupuncture needling is thought to restore healthy energy balance [17]. While data from clinical and experimental studies indicated participation of both the central and peripheral nervous systems, and the involvement of psychological and physiological responses [18], the exact mechanism of action for acupuncture's efficacy has not been elucidated. We previously hypothesized that therapeutic potential of acupuncture was linked to regenerative processes that follow muscle injury induced by needle manipulation, and demonstrated that acupuncture needling of the tibialis anterior (TA) muscle in young male rats produced focal muscle damage that was accompanied by the presence of activated satellite cells [19]. In contrast to the regenerative potential seen in young muscle, the general consensus is that with increasing age there is a decline in skeletal muscle's response to injury. Although satellite cells exist in muscle from birth through senescence [20], their repair capacity [21]-[23], the regenerative potential of satellite cells [24]-[26], and aspects of the regenerative response are impaired in aging muscle [27].

This reduced regenerative capacity of aging muscle has been partially attributed to decreases in the number of available satellite cells [28]-[30]. While most studies, especially those in rodent, suggest a gradual decline in SC number with increasing age [28]-[34], there are inconsistencies. Similar numbers of SC have been reported between the young and old in both humans and animals [22] [35]-[38]; in addition, relative increases in SC numbers have also been observed with aging [24] [39].

There is debate with respect to the functional significance of any change in the number of SCs with increasing age [27]. A reduction in SC number in aged muscle does not appear to affect regeneration or repair, provided that a critical minimum population is present [25] [40] [41]. It is hypothesized that the loss of regenerative potential and generalized atrophy of aged skeletal muscle may be a consequence of an age-related loss of satellite cell function [24] [36]. This loss of functionality may reflect alterations in SC-intrinsic properties, such as erosion of telomere sequences and accumulation of DNA damage [29] [41], diminished responsiveness to intrinsic cues in the niché environment [22] [42], or a decreased responsiveness to systemic signals that govern remodeling and regeneration [24] [27] [41] [43]-[46]. Indeed, the proliferative and regenerative capacities of SC in muscle from old mice are restored after exposure to serum from young mice, or transplantation of aging mouse muscle to a young host [21] [34] [39] [47]-[49]. These observations support the hypothesis that in aging muscle a subset of satellite cells maintains myogenic stem cell properties. Therefore, the purpose of the present study was to assess the effect of manual acupuncture needling on aging tibialis anterior (TA) skeletal muscle by: 1) determining if manual needling produced localized injury to the muscle, and 2) assessing if muscle injury correlated with regeneration processes similar to what was previously observed in young adult rats [19].

2. Material and Methods

2.1. Laboratory Animals

Eight, 17.2 month-old pre-senile female Sprague-Dawley rats (Harlan Sprague-Dawley, Indianapolis, IN), 280 - 360 grams (mean = 324.08 + 10.67 g) were used for this experiment. Female Sprague-Dawley rats gradually cease cycling by 6 - 8 months of age [50] [51], and cease to breed by 15 months of age [52], thus minimizing the influence of estrogen on myogenic satellite cells that has previously been reported [53]-[55]. However, muscle satellite cells from old (>30 months) female rats retain their myogenic potential [56].

Females were housed in groups of 2 in polyethylene shoebox cages (44 × 25 × 30 cm) lined with corncob bedding, under environmentally controlled conditions (0700 hr lights on, 1900 hr lights off, ambient temperature 20˚C - 23˚C, relative humidity 40% - 60%) with *ad libitum* access to Purina Rat Chow and tap water. All procedures were performed with the approval of the Howard University Institutional Animal Care and Use Committee.

2.2. Acupuncture and Muscle Sampling

Rats were lightly anesthetized with sodium pentobarbital (40 mg/kg, i.p.) and a sterile, 0.30 mm diameter stainless steel acupuncture needle (Seirin Co. Ltd., Germany) was inserted perpendicularly into the shaved right hind leg TA muscle, at a point equivalent to human Zusanli (ST 36). The ST 36 acupoint is located 5 mm below and anterior to the tubercle of the tibia [57]. The acupuncture needle was inserted to a depth of 2 mm, and manually twisted from left to right for 20 seconds every 3 min, during the 15 minute session, resulting in 5 needle manipulations. The left TA muscle served as the control; the hind leg was shaved but no needle was inserted [58], in order to avoid the reported controversies associated with the placement of sham needles, which produce biological effects that may complicate interpretation of results [59]. ST 36 is the most commonly targeted acupuncture needle point in both clinical settings [60] and experimental studies [58] [61], and is considered to be more effective in restoring energy balance in humans than other points according to traditional acupuncture medical theory [62].

At 72 hours post-acupuncture, rats were sacrificed and portions of the ST 36 area of the TA muscle (10 × 5 × 4 mm) from both the needled and the contralateral control legs were dissected. Half of the tissue was frozen in liquid nitrogen, and stored at −70˚C. The remaining half of each sample was placed in Prefer fixative (Anatech, Battle Creek, MI), and infiltrated with paraffin [63].

2.3. Histology and Immunohistochemistry

Ten (10) micron paraffin sections of dissected TA muscle were cut and stained with hemotoxylin [64]. Paraffin sections were de-waxed in xylenes, and rehydrated as previously described [63], then treated with sodium citrate buffer (10 mM, pH 6.0) for 30 minutes at 80˚C, and incubated overnight with anti-PCNA antibodies [1:75]. Sections were incubated in biotinylated anti-mouse secondary antibody (Vector Labs), followed by ABC reagent (Vector Labs), and chromogen was developed in 3'3-diaminobenzidine/nickel chloride solution. Fifteen (15) micron cryosections of TA muscle were fixed in 4% paraformaldehyde, incubated overnight with primary antibodies (anti-BrdU, 1U/mL, Roche), (mouse anti-MyoD, 1:30, Dako) followed by FITC labeled secondary antibodies (Dako). All specimens were photographed using a Nikon ES400 microscope.

2.4. Cell Counting

Cell counts were calculated by identifying approximately a 1 square millimeter unit area where labeling was concentrated within the targeted anatomical region. Five to ten sections per animal were analyzed and the average number of counts determined constituted a sample (n = 1).

2.5. Western Blotting

Dissected TA muscle was homogenized in cold buffer (19 mM NaCl, 1.5 mM $MgCl_2$, 20 mM HEPES (pH 7.4), 1 mM dithiothreitol, 20% glycerol, and 0.1% Triton X-100) containing protease inhibitors, sonicated on ice (5 minutes), and centrifuged at 14,000 rpm for 15 minutes at 4˚C. Protein concentrations of supernatants were determined [65]; 40 micrograms of protein was electrophoresed in 12% NuPage Bis-Tris gels (Invitrogen), and transferred to PVDF membranes. Due to the multiplicity of gene expression induced by injury, the choice of a stable gene normalization was limited. Therefore, Ponceau S staining of the Western blot was consistently employed to confirm equal amounts of sample loading and transfer of protein. Membranes were incubated overnight with anti-MyoD1 5.8A monoclonal antibody (1:400, Dako, Carpinteria, CA), followed by peroxidase-conjugated horse anti-mouse secondary antibody (1:1000, Vector Labs). Chemiluminescent signals were densitometrically quantified using NIH Scion Image (version 4.0.3.2) software.

2.6. Statistical Analysis

All quantitative data are expressed as means +/− standard errors. Cell counts and western blot data were analyzed using the paired Student's t test to determine significant differences ($p < 0.05$).

3. Results

3.1. Acupuncture Induces Injury in TA Muscle

Histological signs of injury in TA muscle were assessed by hematoxylin staining. Control TA muscle (**Figure 1(A)**) exhibited a uniform pattern of myofibrils with punctate nuclei. In contrast, acupuncture needling of the TA muscle (**Figure 1(B)**) resulted in a loss of myofibril integrity and accumulation of mononucleated cells.

3.2. Acupuncture Induces a Proliferative Response in TA Muscle

Proliferative activity in response to acupuncture needling was analyzed by quantifying proliferating cell nuclear antigen (PCNA) expression in TA muscles. Compared to control muscle (**Figure 2(A)**), there was a dramatic increase in the number of proliferating cells in needled TA muscle that was consistent with injury and myofiber disruption (**Figure 2(B)**). Quantitation of PCNA in serial sections demonstrated a significant [$t(6) = 4.89$, $p < 0.0001$] 4-fold elevation in needled tissue [194.00 ± 5.12 cells/mm^2] compared to controls [50.55 + 11.88 cells/mm^2 (**Figure 2(C)**). Within the injured tissue, discrete sites of proliferative activity were adjacent to intact fibers that lacked immunoreactivity for PNCA (see **Figure 2(B)**).

3.3. Acupuncture Promotes Myogenic Potential

The sequence of myogenesis in response to injury is well characterized. Specifically, activated satellite cells that undergo differentiation are known to express the myogenic transcription factor, MyoD [7]. MyoD is a transcription factor that is the switch for the cascade of genes associated with remodeling a repair of muscle tissue.

Figure 3(B) demonstrates that acupuncture needling prompted MyoD immunoreactivity, in contrast to little or no expression within controls [**Figure 3(A)**]. Immunoblot analysis showed that there was a 6 and 10 fold increase in two MyoD immunoreactive isoforms (38 and 42 kDa, respectively) at 72 hrs after needling (**Figure 4**), which correlated with results from the *in situ* profile of MyoD expression (**Figure 3**). While the increase in the 38 and 42 kDa species reflects normal MyoD in response to muscle injury, another (~56 kDa) MyoD-immuno-

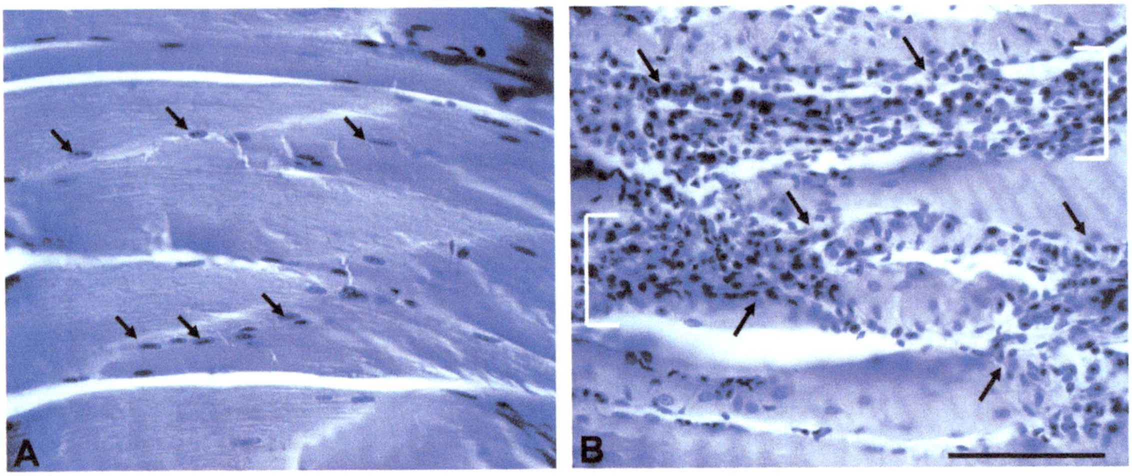

Figure 1. Acupuncture needling-induced signs of TA muscle injury. ((A): Left) Hematoxylin staining of sagittal sections of control TA muscle reveals uniform labeling of compact myofibers and resident nuclei (arrows). ((B): Right) Acupuncture disturbs myofiber integrity of TA muscle, and induces myonecrosis [brackets] and infiltration of mononucleated cells (arrows). Bar = 100 μm.

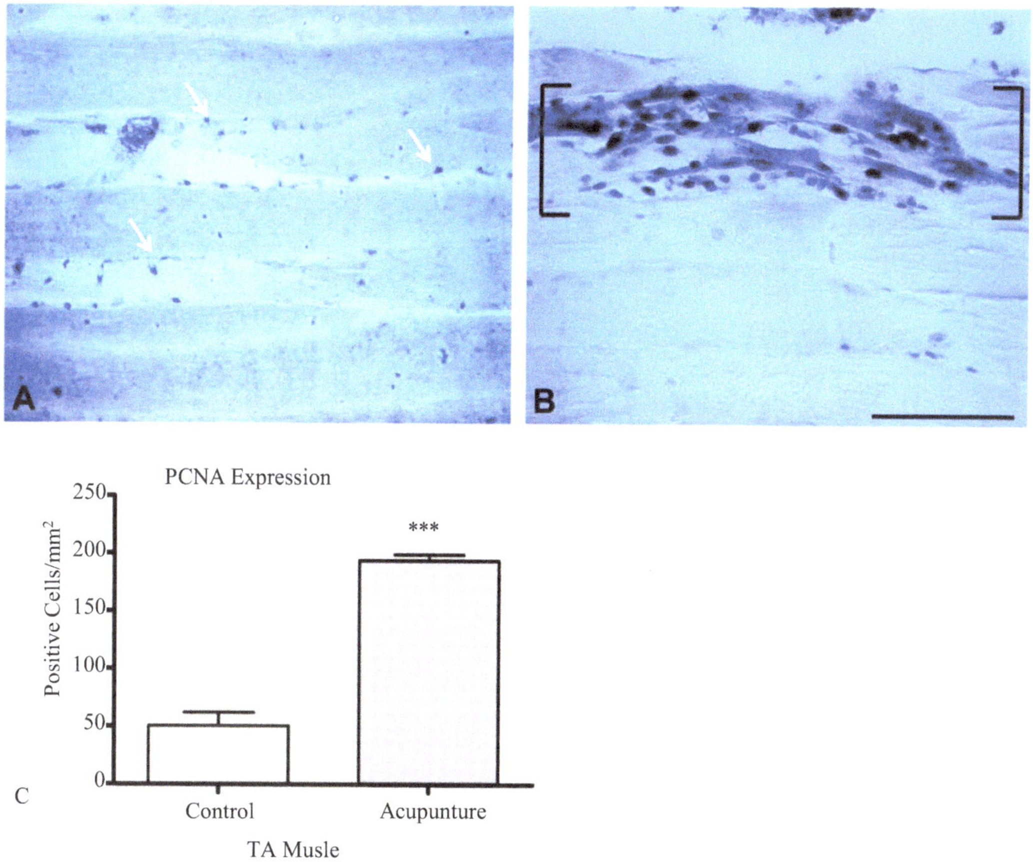

Figure 2. Quantification of proliferation in TA muscle. Sagittal sections of control (A) TA muscle tissue show proliferating cell nuclear antigen (PCNA) expression was limited to superficial regions of the muscle fibers (arrows). (B) Acupunture produced a dramatic accumulation of PCNA-immunoreactive nuclei [brackets] within myofibers (Bar = 100 μm) that resulted in a significant difference from control TA muscle (see histogram in (C)). Data represent means + s.e.m., n = 4/group, $^{***}p < 0.0001$.

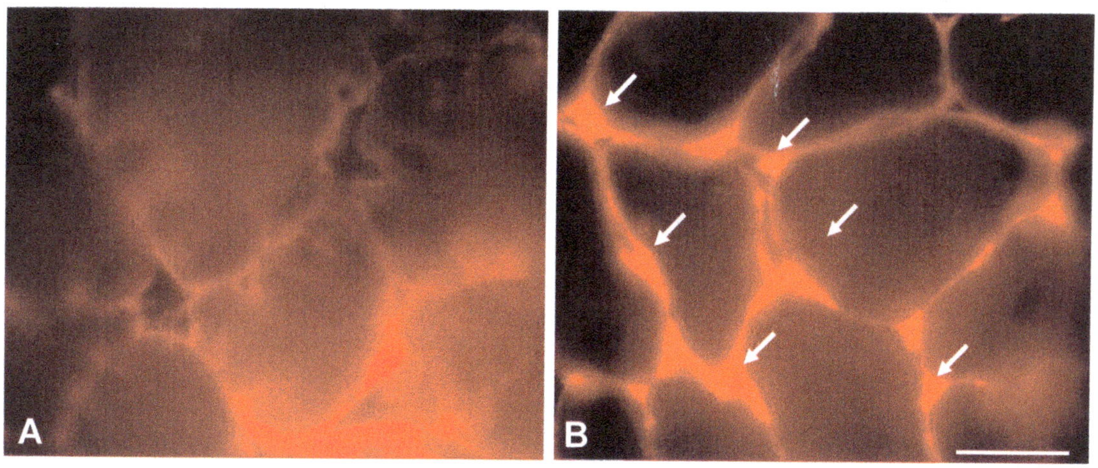

Figure 3. Evidence of myogenic activation in TA muscle. (A) Serial sections of control TA muscle incubated with anti-MyoD antibodies routinely lacked immunoreactivity. (B) Acupunctured TA muscle revealed dense, MyoD-positive immunoreactive profiles within cells at the peripheral membrane of myofibers (arrows). Bar = 50 μm.

reactive species was expressed in two thirds of the controls, and in one third of experimental of the needled TA muscles (**Figure 4(A)**).

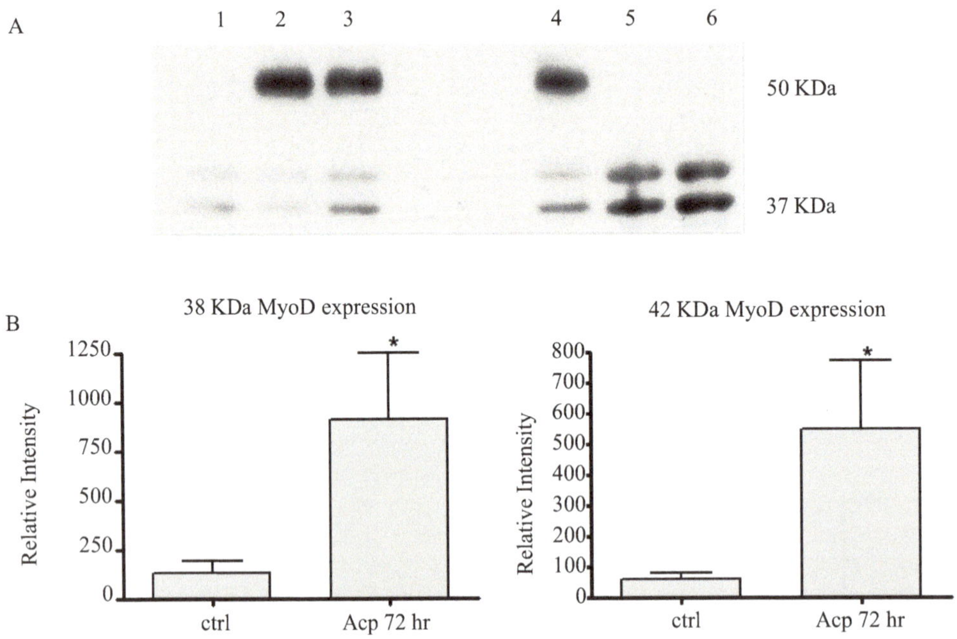

Figure 4. Induction of MyoD expression in TA muscle. Representative Western blot (A) and histograms (B) showing relative levels (mean + s.e.m.) of MyoD-immunoreactivity/expression in control TA muscles (lanes 1 - 3) and acupunctured TA muscles (lanes 4 - 6). MyoD isoforms at ~38 and 42 kD were significantly induced in acupunctured TA muscles. A MyoD-immunoreactive species of approximately 56 kDa (see (A)) was also present within the TA muscles of control and acupunctured samples. Asterisks (*) note significant differences between controls and experimental group means [$t(5) = 3.27$, $p < 0.05$]. Densitometric scans of Ponceau S stained membranes were used to confirmed equivalent protein amounts from control and acupuncture tissues (not shown).

4. Discussion

The present study demonstrates that in the 17-month-old female rat, the TA muscle retains the capacity to express markers that are known to be indicative of mechanisms that promote repair and myogenesis in injured muscle. Acupuncture needling of the TA caused myofibril disorganization that was accompanied by the infiltration of mononucleated cells, increased proliferative activity, and the up-regulation of MyoD transcription factor in SC within 72-hours post-needling. These findings correlate with observations previously reported in 6 week old male rats [19] [66], and are consistent with the results obtained with the use of different muscle injury protocols that promote SC proliferation in young organisms [2] [4] [6] [9] [67] [68].

There are reports, however, of age-related declines in SC-mediated myogenesis in response to acute injury [24] [69] [70]. Myogenic cells from aged muscle show a delayed response to activation cues and an initially reduced proliferative expansion *in vitro* [22] [45]. Despite these shortcomings, there are sufficient populations of SC that retain the myogenic potential for tissue repair [42], which have been shown to be delayed but excellent in old mice [30].

At 72 hrs post-needling, the TA muscle of rats in the present study displayed evidence of myofiber necrosis and mononuclear cell infiltration indicative of muscle injury. The presence of mononuclear cells is considered critical to the process of phagocytosis and clearance of injured muscle debris [71], which is concomitant with induction of the regeneration process [6]. Characteristic features of central nuclei and reorganizing structures have also been reported at similar time points after injury to skeletal muscle, leading to repair and regeneration [72]. Moreover, injury to mouse TA muscle by contractile lengthening results in several fold increase in the number of necrotic fibers concomitant with significant mononuclear infiltration after days [73].

In the present study, increased PCNA expression was localized within the injured TA muscle. PCNA has been used a as prerequisite marker for muscle regeneration and repair, and proliferation of a SC pool [68] [74] [75]. It is important to note that PCNA plays an essential role assisting DNA polymerase δ in processes that involve both DNA replication and repair [76]. Thus, the heightened expression of PCNA within the injured TA muscle in rats in this study may reflect induction of the SC activation/entry into the cell cycle process and/or DNA repair of myofibers. Determination of specific proliferative and immunochemical profiles at earlier post-needling time points within the injured TA muscle will enable further better characterization of myonuclear phenotypes. Preliminary observations of injured TA muscle revealed increased BrdU staining (data not shown).

At cellular and molecular levels, activation of satellite cells in muscle correlates with MyoD expression [40]. MyoD up-regulation during satellite cell activation is documented in response to episodes of myogenic plasticity, adaptation, and regeneration [11] [12] [77]. In proliferating myoblasts, MyoD expression may be critical for their fusion with intact myofibers in response to stimuli produced during muscle injury [78] [79]. In rat skeletal muscle, the molecular weight of MyoD has been reported to range between 33 to 48 kDa [80]. In the current study, two MyoD protein species, at 38- and 42 kDa, were significantly elevated in response to acupuncture needling. In a study with male adolescent rats, acupuncture needling induced the expression of the 38 kDa species [66]. However, their reported approximate 4-fold induction of this 38 kDa species differs from the 6 - 10 fold induction of this protein in aging female rats, and suggests that age- and sex-specific factors may play significant roles to regulate the myogenic response to acupuncture needling.

Recent studies have uncovered the critical impact of systemic and niché factors on stem cell functionality [46]. Selective estrogen receptor-β signaling regulates skeletal muscle regeneration by activating satellite cells and modulating immune responses [68] [81]. Estrogen stimulates skeletal muscle repair and regeneration after trauma [55] [68], and mitigates muscle damage by limiting the inflammatory response [53] [54]. In rodents, sex-related differences in SC number have been reported with aging. The decline in the number of SC in the soleus and extensor digitorium longus muscles with aging has been shown to be more striking in female mice and rats than in their aging male counterparts [82]. However, muscle SC from 30 month old female Long-Evans rats differentiated in culture to form multinucleated myotubules that have the ability to accumulate muscle-specific proteins [56]. Clinically, women have been shown to exhibit faster recovery from exercise-induced muscle damage than men [83]. Although estrogen was not measured in the present experiment, it is likely that in 17-month old pre-senile female rats estrogen levels are lower than in adult females of the species [52], suggesting that alternative systemic factors may influence regeneration seen after acupuncture needling in the aging female. It is possible that age and/or sex may account for the expression of the additional MyoD immunoreactive species which was not observed in young males after a similar acupuncture procedure [66].

The expression of a 56 kDa MyoD-immunoreactive species described here in control and needled TA muscle samples of 17 month-old rats has not been previously reported. However, 55 - 65 kDa MyoD proteins have been reported in both adult and senile rats [84]. In 4-month old male rats, these proteins are expressed in control extensor digitorum longus (EDL), gastrocnemius, and TA muscles, and elevated in response to denervation and injury [84]. In senile male rats, they are expressed in uninjured EDL and gastrocnemius muscle, and between 24 - 32 months of age their expression is steadily enhanced, with total levels in these two muscles showing increases approximately 3 to 11 times higher than at 4 months of age [84]. These high molecular weight MyoD-like species may serve age-related functions that are linked to the homeostatic and regenerative properties of muscle [42].

The 56 kDa species observed in our study may reflect the addition of ubiquitin residues to the native MyoD. Ubiquitination of MyoD has been reported in several types of aging skeletal muscle [84] [85], and while the exact function of this process is unclear, the presence of ubiquitin may influence either the transcriptional activation and/or degradation of MyoD in aged muscle.

5. Conclusion

In conclusion, the results of this study indicate that a single session of manual acupuncture-induced injury to TA (ST36) muscle is sufficient to stimulate cellular and molecular events associated with the myogenic process in skeletal muscle of the aging rat in a manner similar to that seen in younger animals. The novel species of MyoD that are expressed in pre-senile female rats may in part compensate for physiologic changes that occur in aging satellite cells and their niché environment. Understanding the regenerative process that occurs following acupuncture in skeletal muscle of young and old animals may provide important clues about the localized response that underlies the efficacy of this procedure throughout the lifespan.

Acknowledgements

We wish to thank Dr. Kamal Ameis for his expertise and assistance in performing the acupuncture manipulations, Andrea R. Allen for her technical assistance.

Research Support

Funded in part by NIH grant S06 GM 08016-33 to SKS, and the Howard University Medical Alumni Association Endowed Founders Chair in the Basic Sciences to EW.

References

[1] Mauro, A. (1961) Satellite Cell of Skeletal Muscle Fibers. *Journal of Biophysical and Biochemical Cytology*, **9**, 493-498. http://dx.doi.org/10.1083/jcb.9.2.493

[2] Schultz, E. and McCormick, K.M. (1994) Skeletal Muscle Satellite Cells. *Reviews of Physiology, Biochemistry, and Pharmacology*, **123**, 213-257. http://dx.doi.org/10.1007/BFb0030904

[3] Grounds, M.D. (1999) Muscle Regeneration: Molecular Aspects and Therapeutic Implications. *Current Opinion in Neurology*, **12**, 535-543. http://dx.doi.org/10.1097/00019052-199910000-00007

[4] Schultz, E., Jaryszak, D. and Valliere, C.R. (1985) Response of Satellite Cells in Focal Skeletal Muscle Injury. *Muscle and Nerve*, **8**, 217-222. http://dx.doi.org/10.1002/mus.880080307

[5] Seale, P., Asakura, A. and Rudnicki, M.A. (2001) The Potential of Muscle Stem Cells. *Developmental Cell*, **1**, 333-342. http://dx.doi.org/10.1016/S1534-5807(01)00049-1

[6] Chargè, S.B. and Rudnicki, M.A. (2004) Cellular and Molecular Regulation of Muscle Regeneration. *Physiological Reviews*, **84**, 209-238. http://dx.doi.org/10.1152/physrev.00019.2003

[7] Cooper, R.N., Tajbakhsh, S., Mouly, V., Cossu, G., Buckingham, M. and Butler-Browne, G.S. (1999) *In Vivo* Satellite Cell Activation via Myf5 and MyoD in Regenerating Mouse Skeletal Muscle. *Journal of Cell Science*, **112**, 2895-2890.

[8] D'Albis, A., Couteaux, R., Janmot, C., Roulet, A. and Mira, J.C. (1988) Regeneration after Cardiotoxin Injury of Innervated and Denervated Slow and Fast Muscles of Mammals: Myosin Isoform Analysis. *European Journal of Biochemistry*, **174**, 103-110. http://dx.doi.org/10.1111/j.1432-1033.1988.tb14068.x

[9] Fink, E., Fortin, D., Serrurier, B., Ventura-Clapier, R. and Bigard, A.X. (2003) Recovery of Contractile and Metabolic Phenotypes in Regenerating Slow Muscle after Notexin-Induced or Crush Injury. *Journal of Muscle Research and Cell Motility*, **24**, 421-429. http://dx.doi.org/10.1023/A:1027387501614

[10] Neto, H.S. and Marques, M.J. (2005) Microvessel Damage by B. Jararacussu Snake Venom: Pathogenesis and Influence on Muscle Regeneration. *Toxicon*, **46**, 814-819. http://dx.doi.org/10.1016/j.toxicon.2005.08.013

[11] Singh, M.A., Ding, W., Manfredi, T.J., Solares, G.S., O'Neill, E.F., Clements, K.M., Ryan, N.D., Kehayias, J.J., Fielding, R.A. and Evans, W.J. (1999) Insulin-Like Growth Factor I in Skeletal Muscle after Weight-Lifting Exercise in Frail Elders. *American Journal of Physiology*, **277**, E135-E143.

[12] Smith, H.K., Maxwell, L., Rodgers, C.D., McKee, N.H. and Plyley, M.J. (2001) Exercise-Enhanced Satellite Cell Proliferation and New Myonuclear Accretion in Rat Skeletal Muscle. *Journal of Applied Physiology*, **90**, 1407-1414.

[13] Urtizberea, J.A., Fan, Q.S., Vroom, E., Recan, D. and Kaplan, J.C. (2003) Looking under Every Rock: Duchenne Muscular Dystrophy and Traditional Chinese Medicine. *Neuromuscular Disorders*, **13**, 705-707. http://dx.doi.org/10.1016/S0960-8966(03)00116-0

[14] LeBlanc, K.E. and LeBlanc, L.L. (2010) Musculoskeletal Disorders. *Primary Care*, **37**, 389-406. http://dx.doi.org/10.1016/j.pop.2010.02.006

[15] Amezaga, U.M. and Suarez-Almazor, M.E. (2012) Acupuncture in the Treatment of Rheumatic Disease. *Current Rheumatology Reports*, **14**, 589-597. http://dx.doi.org/10.1007/s11926-012-0295-x

[16] Stux, G. (1998) Acupuncture Treatment. In: Pomeranz, B. and Stux, G., Eds., *Basic Acupuncture*, Springer-Verlag, Berlin, 214-271. http://dx.doi.org/10.1007/978-3-642-51433-3_6

[17] MacPherson, H. and Asghar, A. (2006) Acupuncture Needle Sensations Associated with De Qi: A Classification Based on Experts' Ratings. *Journal of Alternative and Complementary Medicine*, **12**, 633-637. http://dx.doi.org/10.1089/acm.2006.12.633

[18] Mao, J.J. and Kapur, R. (2010) Acupuncture in Primary Care. *Primary Care*, **37**, 105-117. http://dx.doi.org/10.1016/j.pop.2009.09.010

[19] Ameis, K.M., Kanaan, Y.M., Das, J.R., George, M. and Sobrian, S.K. (2008) Effect of Manual Acupuncture-Induced Injury on Rat Skeletal Muscle. *Medical Acupuncture*, **20**, 225-230. http://dx.doi.org/10.1089/acu.2008.0641

[20] Yablonke-Reveni, Z. (2011) The Skeletal Muscle Satellite Cell: Still Young and Fascinating at 50. *Journal of Histochemistry and Cytochemistry*, **59**, 1041-1059. http://dx.doi.org/10.1369/0022155411426780

[21] Carlson, B.M. and Faulkner, J.A. (1989) Muscle Transplantation between Young and Old Rats: Age of Host Determines Recovery. *American Journal of Physiology*, **256**, C1262-C1266.

[22] Conboy, I.M., Conboy, M.J., Smythe, G.M. and Rando, T.A. (2003) Notch-Mediated Restoration of Regenerative Potential to Aged Muscle. *Science*, **302**, 1575-1577. http://dx.doi.org/10.1126/science.1087573

[23] Rader, E.P. and Faulkner, J.A. (2006) Recovery from Contraction-Induced Injury Is Impaired in Weight-Bearing Muscles of Old Male Mice. *Journal of Applied Physiology*, **100**, 656-661. http://dx.doi.org/10.1152/japplphysiol.00663.2005

[24] Conboy, I.M. and Rando, T.A. (2005) Aging, Stem Cells and Tissue Regeneration: Lessons from Muscle. *Cell Cycle*, **4**, 407-410. http://dx.doi.org/10.4161/cc.4.3.1518

[25] Dedkov, E.I., Borisov, A.B., Wernig, A. and Carlson, B.M. (2003) Aging of Skeletal Muscle Does Not Affect the Response of Satellite Cells to Denervation. *Journal of Histochemistry and Cytochemistry*, **51**, 853-863. http://dx.doi.org/10.1177/002215540305100701

[26] Liu, L. and Rando, T.A. (2011) Manifestations and Mechanisms of Stem Cell Aging. *Journal of Cell Biology*, **193**, 257-266. http://dx.doi.org/10.1083/jcb.201010131

[27] Biressi, S. and Rando, T.A. (2010) Heterogeneity in the Muscle Satellite Cell Population. *Seminars in Cell and Developmental Biology*, **21**, 845-854. http://dx.doi.org/10.1016/j.semcdb.2010.09.003

[28] Gibson, M.C. and Schultz, E. (1983) Age-Related Differences in Absolute Numbers of Skeletal Muscle Satellite Cells. *Muscle and Nerve*, **6**, 574-580. http://dx.doi.org/10.1002/mus.880060807

[29] Renault, V., Thornell, L.E., Eriksson, P.O., Butler-Browne, G. and Mouly, V. (2002) Regenerative Potential of Human Skeletal Muscle during Aging. *Aging Cell*, **1**, 132-139. http://dx.doi.org/10.1046/j.1474-9728.2002.00017.x

[30] Shefer, G., Rauner, G., Yablonka-Reuveni, Z. and Benayahu, D. (2010) Reduced Satellite Cell Numbers and Myogenic Capacity in Aging Can Be Alleviated by Endurance Exercise. *PLoS ONE*, **5**, Article ID: e13307. http://dx.doi.org/10.1371/journal.pone.0013307

[31] Snow, M.H. (1977) The Effects of Aging on Satellite Cells in Skeletal Muscle of Mice and Rats. *Cell and Tissue Research*, **185**, 399-408. http://dx.doi.org/10.1007/BF00220299

[32] Tajbakhsh, S., Rocancourt, D., Cossu, G. and Buckingham, M. (1997) Redefining the Genetic Hierarchies Controlling Skeletal Myogenesis: *Pax*-3 and *Myf*-5 Act Upstream of *Myo*D. *Cell*, **89**, 127-138. http://dx.doi.org/10.1016/S0092-8674(00)80189-0

[33] Kadi, F., Charifi, N., Christian, D. and Lexell, J. (2004) Satellite Cells and Myonuclei in Young and Elderly Women and Men. *Muscle and Nerve*, **29**, 120-127. http://dx.doi.org/10.1002/mus.10510

[34] Shefer, G., Van de Mark, D.P., Richardson, J.B. and Yablonka-Reuveni, Z. (2006) Satellite-Cell Pool Size Does Matter: Defining the Myogenic Potency of Aging Skeletal Muscle. *Developmental Biology*, **294**, 50-66. http://dx.doi.org/10.1016/j.ydbio.2006.02.022

[35] Hikida, R.S., Walsh, S., Barylski, N., Campos, G., Hagerman, F.C. and Staron, R.S. (1998) Is Hypertrophy Limited to Elderly Muscle Fibers? A Comparison of Elderly and Young Strength-Trained Men. *Basic and Applied Myology*, **8**, 419-427.

[36] Roth, S.M., Martel, G.F., Ivey, F.M., Leemer, J.T., Metter, E.J., Hurley, B.F. and Rogers, M.A. (2000) Skeletal Muscle Satellite Cell Population in Healthy Young and Older Men and Women. *Anatomical Record*, **260**, 351-358. http://dx.doi.org/10.1002/1097-0185(200012)260:4<350::AID-AR30>3.0.CO;2-6

[37] Roth, S.M., Martel, G.F., Ivey, F.M., Lemmer, J.T., Tracy, B.L., Metter, E.J., Hurley, B.F. and Rogers, M.A. (2001) Skeletal Muscle Satellite Cell Characteristics in Young and Older Men and Women after Heavy Resistance Strength Training. *Journals of Gerontology, Series A: Biological Sciences and Medical Sciences*, **56**, B240-B247. http://dx.doi.org/10.1093/gerona/56.6.B240

[38] Wagers, A.J. and Conboy, I.M. (2005) Cellular and Molecular Signatures of Muscle Regeneration: Current Concepts and Controversies in Adult Myogenesis. *Cell*, **122**, 659-667. http://dx.doi.org/10.1016/j.cell.2005.08.021

[39] Brack, A.S., Conboy, M.J., Roy, S., Lee, M., Kuo, C.J., Keller, C. and Rando, T.A. (2007) Increased Wnt Signaling during Aging Alters Muscle Stem Cell Fate and Increases Fibrosis. *Science*, **317**, 807-810. http://dx.doi.org/10.1126/science.1144090

[40] Dedkov, E.I., Borisov, A.B. and Carlson, B.M. (2003) Dynamics of Postdenervation Atrophy of Young and Old Skeletal Muscles: Differential Responses of Fiber Types and Muscle Types. *Journals of Gerontology, Series A: Biological Sciences and Medical Sciences*, **58**, B984-B991. http://dx.doi.org/10.1093/gerona/58.11.B984

[41] Hikida, R.S. (2011) Aging Changes in Satellite Cells and Their Functions. *Current Aging Science*, **4**, 279-297. http://dx.doi.org/10.2174/1874609811104030279

[42] Pannérec, A., Marazzi, G. and Sassoon, D. (2012) Stem Cells in the Hood: The Skeletal Muscle Niche. *Trends in Mole-*

cular Medicine, **18**, 599-606. http://dx.doi.org/10.1016/j.molmed.2012.07.004

[43] Carlson, B.M. and Faulkner, J.A. (1998) Muscle Regeneration in Young and Old Rats: Effects of Motor Nerve Transection with and without Marcaine Treatment. *Journals of Gerontology, Series A: Biological Sciences and Medical Sciences*, **53**, B52-B58. http://dx.doi.org/10.1093/gerona/53A.1.B52

[44] Brack, A.S. and Rando, T.A. (2007) Intrinsic Changes and Extrinsic Influences of Myogenic Stem Cell Function during Aging. *Stem Cell Reviews*, **3**, 226-237. http://dx.doi.org/10.1007/s12015-007-9000-2

[45] Gopinath, S.D. and Rando, T.A. (2008) Stem Cell Review Series: Aging of the Skeletal Muscle Stem Cell Niche. *Aging Cell*, **7**, 590-598. http://dx.doi.org/10.1111/j.1474-9726.2008.00399.x

[46] García-Prat, L., Sousa-Victor, P. and Muñoz-Cánoves, P. (2013) Functional Dysregulation of Stem Cells during Aging: A Focus on Skeletal Muscle Stem Cells. *FEBS Journal*, **280**, 4051-4062. http://dx.doi.org/10.1111/febs.12221

[47] Zacks, S.I. and Sheff, M.F. (1982) Age-Related Impeded Regeneration of Mouse Minced Anterior Tibial Muscle. *Muscle and Nerve*, **5**, 152-161. http://dx.doi.org/10.1002/mus.880050213

[48] Conboy, I.M., Conboy, M.J., Wagers, A.J., Girma, E.R., Weissman, I.L. and Rando, T.A. (2005) Rejuvenation of Aged Progenitor Cells by Exposure to a Young Systemic Environment. *Nature*, **433**, 760-764. http://dx.doi.org/10.1038/nature03260

[49] Collins, C.A., Zammit, P.S., Ruiz, A.P., Morgan, J.E. and Partridge, T.A. (2007) A Population of Myogenic Stem Cells that Survives Skeletal Muscle Aging. *Stem Cells*, **25**, 885-894. http://dx.doi.org/10.1634/stemcells.2006-0372

[50] Freeman, M.E. (1998) The Ovarian Cycle of the Rat. In: Knobil, E. and Neill, J., Eds., *The Physiology of Reproduction*, Raven Press, New York, 1894-1928.

[51] Sokol, R.Z., Okuda, H., Stanczyk, F.Z., Wolfe, G.W., Delaney, J.C. and Chapin, R.E. (1999) Normative Reproductive Indices for Male and Female Adult Sprague-Dawley Rats. *Contraception*, **59**, 203-207. http://dx.doi.org/10.1016/S0010-7824(99)00017-7

[52] Merry, B.J. and Holehan, A.M. (1979) Onset of Puberty and Duration of Fertility in Rats Fed a Restricted Diet. *Journal the Society for Reproduction and Fertility*, **57**, 253-259. http://dx.doi.org/10.1530/jrf.0.0570253

[53] Tiidus, P.M. (2005) Can Oestrogen Influence Skeletal Muscle Damage, Inflammation, and Repair? *British Journal of Sports Medicine*, **39**, 251-253. http://dx.doi.org/10.1136/bjsm.2005.016881

[54] Tiidus, P.M., Deller, M. and Liu, X.L. (2005) Oestrogen Influence on Myogenic Satellite Cells Following Downhill Running in Male Rats: A Preliminary Study. *Acta Physiolgica Scandinavica*, **184**, 67-72. http://dx.doi.org/10.1111/j.1365-201X.2005.01427.x

[55] Enns, D.L. and Tiidus, P.M. (2010) The Influence of Estrogen on Skeletal Muscle: Sex Matters. *Sports Medicine*, **40**, 14-58. http://dx.doi.org/10.2165/11319760-000000000-00000

[56] Allen, R.E., McAllister, P.K. and Masak, K.C. (1980) Myogenic Potential of Satellite Cells in Skeletal Muscle of Old Rats. A Brief Note. *Mechanisms of Ageing and Development*, **13**, 105-109. http://dx.doi.org/10.1016/0047-6374(80)90053-6

[57] Luo, D., Liu, S., Xie, X.P. and Hou, X.H. (2008) Electroacpuncture at Acupoint ST-36 Promotes Contractility of Distal Colon via a Cholinergic Pathway in Conscious Rats. *Digestive Diseases and Sciences*, **53**, 689-693. http://dx.doi.org/10.1007/s10620-007-9929-7

[58] Yim, Y.K., Lee, H., Hong, K.E., Kim, Y.I., Lee, B.R., Son, C.G. and Kim, J.E. (2007) Electro-Acupuncture at Acupoint ST36 Reduces Inflammation and Regulates Immune Activity in Collagen-Induced Arthritic Mice. *Evidence Based Complementary and Alternative Medicine*, **4**, 51-57. http://dx.doi.org/10.1093/ecam/nel054

[59] National Institutes of Health. (1997) Acupuncture. *NIH Consensus Statement*, **15**, 1-34.

[60] Li, X., Hirokawa, M., Inoue, Y., Sugano, N., Qian, S. and Iwai, T. (2007) Effects of Acupressure on Lower Limb Blood Flow for the Treatment of Peripheral Arterial Occlusive Diseases. *Surgery Today*, **37**, 103-108. http://dx.doi.org/10.1007/s00595-006-3347-x

[61] Ameis, K.M. (1991) Analgesic Effect of Captopril and Electroacupunture Stimulation. *Proceedings of* 1*st Guangzhou International Conference of Traditional Chinese Medicine*, Gangzhou, 1991.

[62] Ruchin, I.N. and Burdeiny, A.P. (1987) Auriculo-Electropuncture in Rheumatoid Arthritis (a Double-Blind Study). *Terapevticheskiĭ Arkhiv*, **59**, 26-30.

[63] Walters, E., Buchheit, K. and Maruniak, J.A. (1992) Receptor Neuron Losses Result in Decreased Cytochrome P-450 Immunoreactivity in Associated Non-Neuronal Cells of Mouse Olfactory Mucosa. *Journal of Neuroscience Research*, **33**, 103-111. http://dx.doi.org/10.1002/jnr.490330113

[64] Baker, B.A., Mercer, R.R., Geronilla, K.B., Kashon, M.L., Miller, G.R. and Cutlip, R.G. (2006) Stereological Analysis of Muscle Morphology Following Exposure to Repetitive Stretch-Shortening Cycles in a Rat Model. *Applied Physiology*,

Nutrition, and Metabolism, **31**, 167-179. http://dx.doi.org/10.1139/h05-009

[65] Bradford, M.M. (1976) A Rapid and Sensitive Method for the Quantitation of Microgram Quantities of Protein Utilizing the Principle of Protein-Dye Binding. *Analytical Biochemistry*, **72**, 248-254. http://dx.doi.org/10.1016/0003-2697(76)90527-3

[66] Ameis, K., Jayam Trouth, A., Bond, V. and Kanaan, Y. (2011) Degeneration/Regeneration as a Mechanism Contributing to the Effect of Manual Acupuncture-Induced Injury on Rat Skeletal Muscle, Acupuncture. In: Saad, M., Ed., *Concepts and Physiology*, InTech. http://www.intechopen.com/books/acupuncture-concepts-and-physiology/degeneration-regeneration-as-a-mechanism-contributing-to-the-effect-of-manual-acupuncture-induced-in http://dx.doi.org/10.5772/24801

[67] Rathbone, C.R., Wenke, J.C., Warren, G.L. and Armstrong, R.B. (2003) Importance of Satellite Cells in the Strength Recovery after Eccentric Contraction-Induced Muscle Injury. *American Journal of Physiology, Regulatory, Integrative and Comparative Physiology*, **285**, R1490-R1495.

[68] Velders, M., Schleipen, B., Fritzemeier, K.H., Zierau, O. and Diel, P. (2012) Selective Estrogen Receptors-β Activation Stimulates Skeletal Nuscle Growth and Regeneration. *FASEB Journal*, **26**, 1909-1920. http://dx.doi.org/10.1096/fj.11-194779

[69] Barberi, L., Scicchitano, B.M., De Rossi, M., Bigot, A., Duguez, S., Wielgosik, A., Stewart, C., McPhee, J., Conte, M., Narici, M., Franceschi, C., Mouly, V., Butler-Browne, G. and Musarò, A. (2013) Age-Dependent Alteration in Muscle Regeneration: The Critical Role of Tissue Niche. *Biogerontology*, **14**, 273-292. http://dx.doi.org/10.1007/s10522-013-9429-4

[70] Cousin, W., Ho, M.L., Desai, R., Tham, A., Chen, R.Y., Kung, S., Elabd, C. and Conboy, I.M. (2013) Regenerative Capacity of Old Muscle Stem Cells Declines without Significant Accumulation of DNA Damage. *PLoS ONE*, **8**, Article ID: e63528. http://dx.doi.org/10.1371/journal.pone.0063528

[71] Robertson, T.A., Maley, M.A., Grounds, M.D. and Papadimitriou, J.M. (1993) The Role of Macrophages in Skeletal Muscle Regeneration with Particular Reference to Chemotaxis. *Experimental Cell Research*, **207**, 321-331. http://dx.doi.org/10.1006/excr.1993.1199

[72] Fisher, B.D., Baracos, V.E., Shnitka, T.K., Medbryk, S.W. and Reid, D.C. (1990) Ultrastructural Events Following Acute Muscle Trauma. *Medicine and Science in Sports and Exercise*, **22**, 185-193.

[73] Roche, J.A., Lovering, R.M., Roche, R., Ru, L.W., Reed, P.W. and Bloch, R.J. (2010) Extensive Mononuclear Infiltration and Myogenesis Characterize Recovery of Dysferlin-Null Skeletal Muscle from Contraction-Induced Injuries. *American Journal of Physiology, Cell Physiology*, **298**, C298-C312. http://dx.doi.org/10.1152/ajpcell.00122.2009

[74] Hawk, T.J. and Garry, D.J. (2001) Myogenic Satellite Cells: Physiology to Molecular Biology. *Journal of Applied Physiology*, **91**, 534-551.

[75] Takaoka, Y., Ohta, M., Ito, A., Takamatsu, K., Sugano, A., Funakoshi, K., Takaoka, N., Sato, N., Yokosaki, H., Arizono, N., Goto, S. and Maeda, E. (2007) Electroacupuncture Suppresses Myostatin Gene Expression: Cell Proliferative Reaction in Mouse Skeletal Muscle. *Physiological Genomics*, **30**, 102-110. http://dx.doi.org/10.1152/physiolgenomics.00057.2006

[76] Maga, G. and Hubscher, U. (2003) Proliferating Cell Nuclear Antigen (PCNA): A Dancer with Many Partners. *Journal of Cell Science*, **116**, 3051-3060. http://dx.doi.org/10.1242/jcs.00653

[77] Buonanno, A., Cheng, J., Venepally, P., Weis, J. and Calvo, S. (1998) Activity-Dependent Regulation of Muscle Genes: Repressive and Stimulatory Effects of Innervation. *Acta Physiologica Scandinavica*, **163**, S17-S26. http://dx.doi.org/10.1046/j.1365-201X.1998.1630s3S17.x

[78] Sabourin, L.A. and Rudnicki, M.A. (2000) The Molecular Regulation of Myogenesis. *Clinical Genetics*, **57**, 16-25. http://dx.doi.org/10.1034/j.1399-0004.2000.570103.x

[79] Seale, P., Sabourin, L.A., Girgis-Gabardo, A., Mansouri, A., Gruss, P. and Rudnicki, M.A. (2000) Pax7 Is Required for the Specification of Myogenic Satellite Cells. *Cell*, **102**, 777-786. http://dx.doi.org/10.1016/S0092-8674(00)00066-0

[80] Jones, S.W., Baker, D.J., Gardiner, S.M., Bennett, T., Timmons, J.A. and Greenhaff, P.L. (2004) The Effect of the β_2-Adrenoceptor Agonist Prodrug BRL-47672 on Cardiovascular Function, Skeletal Muscle Myosin Heavy Chain, and MyoD Expression in the Rat. *Journal of Pharmacology and Experimental Therapeutics*, **311**, 1225-1231. http://dx.doi.org/10.1124/jpet.104.071589

[81] Velders, M. and Diel, P. (2013) How Sex Hormones Promote Skeletal Muscle Regeneration. *Sports Medicine*, **43**, 1089-1100. http://dx.doi.org/10.1007/s40279-013-0081-6

[82] Day, K., Shefer, G., Shearer, A. and Yablonka-Reuveni, Z. (2010) The Depletion of Skeletal Muscle Satellite Cells with Age Is Concomitant with Reduced Capacity of Single Progenitors to Produce Reserve Progeny. *Developmental Biology*, **340**, 330-343. http://dx.doi.org/10.1016/j.ydbio.2010.01.006

[83] Clarkson, P.M. and Hubal, M.J. (2001) Are Women Less Susceptible to Exercise-Induced Muscle Damage? *Current*

Opinion in Clinical Nutrition and Metabolic Care, **4**, 527-531. http://dx.doi.org/10.1097/00075197-200111000-00011

[84] Dedkov, E.I., Kostominova, T.Y., Borisov, A.B. and Carlson, B.M. (2003) MyoD and Myogenin Protein Expression in Skeletal Muscles of Senile Rats. *Cell and Tissue Research*, **311**, 401-416.

[85] Puri, P.L. and Sartorelli, V. (2000) Regulation of Muscle Regulatory Factors by DNA-Binding, Interacting Proteins, and Post-Transcriptional Modifications. *Journal of Cellular Physiology*, **185**, 155-173. http://dx.doi.org/10.1002/1097-4652(200011)185:2<155::AID-JCP1>3.0.CO;2-Z

3

Searching Clue of the Relationship between the Alteration of Bioactive Ingredients and the Herbal "Property" Transformation from Raw Rehmanniae Radix (*Sheng-Di-Huang*) to Steam-Heating-Processed Rehmanniae Radix (*Shu-Di-Huang*) by Chromatographic Fingerprint Analysis

Peishan Xie[1*], Longgang Guo[1], Yu Zhao[2], Daniel Bensky[3], Erich Stoeger[4]

[1]Guangdong UNION Biotechnology Development Co., Ltd., Guangzhou, China
[2]Nikyang Enterprise Co., Ltd., Hong Kong, China
[3]Independent Scholar, Seattle, USA
[4]Plantasia GmbH, Oberndorf, Austria
Email: [*]xps340112@gmail.com

Abstract

"*Di-Huang*" (Rehmanniae Radix) is a peculiar Chinese herbal drug, the fresh root named "*Xian-Di-Huang*" ("*Xian*" means fresh; the commerce is now rarely available), mild-baking-dried raw roots "*Sheng-Di-Huang*" ("*Sheng*" means raw) and steam-processed "*Shu-Di-Huang*" ("*Shu*" implies steam-processed). The both kinds of herbal drug exert different efficiencies with different property according to the traditional clinical theory. It would be of interest that searching the clue of why the therapeutic functions of the same drug differ between the pre- and post-processing. To disclose the comprehensive alteration of the iridoids, saccharides and phenylethanoids occurred between the raw and steam-processed "*Di-Huang*", the HPTLC and HPLC chromatographic fingerprint analysis has been carried out. The results showed that in the raw crude drug, the iridoids like catalpol is the major bioactive components, and the oligosaccharides composition kept rather consistent; however, in the steam-processed *Di-Huang*, iridoids was almost disappeared and the oligosaccharides were hydrolyzed gradually through the repeated steam-heating process. The worst case showed only fructose was detected with other minor residual components in the root

[*]Corresponding author.

tuber. It is due to presumably the uncontrollable steaming process in folk workshops. Defining reasonably the boundary between the *"Sheng-Di-Huang"* (mild-baking-dried Rehmanniae radix) and *"Shu-Di-Huang"* (steaming processed Rehmanniae radix) set up by chromatographic fingerprint pattern and standardizing the process would be necessary for assuring the consistent quality of the commercial herbal drugs.

Keywords

Rehmanniae Radix, *Di-Huang*, Processing Incurred Herbal-Property-Change, Chromatographic Fingerprinting, Meaningful Quality Control

1. Introduction

Rehmanniae radix is the fresh or dried tuberous roots of *Rehmannia glutinosa* Libosch, belonging to the family Scrophulariaceae. It has been commonly used in clinics in China for thousands of years. The drug is usually collected in autumn, removed from root stock, rootlet and soil, and used either in fresh state or mild-baked to dryness. The former is known as "*Xian Di-Huang*" (fresh rehmannia root) which is nowadays rarely available in the market because it is hard to store and transport; the latter is known as "*Sheng-Di-Huang*" (dried raw Rehmannia root). Since the Tang Dynasty (618 - 907 AD), according to long historical clinical experience, Chinese medicine practitioners considered the property of *Sheng-Di-Huang* inclined to be used as detoxification for reducing the "*heat*" in blood, and promoting the production of body fluid and saliva, so its property was relatively "cold". For the patients of "*Kidney-Yin*"-deficiency, *Di-Huang* should be transformed to have a "warm" property by repeated steaming process until the crude drug turned black and was called as "*Shu-Di-Huang*" (steam-processed Rehmnania radix or prepared Rehmannia radix). This drug is used to nourish "*yin*" and replenish blood, reinforce the essence of life and marrow and tonify the "*Yin*-deficient *Kidney*" [1] [2].

According to the description of "*Sheng-Di-Huang*" in Chinese Pharmacopoeia [2], the root tuber has brownish-black or brownish-grey external appearance, the texture is heavy, soft and tenacious, fracture surface is brownish black or jet-black, lustrous and viscous. The "*Shu-Di-Huang*", external is black, lustrous, and stickier. Texture is soft and flexible, uneasily broken, fracture surface is jet-black, lustrous.

The transformation of herbal property from "cold" to "warm" through a steaming process implies that some significant alteration of the inherent secondary metabolites in *Di-Huang* roots occurs during the processing cycles. The three kinds of the major bioactive ingredients in *Di-Huang* are iridoids, saccharides and phenylethanols [3]-[7]. For quantitative determination, the current methods are to determine the content of catalpol and rehmannioside D for *Sheng-Di-Huang*; while acteoside and 5-hydroxymethylfurfural (5-HMF) for *Shu-Di-Huang* [2] [8]. Some research focused on the contents of selected constituents [8]-[11]. Those isolated markers' determinations are insufficient for searching the clue of the drug's property change. The unfolded global view of two kinds of chromatographic fingerprints of *Di-Huang* would provide the substantial evidence of dynamic changes of the main bioactive components and possible linkage to the drug properties transformation. The information will serve as the fundamental background for establishing a reliable specification to ensure the meaningful quality control standard.

In this study, the associated fingerprints of High-performance Thin-layer Chromatography (HPTLC) and High-performance Liquid Chromatography (HPLC) complementarily represented the characteristics of *Sheng-Di-Huang* and *Shu-Di-Huang* respectively. According to the fingerprint patterns, the relativity between the dynamic changes of the chemical composition and the drug property transformation from *Sheng-Di-Huang* to *Shu-Di-Huang* is discussed in this paper.

2. Experimental

2.1. Sample and Apparatus

- Samples

39 batches of Rhmannia root (root of *Rehmannia glutinosa* L.; *Di-Huang*) were utilized, 17 batches from He-

nan province, the rests purchased from herbal drug markets in the provinces of Guangdong, Guizhou, Jiangxi, Fujian, Hunan, Anhui, Hebei and Guangxi.

- Chemicals and reagents

Catalptol and acetoside (purchased from Chinese National Institute for the Control of Pharmaceutical and Biological products, Beijing, China); rehmannioside D (provided by State Administration of Traditional Chinese herbal medicine of People's Republic of China, Beijing, China); raffinose (purchased from Sinopharm Chemical Shanghai Chemical Reagent Co. Ltd., Shanghai, China); sucrose (purchased from Tianjin Guangfu Fine Chemical Research Institute, Tianjin, China); D-fructose (Purchased from Sinopharm Chemical Reagent Co. Ltd., Shanghai, China); Stachyose (Purchased from Xi-An Dapeng Biological Technology Co. Ltd., Xi'an, China).

All chemicals and reagents are of analytical grade.

- Apparatus

HPTLC were performed on High performance silica gel pre-coated plate (Merck, Germany), Automatic TLC sampler 4, TLC development twin-trough chamber, TLC scanner 3 with WinCats software, Digistore TLC documentation device and software (all from CAMAG, Switzerland); TLC digiscan-Acquiring software (developed by Franky Du of Nikyang Enterprises Company, Hong Kong).

HPLC were performed on an Agilent 1100 series HPLC system with autosampler and diode array detector (DAD).

HPLC column: ZORBAX SB C18 (4.6 × 250 mm, 5 μm, Agilent).

2.2. Preparation of Sample Solution

- Sample solution for HPTLC analysis

0.1 g of powdered sample were placed in a graduated test tube, add 5 mL of methanol, ultrosonicate at 40°C for 15 minutes, centrifuge for 10 minutes (4000 r/min), use the supernatant as sample solution.

- Sample solution for HPLC analysis

Add 50 mL of 70% ethanol to 2 g of powdered sample, reflux on a 90°C water bath for 30 minutes, filter, evaporate the filtrate to dryness on a 90°C water bath, dissolve the residue in 20 mL of water and transfer to a separating funnel, extract with 30 mL of n-butanol twice, combine the n-butanol, evaporate to dryness on a 90°C water bath, dissolve the residue in 30% ethanol and transfer to a 5 mL of volumetric flask and dilute to volume, mixed well, then filter through 0.45 μm filter membrane, use the final filtrate as sample solution.

2.3. Preparation of Chemical Reference Solution

Dissolve 5 mg of the Chemical Reference Substances (CRS) cataltol and 8 mg of rehmannioside D in 1 mL methanol, respectively. Dissolve 2 mg of raffinose, 2 mg of sucrose and 0.5 mg of D-fructose chemical reagent in 1 mL of 70% ethanol, respectively. Use these as saccharides and iridoids reference solution for HPTLC analysis.

Accurately weight a quantity of acteoside (CRS), dissolve in 30% methanol to produce a solution containing 0.5 mg per 1ml as reference solution for HPLC analysis.

2.4. Experiment Procedure

- HPTLC fingerprint of Rehmannia root (*Di-Huang*) collected from different places

Stationary phase: HPTLC plate (20 × 10 cm; Merck; batch Number: HX604153).

Mobile phase: Dichloromethane-ethyl acetate-methanol-water-glacial acetic acid (8:4:7:1:1).

Saturation: Pre-equilibrate the development chamber with the mobile phase for 15 minutes prior to analysis (add about 8 mL of the solvent mixture into one trough of the chamber).

Sample application: apply 2 μL of sample solution and 1 μL of chemical reference solution as band onto HPTLC plate respectively. The original application position was 8 mm above from the bottom edge.

Development: The plates loaded with sample solution were dried in a vacuum dessicator over phosphorous pentoxide for 2 - 3 hours prior to development. The sufficient dried sample-loaded plate was placed promptly in the chamber, developing distance of the mobile phase reached to 8 cm. The residual solvent on the developed plate was dried with a stream of cold air for 10 minutes. Spray with 2% anisaldehyde in 5% sulphuric acid ethanol solution, heat at 105°C until the bands are clearly visible.

Detection: Observe the fluorescence image under UV light at 366 nm and documentation was done as usual

(**Figure 1**).

- HPLC fingerprint of rehmannia root collected from different place

Column: ZORBAX SB C_{18} (4.6 × 250 mm, 5 μm; Aglient)

Column temperature: 30°C

Gradient of mobile phase: A-acetonitrile; B-0.1% acetic acid in water.

Time(min)	A (%)	B (%)
0	10	90
15	17	83
25	17	83
55	30	70

Flow rate: 1 mL/min

Injection volume: 20 μL

Detection wavelength: 334 nm (for phenylethanol glycosides)

Run time: 55 minutes

Compare the chromatogram of sample solution against the chromatogram of reference solution.

3. Results and Discussion

3.1. HPTLC Fingerprint Analysis

- Characteristics HPTLC fingerprint

The HPTLC fluorescence image of raw dried Rhamannia roots (*Sheng-Di-Huang*) developed four yellow fluorescent bands of saccharides: stachyose (R_f value ac. 0.06), raffinose (R_f value ac. 0.14), sucrose (R_f value ac. 0.26), D-fructose (R_f value ac. 0.35) and two grayish-blue fluorescent bands of iridoids (rehmannioside D (R_f value ac.0.18), catalpol (R_f value ac.0.52). The relative fluorescence abundance of the components in the image can be compared visually (**Table 1**).

The digital scanning profiles of the HPTLC images (**Figure 1**) expressed more clearly the intact view of the fingerprint of *Sheng-Di-Huang*. It can serve as the common pattern of the raw material (**Figure 2**). As a typical *Sheng-Di-Huang*, among saccharides, strachyose is the strongest fluorescence band, raffinose and sucrose gave stronger or weaker fluorescence bands, fructose is the weakest in different samples; As iridoids, catalpol were obviously detected as grey-blue fluorescence bands, but the content (fluorescence abundance) fluctuated widely

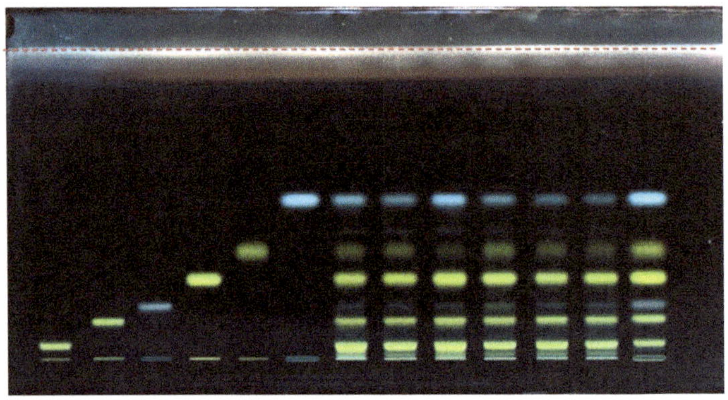

S1 S2 S3 S4 S5 S6 1 2 3 4 5 6 $S_{1\sim6}$

Figure 1. HPTL Cimage of *Di-Huang* (Rehmanniae Radix). (S1)-Stachyose; (S2)-Raffinose; (S3)-Rehmannioside; (S4)-Surcose; (S5)-D-Fructose; (S6)-Catalpol; (1). Reference crude drug; (2)-(6) Commercial samples; ($S_{1\sim6}$) mixed chemical reference substances.

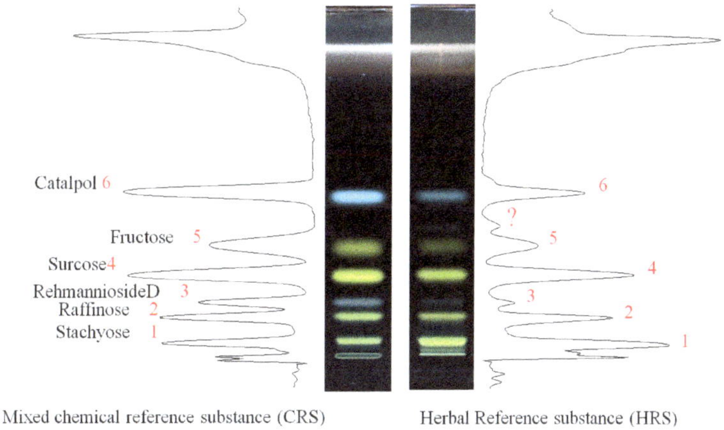

Figure 2. HPTLC images and digital scanning profiles of mixed CRS and HRS of Rehmannia root. Peaks: (1) stachyose; (2) raffinose; (3) rhemannioside D; (4) sucrose; (5) fructose; (6) catalpol, (?) unknown yetsaccharide.

Table 1. Approximate comparison of the fluorescence bands abundance of the saccharides and iridoids in the HPTLC image of *Sheng-Di-Huang* and *Shu-Di-Huang*.

Fluorescent band	Stachyose (Rf ca. 0.06)	Raffinose (Rf ca. 0.14)	Rehmannioside D (Rf ca.0.18)	Sucrose (Rf ca. 0.26)	D-fructcose♠ (Rf ca. 0.35)	Catalpol (Rf ca. 0.52)
Sheng-Di-Huang	+++	++	+	++/+++	+/++	+/++/+++
Shu-Di-Huang	++/+	minor/−	+/trace	+++/++	++/+++	minor/−

♠: glucose overlapped with fructose.

in different commercial samples (The literature reported catalpol is the highest content among the iridoids glycosides [11]). Briefly, the intact image and the scanning profile (number of bands, location and order, fluorescence/visible color, strength of the fluorescence abundance, peak height/area ratio between bands) constructed the unique fingerprint pattern of *Sheng-Di-Huang*.The digital scanning profiles of the HPTLC images (**Figure 1**) provided more clear intact view of the fingerprint. It can serve as the common pattern of *Sheng-Di-Huang* (**Figure 2**).

With regard to the HPTLC image pattern of *Shu-Di-Huang*, comparison with of *Sheng-Di-Huang*, the prominent feature is iridoids represented by catalpol were decomposed seriously, even radically disappeared. Secondly, the oligosaccharides were hydrolyzed at different degrees, consequently sucrose, even fructose increased accordingly (**Table 1**). Therefore the HTPLC image of *Shu-Di-Huang* showed a rather different visage from *Sheng-Di-Huang*. Glucose almost dehydrated to 5-hydrxoy-methyl furfural (5-HMF) (vide infra).

- Dynamic alteration of the active ingredients of the root tuber of Rehmannia subjected to the steaming process

For the sake of investigation of the dynamic alteration of the compounds in *Di-Huang*, a quantity of "*Sheng-Di-Huang*" was steamed in a small bamboo steamer placed in a wok filled with boiling water, heated for 0, 2, 4 and 8 hours; and then a given quantity was taken out as samples, dried under reduced pressure at 60°, powdered, then prepared the sample solutions as described in section 2.2. for HPTLC analysis. The experiment demonstrated the steam-heating tolerance test of oligosaccharides and catalpol. The results indicated that stachyose, raffinose and sucrose in the roots were at rather stable till 4 hours. After that, those all gradually hydrolyzed drastically in different extent, and the D-fructose proportional increased, but stachyose was relatively rather stable against steam-heating (**Figure 2**). It means that the majority of the oligosaccharides were hydrolyzed to monosaccharide—D-fructose and glucose, only stachyose still exist. Catalpol—the main iridoid glycoside seriously decreased, even radically disappeared (**Figure 3**).

On the other hand, the chain-structured monosaccharide like glucose would be decomposed to be 5-hydroxymethylfurfural (5-HMF). The increase trend of 5-HMF along with the steaming period was occurred simultaneously (**Figure 4**).

- Application of fingerprint to the commercial samples analysis

Generally the commercial samples of *Sheng Di-Huang* and *Shu-Di-Huang* collected from various markets, the

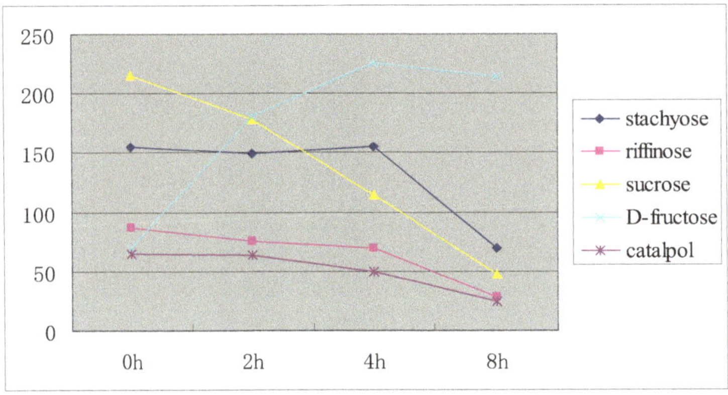

Figure 3. Comparison of peak area of several active components of Di-Huang (Rehmanniae Radix) steamed in persistently prolonged heating.

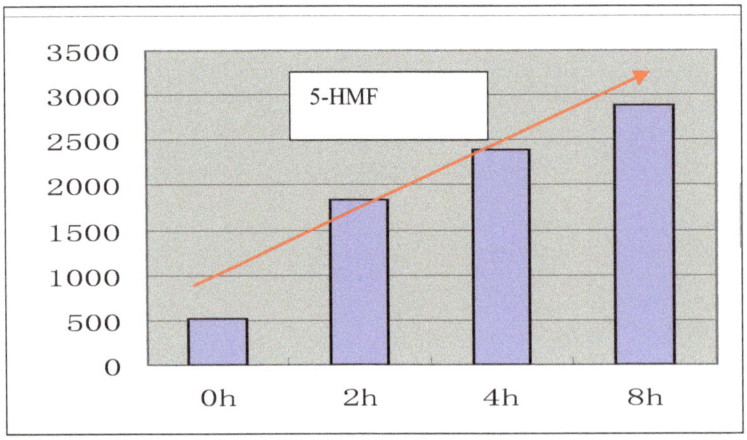

Figure 4. Peak area of 5-hydroxy-methylfurfural (5-MHF) inDi-Huang which was generated from decomposition of glucose when steamed in persistently prolonged heating.

labeled names rely solely on the claims of the suppliers. From the chromatographic fingerprints it is apparent that the ingredients in various samples exhibited some fluctuation which caused by variations in determining methods, sample habitats and uncontrolled steam-heating process [12] [13].

Based on the extent of decomposition of the ingredients, there are four grades of the patterns in the collected commercial samples as shown in the HPTLC fingerprints (images combined with the corresponding scanning profiles) (**Figure 5**). It is noteworthy that the most important tetra-oligosaccharide—stachyose [14] seems relatively more stable than the other oligosaccharides (**Figure 5** and **Figure 6**).

The project plot of Principle Component Analysis (PCA) of "*Di-Huang*" disclosed that while some of the commercial samples of "*Sheng-Di-Huang*" were closely distributed around the common pattern, (Grade I), others spread a distance from the common pattern, located at the upper part (Grade II) which have the typical character of of "*Sheng-Di-Huang*" common pattern, but catalpol was hard to be detected. Grade III and Grade IV those in the right side belonging to "*Shu-Du-Huang*". An exceptional example of *Shu-Di-Huang* (21#) showed only fructose. (The intact root tuber is of "as black as Chinese lacquer" (e.g., #21 sample) and always being considered as superior entity in the description of ancient herbal compendia). Obviously in fact such sample suffered from over-steaming (**Figures 5-7**).

3.2. HPLC Fingerprint Analysis

- HPLC fingerprint of *Di-Huang*

For analysis of the phenylethanol derivatives in *Di-Huang*, the HPLC-DAD experiment was carried out, the

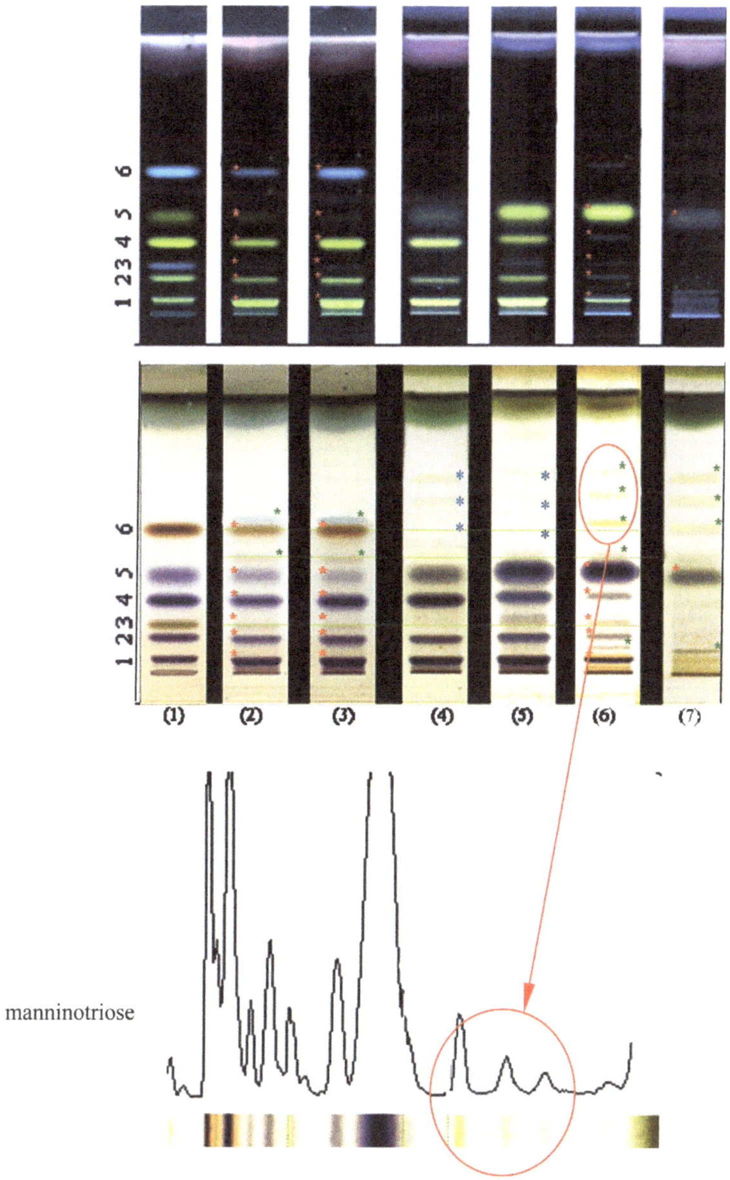

Figure 5. The HPTLC images of "*Di-Huang*" are divided four grades. (The figure below is the inverted color image from the upper fluorescence figure for more easy comparison), Track (1) Chemical reference substances: (1) stachyose, (2) raffinose, (3) rehmannioside D, (4) sucrose, (5) fructose, (6) catalpol Track (2) authentic sample of "*Sheng-Di-Huang*"; Track (3) commercial sample of "*Sheng-Di-Huang*" Track (4) similar appearance of the crude drug with the authentic sample (2) pattern, but catalpol exceptionally disappeared and the rehmanioside D was very weak. (cf. **Figure 7**). Track (5)-(6) the crude drugs appearances and the HPTLC pattern of the commercial samples were up to the description of "*Shu-Di-Huang*" in Chinese Pharmacopoeia, but the extent of hydrolysis of the saccharides differ, the monosaccharide-fructose increased drastically. Note that the stachyose (band 1) was relatively more stable than the others. Track (7) an over-steaming-processed sample of "*Shu-Di-Huang*", almost all the major ingredients disappeared or only residual amounts remained, but fructose being abundant. The blue stars marked in the invert color images (the figure below) showed some weak chemicals which are almost hard to be recognized under deep color background in the original fluorescence image.

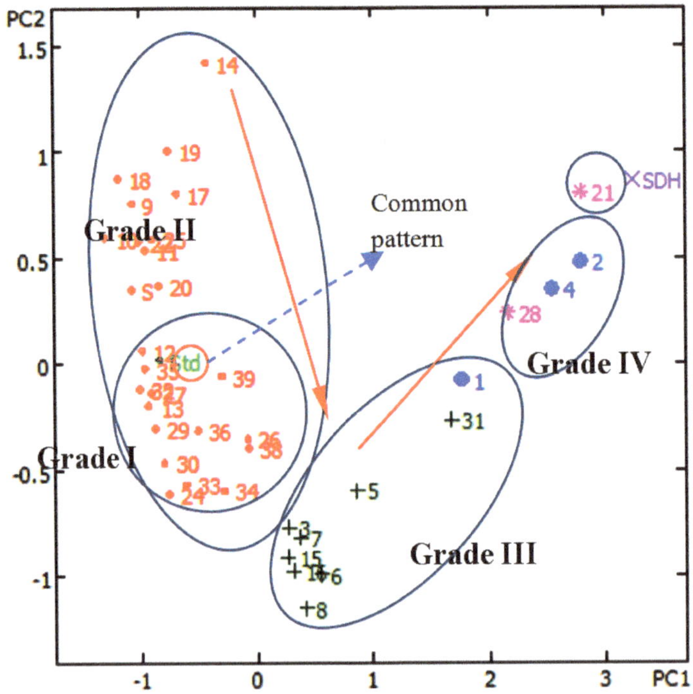

Figure 6. PCA projection plot of HPTLC fingerprint of *Di-Huang*. The Grade I and Grade II belong to "*Sheng-Di-Huang*", but the samples in Grade II, catapol was hard to be detected. Grade III and IV expressed the feature of "*Shu-Di-Huang*", but the samples in Grade IV contain minor amount of catalpol. The dynamic change of the oligosaccharides accompanying the steam processing caused some samples ("Shu-Di-Huang") distance from the common pattern. The longer the steam-heating time, the more severe the hydrolysis of raffinose and sucrose transforming them into fructose and glucose will occur. Stachyose was rather stable than the other oligosaccharides. (cf. **Figure 5**). Sample #21("SDH") showed only fructose (+ glucose) dominated in the fingerprint due to over-steam-heating led almost all oligosaccharides hydrolyzed to monosaccharide.

detection wavelength set at UV 334 nm to meet the maximum absorbance of this kind of components. The HPLC common pattern of "*Sheng-Di-Huang*" consisted of 11 characteristic peaks including acteoside and other phenylethanols (**Figure 8**).

- Applied Fingerprint to commercial sample analysis

Similarity of commercial samples has been calculated based on correlation coefficient for comparison with the common pattern (CP) (see **Figure 9**).

Since the concentration, distribution and proportion between the active components differ from reference crude drug, some samples of relative lower similarity (below 0.85) compared with the common pattern. Samples q#14 and #30 are two examples with unusual profiles individually. The supernormal strong peak of acetoside in HPLC profile of sample #14 also led to lower similarity (correlative coefficient 0.83) and oppositely a severe decline peak of acetoside as well as the peak (3) and (4) in the HPLC profile of sample #30 caused the lowest similarity of 0.24 (**Figure 10** and **Figure 11**).

- Comparison of HPLC fingerprints between *Sheng-Di-Huang* and *Shu-Di-Huang*

In HPLC fingerprint of the phenylethanols derivatives of *Shu-Di-Huang* are also decomposed in some extent by comparison with "*Sheng Di-Huang*", and increased some of the higher polarity compounds in the region of ca. Rt 4 min to 14 min (**Figure 12**).

4. Discussion

Combining the HPTLC fingerprint (fluorescence images plus the corresponding digital scanning profiles) and

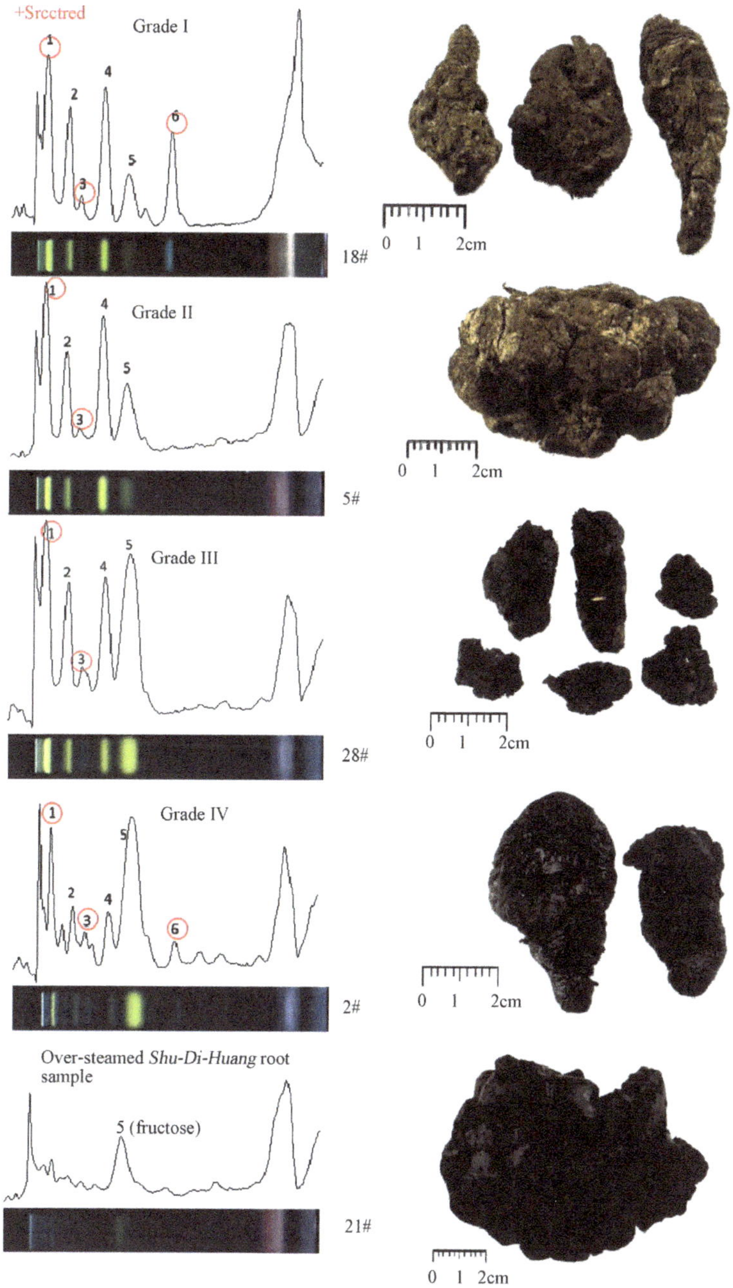

Figure 7. The changes of the HPTLC fingerprints of various commercial Di-Huang sample. (1)-Stachyose; (2)-Raffinose; (3)-Rehmannioside D; (4)-Surcose; (5)-D-Fructose; (6)-Catalpol.

the HPLC-DAD fingerprints of "*Di-Huang*" constructs an integrative view on the characteristics distributions of ingredients in "*Sheng-Di-Huang*" and "*Shu-Di-Huang*". The HPTLC fingerprint showed a whole range of detectable iridoids and saccharides. HPLC gave the profile of phenylethanol derivatives. The fingerprints provided useful information to distinguish Di-Huang by means of dual chromatographic analysis. It was revealed that all the bioactive ingredients in *Di-Huang* are steam-heating-labile. The fingerprint of *Sheng-Di-Huang* consists of catalpol, rehmannioside D, stachyose, raffinose, sucrose, and fructose as well as some minor unknown components. But those chemical ingredients led to decompose during the steaming process. The loss of catapol and other iridoids and varying degrees of decomposition of saccharides exhibited in the fingerprints of *Shu-Di-Huang*. The dynamic change of the saccharides in HPTLC fingerprint can possibly be traced to the extent of the

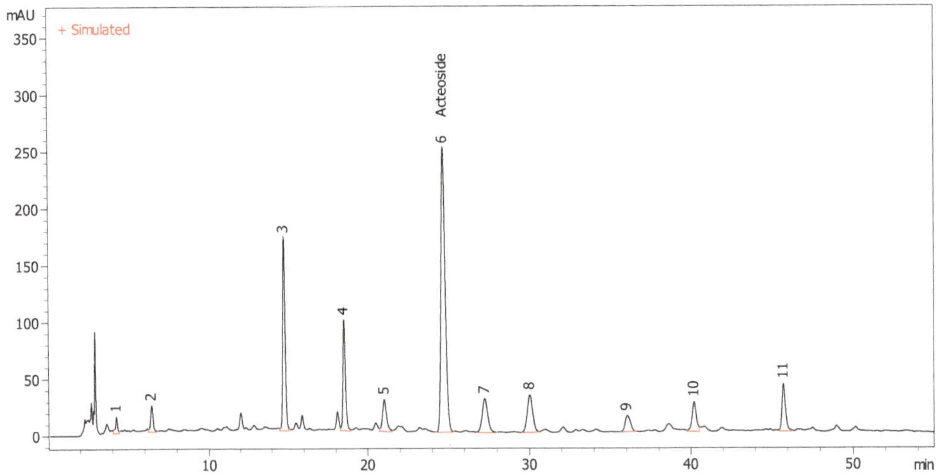

Figure 8. HPLC fingerprint common pattern of dried raw Rehmmaniae radix (*Sheng-Di-Huang*).

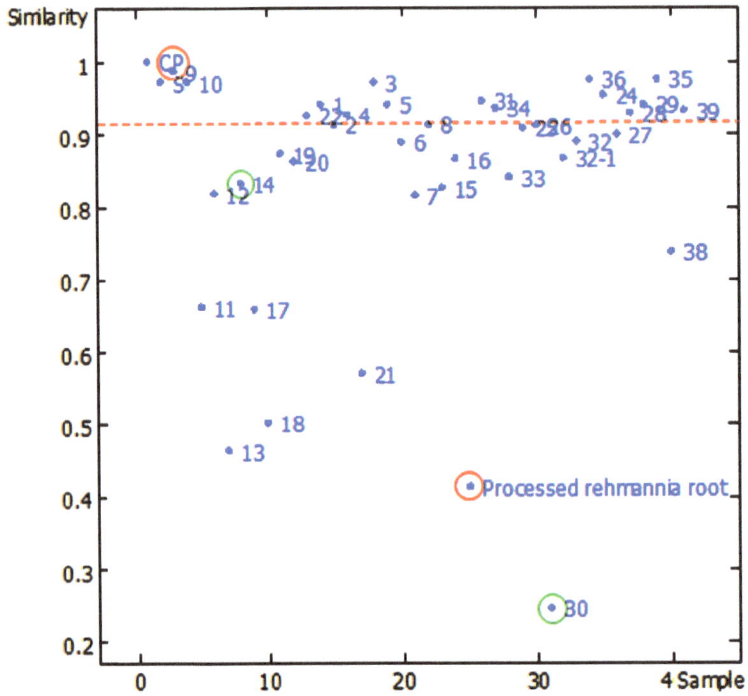

Figure 9. Similarity results of HPLC fingerprint of all samples of *Di-Huang*.

steaming process. It is noteworthy that stachyose seemed rather stable than the other oligosaccharides as expressed in the fluorescence images of various samples of "*Shu-Di-Huang*".

Referring to phenylethanol derivatives, acteoside which dominated in the HPLC fingerprint of "*Sheng-Di-Huang*" also decline gradually in *Shu-Di-Huang* as the steaming process went on.

In a word, "*Shu-Di-Huang*" cannot preserve the intact appearance of the fingerprint like that of *Sheng-Di-Huang*, either HPTLC (iridoids and oligosaccharides) or HPLC (phenylethanol derivatives) due to instability of the said bioactive metabolites. On the other hand, an ensuing rising of 5-HMF derived from glucose was also a complementary feature of *Shu-Di-Huang* (**Figure 4**). Recent studies claimed that 5-HMF is likely also an important bioactive component which exists in many herbal drugs with the function of antioxidant and nourishing kidney *Yin* deficiency [15]. So its influence to the drug property is also worth considering.

As iridoids and hydrolysable oligosaccharides are unstable, it brought up the possibility of developing a line

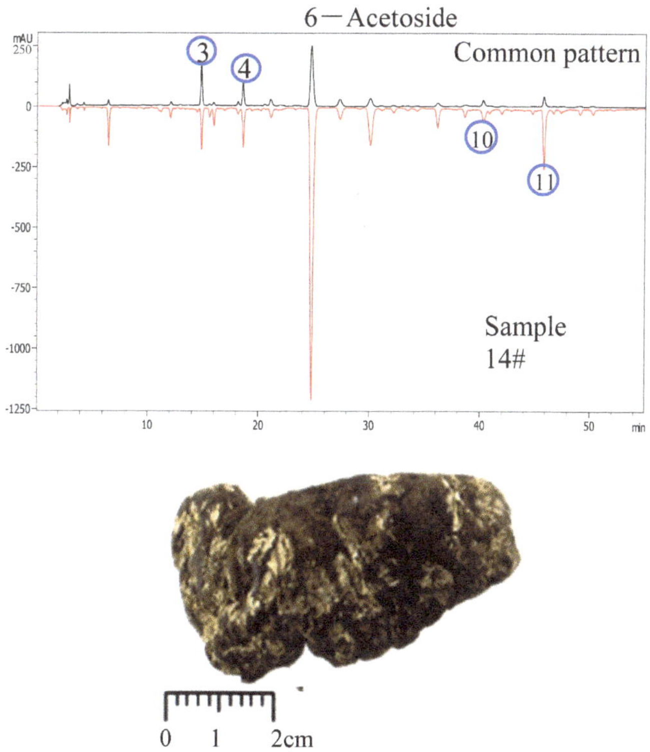

Figure 10. Comparison of HPLC profiles of commercial sample 14# with common pattern of "*Sheng-Di-Huang*". the content of acteoside is much higher than that in the common pattern.

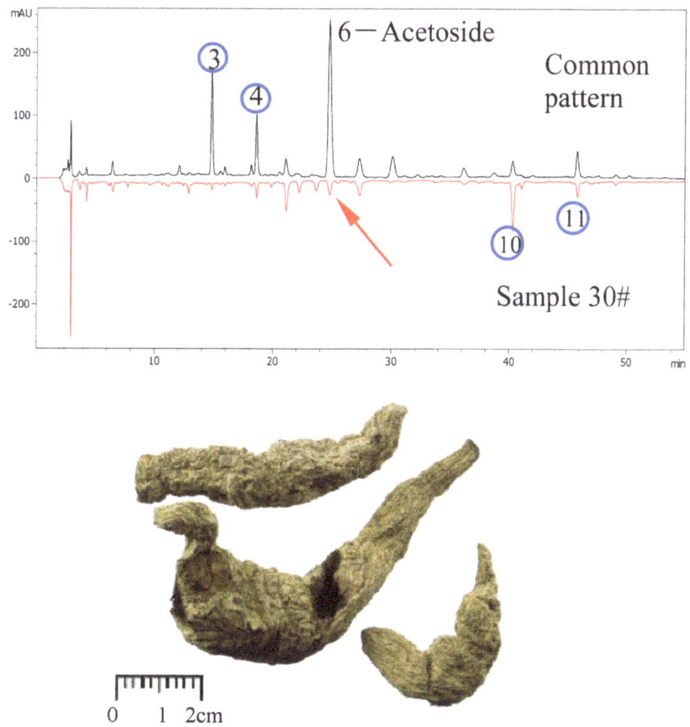

Figure 11. Comparison of HPLC profiles of sample 30# and the common pattern. The acteoside and other phenylethanol compounds severely declined in sample 30#,the appearance of which looked as *Sheng-Di-Huang*.

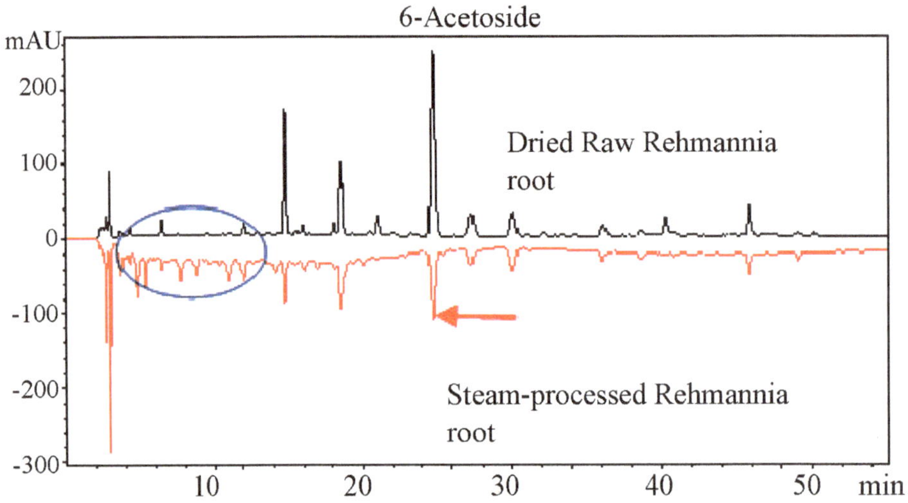

Figure 12. Comparison of HPLC profiles of *Sheng-Di-Huang* and *Shu-Di-Huang*.

to divide *Di-Huang* from "*Sheng*-" (raw, dried) to "*Shu*-" (processed, steam-heated). The dynamic alteration of the bioactive ingredients provided some clue on the correlation with the herbal drug's "property" transformation. It might presume from the fingerprint that the iridoids (catalpol is the highest content [8]), in particular, with "cold" property in *Sheng-Di-Huang* to exert the principle role for "cooling the hot of the blood", etc.; oligosaccharides, fairly stable stachyose with "warmer" property in *Shu-Di-Huang* to exert the function of nourishing "yin" of the "kidney", etc. It cannot certainly be neglected that the holistic role with the other chemical components, *i.e.*, phenylethanol glycosides, polysaccharides, etc.; in addition, the 5-HMF derived from dehydration of glucose and fructose during processing has also its contribution to the property transformation in *Shu-Di-Huang*. But the obvious different distributions of the detectable bioactive constituents in the two kinds of Di-Huang demonstrated in the chemical fingerprints are inferable that the properties of the both Di-Huang have their own individual focus and cannot be considered equivalent based on bioactivity. Modern pharmacological studies have also disclosed the various bioactive functions of different constituents in *Di-Huang* [15] [21]. The analysis result confirmed that too long steam-heating for getting the root tuber black as lacquer recorded in the historic herbal books cannot be considered the effective bioactive ingredients composition retained. Hence, standardizing the process procedure is necessary. Supposedly, it would be feasible to steady the quality of *Shu-Di-Huang* with the measures like cutting the root tuber into small pieces, improving the facilities, fix the time of steaming, enhancing the in-process quality control. Further in-depth investigation on the causal relationship between the chemical fingerprints and the traditional recorded Chinese medicine uses in a holistic way can be expected in the future.

5. Conclusion

The inconsistent chemical profiles of *Shu-Di-Huang* demonstrate that traditional processing methods can sometimes be of questionable value. Traditionally, nine cycles of "steam-heating and drying" process would be carried out turning the color to be as black as lacquer to obtain "the best quality" of *Shu-Di-Huang* according to traditional descriptions in the ancient Compendium Materia Medica. However there was no standardized procedure to regulate the operation and no real criteria for evaluation in spite of the request of the root tuber's color. The results of chromatographic fingerprint analysis confirmed that the uncertainty of the total steam-heating procedure makes the quality of the final product inconsistent, even some over-steamed *Shu-Di-Huang* caused a loss of almost all bioactive components and only fructose remained. It is appealed to the manufacturer the significance for defining the appropriate standard for both *Sheng-Di-Huang* and *Shu-Di-Huang*. Referring to the pattern of chromatographic fingerprints, the iridoids should be preserved as more as possible in "*Sheng-Di-Huang*", and the oligosaccharides, stachyose in particular, should be kept as consistent as possible in "*Shu-Di-Huang*", the increment of 5-HMF caused by dehydration of glucose in processing period should also be measured as it has its bioactive contribution.

Acknowledgements

The corresponding author thanks Professor Du Hengqing for her help in obtaining authentic samples of *Di-Huang*.

References

[1] Xiao. P.G. (2002) Modern Chinese Materia Medica, Vol. 2, Chemical Industry Press, Beijing, 390.

[2] The Commission of the PPRC (2005) Pharmacopoeia of People's Republic of China, Vol. 1, Chinese Medicinal Science and Technology Press, Beijing, 115-117.

[3] Tomoda, M., Kato, S. and Onuma M. (1971) Water Soluble Constituents of Rhemanniae Radix I. Carbohydrates and Acids of *Rehmannia glutinosa* f. *hueichingensis*. *Chemical & Pharmaceutical Bulletin* (Tokyo), **19**, 1455-1460. http://dx.doi.org/10.1248/cpb.19.1455

[4] Tomoda, M., Tanaka, M. and Kondo, N. (1971) Water Soluble Constituents of Rehmanniae Radix II: On the Constituents of Roots of *Rehmannia glutinosa* var. purpurea. *Chemical & Pharmaceutical Bulletin*, **19**, 2411-2413. http://dx.doi.org/10.1248/cpb.19.2411

[5] Oshio, H. and Inouye, H. (2008) Iridoid Glycosides of *Rehmannia glutinosa*. *Phytochemistry*, **21**, 133-138. http://dx.doi.org/10.1016/0031-9422(82)80029-0

[6] Tang, W.C. and Eisenbrand, G. (1992) Chinese Drugs of Plant Origin, Subtitle: Chemistry, Pharmacology and Use in Traditional and Modern Medicine, Springer Berlin Heidelberg, 849-854. http://dx.doi.org/10.1007/978-3-642-73739-8_106

[7] Liu, C.H., Zhang, L.J. and Li, G.S. (2002) Determination of Rehmannioside A in Root Tuber of *Rehmannia glutinosa*. *Chinese Traditional and Herbal Drugs*, **33**, 706-707.

[8] Zhu, M.F., Liu, X.Q., Ju-hee, O., Chang-soo, Y. and Je-Hyun, L. (2007) Effect of Concentration of Catalpol and 5-Hydroxymethyl-2-Furaldehyde from Processing of Rehmanniae Radix. *Zhongguo Zhong Yao Za Zhi*, **32**, 1155-1157.

[9] Zhang, H.-F. (2009) Survey on the Influence of Different Processing Methods to the Contents of Saccharids and Catalpol (in Chinese). *Journal of Practical Traditional Chinese Medicine* (*Zhongguo Shiyan Zhongyao Zazhi*), **25**, 501-502.

[10] Li, G.S., Liu, C.H. and Wang, H.S. (2002) Comparison of the Content of Catalpol of Dihuang in Different Habitats. *Zhong Cao Yao*, **33**, 12.

[11] Zhang, K., Guo, J.H., Tian, C.W. and Zhang, T.J., (2013) Effects of Various Treatments and Influencing Factors on Catalpol in *Rehmannia glutinosa*. *Chinese Traditional and Herbal Drugs*, **44**, 896-899.

[12] Chang, W.-T., Choi, Y.H., Van Der Heuden, R., Lee, M.-S., Lin, M.-K., Kong, H.W., Kim, H.K., Verpoorte, R., Hankemeier, T., Van Der Greef, J. and Wang, M. (2011) Traditional Processing Strongly Affects Metabolite Composition by Hydrolysis in *Rehmannia glutinosa* Roots. *Chemical and Pharmaceutical Bulletin*, **59**, 546-552. http://dx.doi.org/10.1248/cpb.59.546

[13] Wen, X.-S., Yang, S.-L., Ma, X.-J. and Zheng J.-H. (2004) HPLC Chromatogram Changes with Processing for Roots of Radix Rehmanniae. *Chinese Traditional and Herbal Drugs* (*Zhong Cao Yao*), **35**, 153-154.

[14] Lai, P.K.-K., To, M.-H., Lau, K.-M., Liu, C.-L., Cheng, L., Fung, K.-P., Leung, P.-C. and Lau, C.B.-S. (2012) Stachyose: One of the Active Fibroblast-Proliferating Components in the Root of Rehmanniae Radix (Dìhuáng). *Journal of Traditional and Complementary Medicine*, **2**, 227-234

[15] Li, D.Q., Duan, Y.L., Bao, Y.M., Liu, C.P., Liu, Y. and An, L.J. (2004) Neuroprotection of Catalpol in Transient Global Ischemia in Gerbils. *Neuroscience Research*, **50**, 169-177. http://dx.doi.org/10.1016/j.neures.2004.06.009

[16] Li, D.Q., Li, Y., Liu, Y., Bao, Y.M., Hu, B. and An, L.J. (2005) Catalpol Prevents the Loss of CA1 Hippocampal Neurons and Reduces Working Errors in Gerbils after Ischemia-Reperfusion Injury. *Toxicon*, **46**, 845-851. http://dx.doi.org/10.1016/j.toxicon.2004.09.007

[17] Tian, Y.Y., An, L.J., Jiang, L., Duan, Y.L., Chen, J. and Jiang, B. (2006) Catalpol Protects Dopaminergic Neurons from LPS-Induced Neurotoxicity in Mesencephalic Neuron Glia Cultures. *Life Sciences*, **80**, 193-199. http://dx.doi.org/10.1016/j.lfs.2006.09.010

[18] Jiang, B., Liu, J.H., Bao, Y.M. and An, L.J., (2004) Catalpol Inhibits Apoptosis in Hydrogen Peroxide-Induced PC12 Cells by Preventing Cytochrome *c* Release and Inactivating of Caspase Cascade. *Toxicon*, **43**, 53-59. http://dx.doi.org/10.1016/j.toxicon.2003.10.017

[19] Yu, Z., Wang, J., Li, G.S. and Wang, Y.S. (2001) Experimental Study on Rehmannioside D in the Action of Nourishing Yin, Enriching the Blood and Reducing the Blood Sugar. *Liaoning Journal of Traditional Chinese Medicine* (*Liaoning Zhongyi Zazhi*), **28**, 240-242.

[20] Guo, X.N., Zhang, R.X., Jia, Z.P., Li, M.X. and Wang, J. (2006) Effects of *Rehmannia glutinosa* Oligosaccharides on

Proliferation of 3T3-L1 Adipocytes and Insulin Resistance. *Chinese Journal of Chinese Materia Medica* (*Zhongguo Zhongyao Zazhi*), **31**, 403-407.

[21] Ding X., Wang, Mi.-Y., Yu, Z.-L., Hu, W. and Cai, B.-C. (2008) Stuides on Separation, Appraisal and the Biological Activity of 5-HMF in Cornusofficinalis. *Chinese Journal of Chinese Materia Medica* (*Zhongguo Zhongyao Zazhi*), **33**, 392-396.

4

Effects of *Nigella sativa* L. Seed Extract on Fatigue, Blood Biochemical Parameters and Thyroid Function in Male Mice

Azadeh Shariatifar, Mahdieh Riazi, Mona Ebnolelm, Mahsa Hadipour Jahromy*

Department of Pharmacology, Medical Sciences Research Center, Tehran Medical Sciences Branch, Islamic Azad University, Tehran, Iran
Email: *jahromymh@yahoo.com

Abstract

***Nigella sativa* L. (Black seed), is a traditional herbal medicine that has been used for many purposes. The present study was designed to investigate the effects of hydro-alcoholic extract of *nigella sativa* L. (NS) on performance of Forced Swimming Test (FST), blood biochemical parameters related to fatigue and thyroid functions. Therefore, Blood Urea Nitrogen (BUN), Creatine Kinase (CK), Lactic Dehydrogenase (LDH), and Total Protein (TP), triiodothyronine T3, thyroxin T4 and TSH tests were investigated. Thirty five male adult mice were randomly divided into five groups: three NS-fed groups, one fluoxetine treated group and one control group. Three NS experimental groups received hydro-alcoholic extract of NS at doses of 50, 100 and 200 mg/kg orally for two weeks. Immobility time decreased in all NS groups compared with control group. Administration of NS significantly increased the concentration of T3 and T4 of the treatment groups. On the contrary, the amount of BUN, CK, LDH, TP and TSH decreased. In conclusion, black seed extract at the experimented doses showed anti-depressant, anti-fatigue and hyperthyroid effects.**

Keywords

***Nigella sativa* Hydro-Alcoholic Extract; Black Seed; Thyroid Functions; Forced Swimming Test; Blood Biochemical Parameters Related to Fatigue**

1. Introduction

The genus Nigella is an annual plant that belongs to the *Renunculaceae* family and comprises about eight species [1].

*Corresponding author.

Nigella sativa L. is one of the spices that commonly known as black seed. It is native to many areas such as southern Europe and western Asia [2] which has been used as an herbal medicine for more than 2000 years.

Compound of black seed contains fixed and essential oils alkaloid, steroids, proteins, carbohydrates, fatty acids, and flavonoids. Also, it contains many bioactive constituents such as thymoquinone, thymohydroquinone, pinene, p-cymene, dithymoquinone [3] [4] that have been shown to possess biological, pharmacological and biochemical actions, including antibacterial [5], bronchodilator [6]. Besides it has activity against diabetes [7] and prevents lipid peroxidation [8]. Moreover, in some studies, NO exhibits anti-oxidant and immune-potentiating effects [9] [10].

Forced Swimming Test (FST) is a behavioral test for rodents, which evaluates the efficacy of antidepressant treatment and physical stamina [10]-[13]. Blood urea nitrogen (BUN), lactic dehydrogenase (LDH), creatine kinase (CK), and total protein (TP) are blood biochemical parameters related to fatigue. The BUN test is a routine test used primarily for evaluating renal functions. Serum CK and LDH in the body normally exist in muscle, and an increase in the amount of serum CK and LDH in the blood indicates that muscle damage has occurred [14]. TP is a rough measure of serum protein. Protein measurements can reflect the nutritional state, liver disease, kidney disease, and many other conditions [15]. Serum levels of Triiodothyronine (T3), thyroxin (T4) and thyroid stimulating hormones (TSH) are usually used to assess thyroid functions. Regarding NS, different kinds of extraction have been used on different animals and effects on blood biochemical parameters and thyroid function have been reported. So far however, the results are controversial [16]-[18].

The present study was undertaken to determine the effects of *Nigella sativa* L. hydro-alcoholic extract on FST performance, plasma concentration of BUN, CK, LDH, TP and thyroid functions.

2. Materials and Methods

2.1. Animals

35 Male adult mice Balb/c weighing 23 ± 5 g (Pasteur Institute, Karaj Production and Research Center, Iran) were used in this study. The animals were randomly divided into 5 groups of 7 each and treated according to the experimental protocol for 2 weeks. Animals housed under the following laboratory conditions: temperature 22˚C ± 1˚C, humidity 40% - 60%, 12 h Light/Dark cycle, lights on at 07:00 h. Mice were maintained in polyethylene cages with enough food and water available *ad libitum*. All measurements were performed between 10:00 and 14:00 h in the animal testing room. Mice were treated by the current law of Medical Sciences Research Center, Tehran Medical Branch, Islamic Azad University, Tehran, Iran, in accordance with the National Institutes of Health (NIH) Guide for Care and Use of Laboratory Animals. Control Group administrated distilled water orally. One group administered Fluoxetine, 10 mg/kg/day and three other groups administered NS at doses 50, 100 and 200 mg/kg/day.

2.2. Drugs

Black seeds were purchased from a local herb market, cleaned, dried, mechanically powdered, extracted with 70% ethanol and dried, with rotary evaporator to render the extract alcohol free and kept in refrigerator at 4 degree centigrade until used. The NS seeds extract was provided at doses of 50, 100, 200 mg/kg.

2.3. Forced Swimming Test

FST is generally used for evaluating anti depressive effects. Recently, the FST has also been used as an anti-fatigue test. During the FST, the animals were placed in a Plexiglas cylinder with 25 cm height and 10 cm width, which was filled with water (25˚C ± 0.5˚C).

The total duration of immobility was measured during a period of 4 min, after a delay of 2 min [19]. Each mouse was consider to be immobile when it ceased struggling and remained floating in the water, making only these movements necessary to keep its head above water.

2.4. Sample Collection

At the end of the experimental period (2 weeks) animals in all 5 groups were killed with chloroform and the blood samples were taken from the heart. Plasma was separated by centrifugation at speed 3000 rpm for 5 minutes and placed in plain Containers and stored at −10°C until analysis.

2.5. Hormones Estimation

T3, T4 and TSH levels were measured by electrochemiluminescence method (Elecsys2010). In order to clarify its anti-fatigue mechanisms, we assessed the levels of several blood biochemical parameters in mice after FST. Contents of BUN, LDH, CK and TP were determined by an auto analyzer (Hitachi 747, Hitachi Japan).

2.6. Statistical Analysis

To evaluate significance differences among treatment groups with control groups, one-way analysis of variance (ANOVA) was applied. The data were expressed as mean ± standard error of the mean (SEM). A value of $p < 0.05$ or less was considered to show statistical significance.

3. Results

3.1. Forced Swimming Test

Immobility time or exhaustion of the control and Fluoxetine group was measured 95.28 ± 19.81 s, 31.66 ± 2.94, respectively. Data of the FST test (**Figure 1**) demonstrated that administration of NS were significantly decrease the immobility time of the treatment groups which were 49.00 ± 6.03 s, 40.83 ± 6.17 s, 50.66 ± 3.88 s respectively ($p < 0.01$, $F = 36.89$).

3.2. Effect of NS on Biochemical Parameters

In order to clarify its anti-fatigue mechanisms, we assessed the levels of several blood biochemical parameters in mice after FST (**Table 1**). All the biochemical parameter such as BUN, LDH, CK and TP levels significantly tended to decrease in compared with control group ($p < 0.001$).

3.3. Thyroid Function Tests

These results of T3, T4 and TSH serum level of control and treatment groups are shown in **Table 2**. The plasma concentration of T3 and T4 are significantly ($P \leq 0.001$) increased and TSH serum level significantly ($p < 0.001$) decreased in treatment groups compared with control groups.

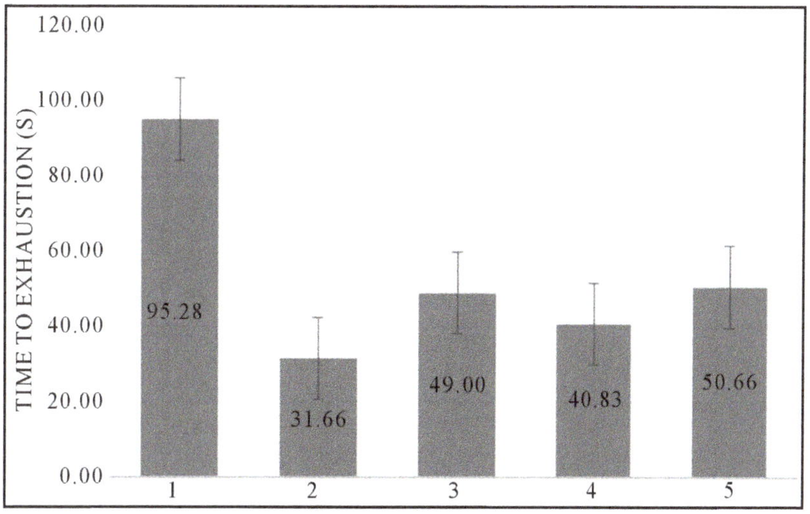

Figure 1. Time to exhaustion in swimming test (n = 7). Group 1: control mice administered distilled water, Group 2: administered Fluoxetine 10 mg/kg/day, Group 3: administered NS 50 mg/kg/day, Group 4: administered NS100 mg/kg/day, Group 5: administered NS 200 mg/kg/day. Values are means ± S.D.

Table 1. Effect of NS on blood biomedical parameters in mice treated with NS after FST.

	BUN (mg/dl)	TP (mg/dl)	CK (U/l)	LDH (U/l)
Group I	42.44 ± 3.18	11.61 ± 1.99	1058.50 ± 427.72	5288.50 ± 2288.27
Group II	29.93 ± 7.96**	8.04 ± 1.97**	481.42 ± 334.58*	2561.28 ± 392.66*
Group III	23.42 ± 2.36**	6.75 ± 0.49**	55.16 ± 12.38**	1659.20 ± 346.36**
Group IV	16.26 ± 3.80**	6.05 ± 1.25**	90.14 ± 87.02**	1198.66 ± 370.65**
F	31.33	13.97	18.10	13.97
P	<0.001	<0.001	<0.001	<0.001

Values are the means ± S.D. (n = 7). *p < 0.05 indicates significant difference from the control group and **p < 0.001 indicates significant difference from the control group. Group I: control mice administered distilled water, Group II: administered NS 50 mg/kg/day, Group III: administered NS100 mg/kg/day, Group IV: administered NS 200 mg/kg/day.

Table 2. Thyroid function tests before and after supplementation of NS.

	TSH	T3	T4
Group I	0.30 ± 0.10	1.24 ± 0.20	67.66 ± 1.52
Group II	0.08 ± 0.02	1.75 ± 0.19*	74.33 ± 5.13
Group III	0.005 ± 0.01**	1.63 ± 0.12*	76.80 ± 8.07
Group IV	0.005 ± 0.01*	1.95 ± 0.05*	102.33 ± 7.50*
F	29.21	11.96	16.24
P	<0.001	<0.001	<0.001

Values are the means ± S.D. (n = 7). *p < 0.05 indicates significant difference from the control group and **p < 0.001 indicates significant difference from the control group. Group I: control mice administered distilled water, Group II: administered NS 50 mg/kg/day, Group III: administered NSv100 mg/kg/day, Group IV: administered NS 200 mg/kg/day.

4. Discussion

First, we investigated the effect of NS on FST, which is commonly accepted an experimental exercise model used for assessing anti-depressive and anti-fatigue effects. Increases in concentrations of NS treated mice showed significant improvement in the swimming test. It suggests that the decreased duration of immobility in mice is related to change of certain metabolites in the system. These results agree with Roshan, who reported feeding NS could protect neural cell against oxidative stress [20]. In addition, there is evidence suggesting that the anti-depressant effect of NS was most probably related to its anti-oxidant effects [8] [17].

In order to investigate its mechanisms, we assessed biochemical serum markers after FST. BUN, CK, LDH and TP levels are related to fatigue. In the present study, CK level which is known to be an accurate indicator of muscle damage tended to decrease and less leakage of CK occurring during the swimming exercise. These results indicated that muscle damage in the treated groups, as reflected by the serum CK levels, was minimized by NS. Moreover, LDH is known to be an accurate indicator of muscle damage [21]. Therefore, the LDH serum level increases after exercise. In this study, however, the LDH level tended to decrease; thus, our results indicate that NS could influence the fatigue metabolism. Also, NS could significantly reduce BUN level which may be due to inhibition of stimulation of sympathetic nervous system. In fact, further studies are needed to clarify the detailed mechanisms involved in the anti-fatigue-like properties of NS in order to support present results.

The main findings of our study were that NS significantly increases the concentration of T3 and T4 and decreases the TSH in experimental groups compared to untreated mice. These results are in agreement with previous studies by Sharif *et al.* who indicated that treatment with oral administration of NS increased T4 levels in rabbits [18]. These results indicated that oral administration of NS lead to hyperthyroidism in mice; likewise, other study reports that the oral administration of NS not only increased serum T3 and decreased TSH but also has an anti-oxidant effect [22]. Yet, Marel reported that treatment oral administration with NS could raise T3 level without changing T4 and TSH serum concentration levels [23]. Further work is suggested for evaluating the effect of NS on the serum concentration of thyroid hormones to clarify the possible mechanism of action.

5. Conclusion

In brief, in the present study, swimming time in NS-fed groups increased during FST. NS also increased the blood concentration of T3 and T4, leading to the decrease of TSH serum level. Taken together, it is suggested that NS not only has anti-depressive effect and anti-fatigue like effects that might be useful in the development of physical strength, but also leads to hyperthyroidism in mice, so it can be tested in thyroid function disorders.

References

[1] Mozaffarian, V.A. (1998) Dictionary of Iranian Plants Names. Moaser Publisher, Tehran Farhang.

[2] Boskabady, M.H., Shirmohammadi, B., Jandaghi, P. and Kiani, S. (2004) Possible Mechanism(s) for Relaxant Effect of Aqueous and Macerated Extracts from *Nigella sativa* on Tracheal Chains of Guinea Pig. *BMC Pharmacology*, **4**, 3. http://dx.doi.org/10.1186/1471-2210-4-3

[3] Winkler, C., Houcher, B., Schoroechsnadelk, S.H. and Fuchs, D. (2005) Nigella Sativa Seeds (Balck Cumin) Conteract Cytokine Induced Neopterinproduction and Tryptophan Degradation *in Vitro. Pterins*, **16**, 152-153.

[4] Liu, X., Abd El-Aty, A.M. and Shim, J.H. (2011) Various Extraction and Analytical Techniques for Isolation and Identification of Secondary Metabolites from Nigella Sativa Seeds. *Mini-Reviews in Medicinal Chemistry*, **11**, 947-955. http://dx.doi.org/10.2174/138955711797068472

[5] Hanafy, M.S.M. and Hatem, M.E. (1991) Studies on Theantimicrobial Activity of Nigella Sativa Seed (Black Cumin). *Journal of Ethnopharmacology*, **34**, 275-278. http://dx.doi.org/10.1016/0378-8741(91)90047-H

[6] El-Tahir, K.E.H., Ashour, M.M.S. and Al-Harbi, M.M. (1993) The Respiratory Effects of the Volatile Oil of the Black Seed (Nigella Sativa) in Guinea-Pigs: Elucidation of the Mechanism(s) of Action. *General Pharmacology*, **24**, 1115-1122. http://dx.doi.org/10.1016/0306-3623(93)90358-5

[7] El-Dakhakhny, M., Mady, N., Lembert, N. and Ammon, H.P. (2002) The Hypoglycemic Effect of Nigella Sativa Oil Is Mediated by Extrapancreatic Actions. *Planta Medicine*, **68**, 465-466. http://dx.doi.org/10.1055/s-2002-32084

[8] Perveen, T., Haider, S., Kanwal, S. and Haleem, D.J. (2009) Repeated Administration of Nigella Sativa Decreases 5-HT Turnover and Produces Anxiolytic Effects in Rats. *Pakistan Journal of Pharmaceutical Sciences*, **22**, 139-144.

[9] El-Kadi, A. and Kandil, O. (1987) The Black Seed (Nigella Sativa) and Immunity: Its Effect on Human T Cell Subset. *Federation Proceedings*, **46**, 1222.

[10] Estrada-Camarena, E., Contreras, C.M., Saavedra, M., Una-Baltazar, I. and López-Rubalcava, C. (2002) Participation of the Lateral Septal Nuclei (LSN) in the Antidepressant-Like Actions of Progesterone in the Forced Swimming Test (FST). *Behavioural Brain Research*, **134**, 175-183. http://dx.doi.org/10.1016/S0166-4328(02)00023-2

[11] Griebel, G., Simiand, J., Serradeil-Le Gal, C., Wagnon, J., Pascal, M., Scatton, B., Maffrand, J.P. and Soubrie, P. (2002) Anxiolytic- and Antidepressant-Like Effects of the Non-Peptide Vasopressin V1b Receptor Antagonist, SSR149415, Suggest an Innovative Approach for the Treatment of Stress-Related Disorders. *Proceedings of the National Academy of Sciences of the USA*, **99**, 6370-6375. http://dx.doi.org/10.1073/pnas.092012099

[12] Tejani-Butt, S.M., Kluczynski, J. and Paré, W.P. (2003) Strain-Dependent Modification of Behavior Following Antidepressant Treatment. *Progress in Neuro-Psychopharmacology & Biological Psychiatry*, **27**, 7-14. http://dx.doi.org/10.1016/S0278-5846(02)00308-1

[13] Koo, H.N., Um, J.Y., Kim, H.M., Lee, E.H., Sung, H.J. and Kim, I.K. (2008) Effect of Pilopool on Forced Swimming Test in Mice. *International Journal of Neuroscience*, **118**, 365-374. http://dx.doi.org/10.1080/00207450701593145

[14] Koo, H.N., Lee, J.K. and Hong, S.H. (2004) Herbkines Increases Physical Stamina in Mice. *Biological & Pharmaceutical Bulletin*, **27**, 117-119. http://dx.doi.org/10.1248/bpb.27.117

[15] Dorchy, H. (2002) Sports and Type I Diabetes: Personal Experience. *Revue Médicale de Bruxelles*, **23**, A211-A217.

[16] Farah, K.M., Atoji, Y., Shimizu, Y., Shiina, T., Nikami, H. and Takewaki, T. (2004) Mechanism of Hypoglycemic Immune Potentiating Effects of *Nigella sativa* L. Oil in Streptozotocin-Induced Diabetic Hamster. *Research in Veterinary Science*, **77**, 123-129. http://dx.doi.org/10.1016/j.rvsc.2004.03.002

[17] Hosseini, M., Zakeri, S., Khoshdast, S., Yousefian, F.T., Rastegar, M., Vafaee, F., Kahdouee, S., Ghorbani, F., Rakhshandeh, H. and Kazemi, S.A. (2012) The Effects of Nigella Sativa Hydro-Alcoholic Extract and Thymoquinone on Lipopolysaccharide-Induced Depression Like Behavior in Rats. *Journal of Pharmacy and Bioallied Sciences*, **4**, 219-225.

[18] Sharif, S.H., Elmahdi, B.M., Ali Mohammed, A.M. and Mohammed, A.H. (2012) The Effects of Nigella Sativa L. Ethanolic Extract on Thyroid Function in Normal and Alloxan-Induced Diabetic Rats. *Thyroid Research and Practice*, **9**, 48-54. http://dx.doi.org/10.4103/0973-0354.96044

[19] Porsolt, R.D., Bertin, A. and Jalfre, M. (1997) Behavioral Despair in Mice: A Primary Screening Test for Antidepres-

sants. *Archives Internationales de Pharmacodynamie*, **229**, 327-336.

[20] Roshan, S., Abdullah, K., Tazneem, B. and Sadath, A. (2010) To Study the Effect of Nigella Sativa on Various Biochemical Parameters on Stressed Induced in Albino Rats. *International Journal of Pharmacy and Pharmaceutical Sciences*, **4**, 185-189.

[21] Coombes, J.S. and McNaughton, L.R. (2000) Phys. Fitness. *Journal of Sports Medicine*, **40**, 240-246.

[22] Khalawi1, A.A., Al-Robai, A.A., Khoja, S.M. and Shaker, A.S. (2013) Can Nigella Sativa Oil (NSO) Reverse Hypothyroid Status Induced by PTU in Rat? Biochemical and Histological Studies. *Life Science Journal*, **10**, 802-8011.

[23] Meral, I., Yener, Z., Ozbek, H. and Ustun, R. (2001) Effects of *Nigella sativa* L. on Serum Concentrations of Thyroid Hormones, Thyroid Stimulating Hormone and Glucose in Alloxan-Induced Diabetic Rabbits. *Journal of Veterinary Medicine. A Physiology, Pathology, Clinical Medicine*, **48**, 593-599.
http://dx.doi.org/10.1046/j.1439-0442.2001.00393.x

5

Design, Development and Phytochemical Evaluation of a Poly Herbal Formulation Linkus Syrup

Zeeshan Ahmed Sheikh[1], Aqib Zahoor[1*], Saleha Suleman Khan[1], Khan Usmanghani[1,2]

[1]Department of Research and Development, Herbion Pakistan (Pvt.) Limited, 30/28 Korangi Industrial Area, Karachi, Pakistan
[2]Faculty of Pharmacy, Jinnah University for Women, Karachi, Pakistan
Email: *aqib.zahoor@herbion.com

Abstract

The present work has been carried out on polyherbal formulation named as Linkus Syrup. The herbal formulation consists of *Glycyrrhiza glabra, Hyssopus officinalis, Piper longum and Alpinia galangal.* The Linkus syrup physico-chemical evaluation such as pH, density, identification of polysaccharide, tanning agents, ascorbic acid and shelf life was complied. The TLC and quantitative determination of alkaloid were quantified. Determination of biomarker has been validated for the analysis of vasicine. The study result revealed that Linkus syrup formulation was well standardized at different levels such as physic-chemical consistency and assay of bio marker compound.

Keywords

Syrup, Crude Herb, Anti-Tussive, Anti-Bronchitis, Anti-Pharyngitis, Sore Throat, Tracheitis, HPLC

1. Introduction

Cough is one of the most common symptoms for which patients seek medical attention from primary care physicians and pulmonologists [1]. These studies were carried out for the design, development and phytochemical evaluation of a poly herbal formulation named as Linkus syrup. The syrup consists of leaves of *Adhatoda vasica* used in the treatment of coughs, bronchitis, asthma, common cold, expectorant and antispasmodic (bronchodilator). The active components are vasicine (aka peganine) and vasicinone [2]. The root and rhizome of *Glycyrrhiza glabra* contain glycyrrhizin that inhibit growth and cytopathology of cytomegalovirus and are utilized in

*Corresponding author.

cough, catarrhal infections, asthma, bronchitis, coughs, arthritis and allergic complaints [3]-[5]. *Hyssopus officinalis* contains pinocamphone, camphone, pinocampheol, cineole used as an expectorant, bronchitis, respiratory infections, upper respiratory tract infections, coughs [3] [6]-[8]. The fruits and roots of *Piper longum* are attributed for diseases of respiratory tract, such as cough, bronchitis, asthma [9] and contain piperine, piperlongumine, piperlonguminine, methyl 3,4,5-trimethoxycinnamate [9]. *Alpinia galanga* has a bronchodilator and anti-inflammatory effect on bronchioles [10] [11] and the main components isolated from its rhizomes were galangoisoflavonoid, methyleugenol, galangin, acetoxychavicol acetate (ACA) and hydroxychavicol acetate In the standard German text, *Hager's Handbuch der Pharmazeutischen Praxis*, *Zingiber officinale* has been listed as being used against nervousness, chronic inflammation of the intestine, coughing, conditions of the urinary tract and lower abdomen, rheumatism, and a sore throat [12] and the chemical constituents are zingerone, shogaols and gingerols, zingiberene, bisboline and cineol. The leaves and flower of *Althea officinalis* have demulcent, expectorant, diuretic, and emollient properties and generally used to treat ailments of the lungs and the urinary system [13]. The active constituents are Pectin, disaccharide sacharose, mucilage, Hypolaetin-8-glucoside, isoquercitrin, kaempferol, caffeic, *p*-coumaric acid, scopoletin, asparagines and many amino acids.

Cordia latifolia [14] is used to treat gastrointestinal, respiratory and dermatological disorders and the constituents cited were cordinoic acid, cordicilin, cordinol and cordicinol [15]. *Zizyphus jujuba* used for colds and coughs; they also have antifungal, antibacterial, antiulcer, anti-inflammatory, sedative and antiseptic properties [16] [17] and it possesses mauritine-A; amphibine-H, jubanine-A, jubanine-B; mucronine-D, and nummularine-B, sativanine-E, frangufoline, ziziphines jujubosides [17]. *Onosma bracteatum* leaves and stems are used to treat bronchitis and asthma [18] and main phytochemicals present are naphthazarins, naphthoquinones, alkannins and Shikonins [19].

2. Material and Method

Herbs were bought through Supply Chain Department of the Herbion Pakistan (Pvt.) Limited, Karachi from the local market. All samples were stored in dark at 23˚C. The herbs utilized in Linkus syrup were morphologically compared with the authentic specimen available at QC department of Herbion Pakistan Pvt. Ltd., they details are as follows, *Adhatoda vasica* reference No. B18, *Glycyrrhiza glabra* reference No.M4, *Piper longum* reference No. F1, *Viola odorata* reference No. B2, *Hyssopus officinalis* reference No.Z1, *Alpinia galangal* reference No. A2, *Cordia latifolia* reference No. S9, *Althea officinalis* reference No. K3, *Zizyphus vulgaris* reference No.U3, *Onosma bracteatum* reference No. B1. These herbs have also been authenticated and verified by Prof. Dr. Iqbal Azhar, Department of Pharmacognosy, Faculty of Pharmacy, University of Karachi. and chemically for biomarker of some herbs. All the other chemicals and reagents were of pure analytical grade and obtained from local supplier.

2.1. Development of Linkus Syrup

With extensive literature review and traditional knowledge research and development department of Herbion Pakistan Pvt. Limited was successfully developed the formulation for cough and cold which named as Linkus Syrup.

2.1.1. Selection and Evaluation of Herbs

Table 1 represents the quantity and pharmacological action of herbs used in this preparation.

All herbs were tested for their prescribed part, macro and microscopic descriptions, identification, chemical assays, foreign matter, total ash, Acid insoluble ash, alcohol and water soluble part of extract. These properties with specifications were listed in **Table 2**.

2.1.2. Preparation of Extracts

Each herb was extracted individually in vacuum jacketed extractor with water five times to the amount of herb taken. Stir for 10 minutes and then start heating. Heat to boil. The temperature should be from 100˚C - 110˚C. Then slow down the temperature to 80˚C - 90˚C. Amount of the herb, extraction time and percent yield are mentioned in the **Table 3**.

2.1.3. Preparation of Linkus Syrup

625 liter deionized water was took in manufacturing tank. Heated and boil for 40 to 45 minutes. When boiling

Table 1. The herbs used, quantity and pharmacological actions.

S.No	Active ingredients	Common name	Quantity*	Pharmacological Action
01	*Adhatoda vasica* (dry leaves Extract)	Arusa	600 mg	Bronchodilator and expectorant, use in breathlessness
02	*Glycyrrhyza glabra* (Dry root extract)	Mulaithi	75 mg	Anti-inflammatory and it reduces inflammation of the respiratory tract, relieve a spasmodic cough
03	*Piper longum* (Dry fruit extract)	Piplamol	100 mg	Prevents recurrent attacks of bronchial asthma, immune-modulator activity, anti-allergic
04	*Viola odorata* (Dry fruit extract)	Banafsha	25 mg	Expectorant
05	*Hyssopus officinalis* (Dry leaves extract)	Zufa	50 mg	antiseptic, cough reliever, and expectorant, soothing and cough suppressant properties. antibacterial activity against *S. aureus*
06	*Alpinia galanga* (Dry root extract)	galangal	50 mg	Cough and respiratory troubles, cold, flu, lung diseases, phlegm
07	*Cordia latifolia* (Dry fruit extract	Lasorda	100 mg	against *H. influenzae*
08	*Althea officinalis* (Dry extract of flower)	Khatmi	100 mg	cough suppression, bronchodilator activity
09	*Zizyphus jujuba* (Dry fruit extract)		100 mg	colds and coughs, antibacterial, antiseptic properties, produced sound sleep
10	*Onosma bracteatum* (Dry leaves Extract)		100 mg	bronchitis and asthma, restlessness antibacterial activity against *S. aureus*

*amount of herb used in the preparation of 10 ml syrup.

Table 2. Specification and analytical method of raw material used in Linkus syrup by quality operation.

Name of the Herbs	Drug Parts	Description	Identification	Assay	Foreign Matter	Total ASH	Acid Insoluble Ash	Alcohol Soluble Extraction	Water Soluble Extraction
Adhatoda vasica	dried leaves	Macroscopic and Microscopic	By TLC Spot observed	About 1.3% of alkaloids as vascine by HPLC	NMT 2.0%	NMT 17.0%	NMT 1.0%	NLT 6.0%	NLT 27.0%
Glycyrrhyza glabra	Rhizome dark brown to black brown extract	Soluble in Water	Through taste: Sweetish bitter (Organoleptic)	Glycyrrhizin content present in Gylcyrrhiza glabra by HPLC	---	---	---	---	---
Piper longum	Fruiting spikes	Macroscopic	Spot observed by TLC	NLT 5% of Piperinre by HPTLC	NMT 2.0%	NMT 8.0%	NMT 1.0%	NLT 9.0%	NLT 35.0%
Viola odorata	Dried leaves	Viola has characteristic odor	Macroscoipc (As per Flora of Pakistan page # 4)	---	NMT 3.0%	NMT 15.0%	---	---	---
Hyssopus officinalis	Flowering tops	Macroscopic. Microscopic	Spot observed by TLC	---	NMT 2%	NMT 10%	NMT 2.5%	water soluble extractive: NLT 10%	---
Alpinia galanga	Dried rhizome	Macroscopic and Microscopic	----	---	NMT 2.0%	NMT 2.0%	----	NLT 6.0%	NLT 13.0%
Cordia latifolia	Ddried fruit	Macroscopic	----	---	NMT 2.0%	NMT 3.0%	NMT 1.0%	---	---
Althea officinalis	Dried seeds	Macroscopic and Microscopic	---	---	NMT 2.0%	NMT 8.0%	NMT 1.5%	NLT 10.0%	NLT 18.0%
Zizyphus jujuba	Dried mature fruit of	Macroscopic and Microscopic	---	----	NMT 1.0%	NMT 4.5%	NMT 0.2%	NLT 25.0%	NLT 45.0%
Onosma bracteatum	Ddried leaves and stem	Macroscopic and Microscopic	---	---	NMT 2.0%	NMT 26.0%	NMT 4.0%	NLT 1.0%	---

Table 3. Extraction of Linkus syrup herbs.

Herb	Herb Quantity	Quantity of Thick Extract	Extraction Time	Percent Yield
Adhatoda vasica Nees.	18.0 kg	3.60 kg	1 hour	20.0%
Piper longum L.	3.0 kg	0.75 kg	20 minutes	25.00%
Cordia latifolia L.	3.0 kg	0.75 kg	20 minutes	25.00%
Althaea officinalis L.	3.0 kg	0.75 kg	20 minutes	25.00%
Zizyphus vulgaris Lam.	3.0 kg	0.75 kg	20 minutes	25.00%
Onosma bracteatum Wall	3.0 kg	0.75 kg	20 minutes	25.00%
Glycyrrhiza glabra L.	2.3 kg	0.56 kg	15 minutes	24.30%
Alpinia galanga (L.) Wild.	1.5 kg	0.37 kg	10 minutes	24.60%
Hyssopus officinalis L.	1.5 kg	0.37 kg	10 minutes	24.60%
Viola odorata L.	0.8 kg	0.19 kg	10 minutes	23.70%

was started, add 1750 kg sugar slowly with constant stirring. Continue heating with constant stirring till it became homogenize syrup. Separately dissolved Methyl Paraben, Propyl Paraben, Citric acid and Glycerin in 83 liter deionized Water, mixed, heat and boiled thoroughly. Mix this solution to the homogenized syrup and stirred for 20 minutes. Took 416 Liters of Purified water in jacketed kettle and add to it 73.75 kg combine extract. Heat till it was fully dissolved and then filter the solution. Add the filtered solution to homogenized syrup prepared previously, stirred and mix for 20 min. After mixing, allow the syrup to cool down by chilled water circulation. Circulation was continued until the temperature of the syrup reached to "room temperature". Mixed the flavors like Peppermint Oil, Clove Oil and Propylene glycol, then made up the volume of syrup to 1250 liters with deionized water. Afterward allow final mixing by stirring for half an hour. This process represented here in **Table 4**.

3. Phytochemical Evaluations

Brown color syrup was prepared with characteristic odor, having pH in between 3.0 - 6.0, and density 1.25 - 1.35 g/cm^3. Identification of polysaccharides, tanning agent, and ascorbic acid were performed by test tubes method. While the identification of vasicine was done by TLC.

3.1. Physical Evaluation

3.1.1. Appearance

Brown color viscosity syrup with characteristic odor, Determination was conducted visually.

3.1.2. pH Determination

Dissolved 10 ml of syrup in 100 ml of water. Filtered and determine pH potentiometrically Standard: 3.0 - 6.0

3.1.3. Density

Determination was conducted by SP XII method 3 and it was according to Standard: 1.25 to 1.35 g/cm^3.

3.1.4. Qualitative Identification Reactions

Placed 5 ml of the preparation to a flat-bottomed 50 ml flask. Added 20 ml of 96% spirit and mixed; precipitated suspension was formed **(polysaccharides)**. Left the obtained solution for 1 hour for layer separation and filter carefully through the folded paper filter (Solution A).

Added 3 drops of Ferric chloride solution to 3 ml of the solution A. After shaking greenish-yellow coloring appears **(tanning agents)**. To 3 ml of A solution added 3 drops 0.1% spirit solution of sodium 2.6-dichlorfeno-lindofenolite solution had a reddish-violet coloring at mixing **(ascorbic acid)**.

Table 4. Manufacturing of Linkus syrup.

Ingredients for 1 lot	Quantity	Unit
	Active	
Thick combined Extract	73.75	Kg
	Excipient	
Sucrose	1750	Kg
Anhydrous citric acid	5	Kg
Methyl Paraben	2.5	Kg
Propyl Paraben	0.5	Kg
Glycerin	25	Lit
Propylene glycol	2.5	Lit
Peppermint oil	0.9375	Lit
Clove oil	0.3125	Lit
Purified water	Up to 1250	Lit

Preparation of 0.1% Alcohol Solution of Sodium 2, 6-Dichlorphenolindophenolat
Placed 0.1 g of sodium 2, 6-dichlorphenolindophenolyat in 100 ml of measuring retort and dissolve it in 30 ml of 96% ethyl alcohol and then made up the volume with 96% ethyl alcohol. Shelf life of solution was 1 month

3.1.5. Qualitative Identification by TLC

Applied 0.05 ml of solution I to chromatographic plate "Silica gel 60 F_{254}" (size 10 × 20 cm manufactured by Merck) in the form of spot. Dry the plate in hot air for 5 minutes and placed it in the chamber preliminary saturated for 1 hour with a mixture of the following solvent: 96% alcohol : chloroform : hydrous ammonia (30:19:1).

When the front of solvents was reached the plate edge, took it out from the chamber and dried in a drying oven for 3 minutes at 100°C. Then apply Dragendorff reagent to the plate. 1 reddish pink color spot (vasicine) was shown on the plate in UV light at wave length 254 nm R*f* (0.4).

The physicochemical and organoleptic parameters so generated for standardization were further determined by HPLC and UV spectrophotometers as mentioned by using colorimeter.

3.2. Quantitative Determination of Total Alkaloids

About 12 g (exact weight, with accuracy to 0.0001 g) (about 10 ml) of preparation was placed in a 100 ml dividing funnel. Added 1 ml of hydrous ammonia, mixed then adds 20 ml of water and mixed again. Added 25 ml of chloroform to the obtained solution in the funnel. Shake carefully for 3 minutes. After full division of layers. Filtered lower chloroform layer through the paper filter with anhydrous sodium sulfate (about 10 g) in 500 ml round-bottomed flask.

Repeated extraction procedure 4 times more using 25 ml portions (5 times in total). Collected chloroform layers in 500 ml round bottom flasks... Combined chloroform extraction steamed to dryness on a water bath under vacuum. The dry residue was dissolved in 3 ml of 96% alcohol (Solution 1).

Transferred 1 ml of solution 1 to 50 ml volumetric flask. Added 1 ml of hydrous ammonia and made up the mixture volume with 96% alcohol to the mark. To 2 ml of the obtained solution add 10 ml of 96% alcohol and mixed.

Absorbance was measured on 302 nm by using 96% spirit as blank solution.

Total alkaloids were calculated as vasicine in percentage (X) through below formula:

$$X = \frac{10 \times 12 \times 50 \times 3 \times D \times 100}{2 \times 1 \times m \times 1000 \times 430} = \frac{900 \times D}{430 \times m}$$

where:

D = Optical density of the tested solution;
m = weight of preparation in grams;
430 = Specific parameter of vasicine absorption.

3.3. Determination of Vasicine by HPLC

3.3.1. Sample Preparation

About 12 g (exact weight) of preparation placed in a 100 ml dividing funnel. Added directly 20 ml of water, and 3 ml of hydrous ammonia, then carefully mixed the contents. The organics were extracted with 50 ml of chloroform (3 times in total). Combined chloroform extraction evaporated to dryness under vacuum. Dissolved the dry residue in 20 ml of mobile phase and transferred quantitatively into a 25 ml volumetric flask. The solution makeup to the mark with mobile phase. Filtered the obtained solution through a filter with pore size 0.45 μm and used for chromatography.

3.3.2. Vasicine Standard Solution Preparation

Placed about 50 mg (exact weight) of RSO vasicine standard solution in a 50 ml volumetric flask and dissolved in mobile phase.

The volume of the solution was brought up to the mark with mobile phase. Placed 1 ml of the obtained solution in a 25 ml volumetric flask and diluted with mobile phase to the mark. Filtered the obtained solution if necessary. Used fresh solution.

Chemical analysis

HPLC was performed using Agilent 1260 HPLC system (Agilent Technologies, Santa Clara, CA). Chromatographic separation and detection of samples were performed.

Chromatography conditions—liquid chromatograph with UV detector.

Column—chromatography column μ Bondapak^{TM} C18 10 μm 125°A 3.9 × 300 mm or equivalent.

Mobile phase—degassed mixture consisting of acetonitrile: 0.1 M phosphate buffer: glacial acetic acid (15: 85: 1 v/v).

Flow rate—0.7 ml/min.

Wave length—300 nm.

Column temperature—room temperature.

Vasicine content in Linkus Syrup should not be less than 0.3 mg per 10 ml was calculated by the following formula:

$$X = \frac{A_{smp} \times W_{std} \times f \times Smp - \text{dilution} \times P \times D \times 10}{A_{std} \times W_{smp} \times Std - \text{dilution} \times 100}$$

f—0.838 conversion factor of vasicine Hydrochloride to vasicine
A_{SMP}—Mean value of peak area of tested solution samples
A_{STD}—Mean value of peak area of standard solution samples
W_{SMP}—Preparation weight, mg
W_{STD}—Standard weight, mg
P—Percent purity of standard sample, %
D—Density of syrup

3.3.3. Preparation of Phosphate Buffer

5.68 gm of sodium di-hydrogen phosphate and 3.63 gm potassium di-hydrogen phosphate transferred to 1000 ml volumetric flask, added 100 ml of water and mixed. Brought the solution volume to the mark with water [20]. Other parameters and norms of developed Linkus syrup were summarized in **Table 5**.

After evaluating the above parameters the preparation of Linkus syrup was established.

4. Results and Discussion

Standardization of biologically active material in the poly herbal formulation and quantitative analysis cover identification of chemical components where as quantitative assay measure the identification and level of bio-

Table 5. Different physico-chemical parameters.

Parameters	Method/Norms
Appearance	Brown color viscosity syrup with characteristic odor. Determination was conducted visually.
PH	3.0 - 6.0
Density	1.25 to 1.35 g/cm^3
	Originality
Polysaccharides	Qualitative reactions with: With of 96% spirit Should be precipitate suspension was formed
Tanning agents	With of Ferric chloride solution 3% Should be appears of greenish-yellow coloring
Ascorbic acid	With of spirit solution of sodium 2.6-dichlorfenolindofenolite Appeared reddish-violet coloring
Alkaloid vasicine determination	TLC, 1 reddish pink color spot (vasicine) was shown on the plate after treatment with Dragendorff reagent in UV light at wave length 254 nm
Methylparahydroxybenzoat Propylparahydroxybenzoat	HPLC, Periods of 2 main peaks retention should match to peaks retention periods of on standard solutions
	Quantitative determination
Total alkaloids	Spectrophotometric determination , Total alkaloids calculated as vasicine should not be less than 0.035% and not more than 0.07%
Methylparahydroxybenzoat Propylparahydroxybenzoat	HPLC, Methylparahydroxybenzoate 9.0 - 11.0 mg/10 ml of preparation Propylparahydroxybenzoate 1.8 - 2.2 mg/10 ml of preparation

marker in the extract establish the standard of that particular compound for validation. Linkus is a poly herbal formulation manufactured by Herbion Pakistan (Pvt.) Limited. In order for the standardization of the procedure of the finished product and there in the five different herbal drugs of different batches were analyzed for physico-chemical parameters. The drugs in the Linkus are *Glycyrrhiza glabra*, *Hyssopus officinalis*, *Piper longum* and *Alpinia galangal.* The formulation organoleptic characteristics such as identification by TLC, assay of alkaloid content, foreign matter, total ash, acid insoluble ash, alcohol; soluble extraction and water soluble extraction are adequately presented in **Table 2**. Thereafter the extraction of different herbal drugs is given in **Table 3**, giving details of quantity used, quantity of thick extract, extraction time taken and percentage yield of the extract. Preparation of manufacturing of the syrup is depicted in **Table 3**. Physico-chemical evaluation such as appearance, pH determination plays a significant role in the quality assessment. The identification with quantitative reaction and preparation of 0.1% alcohol solution exhibit the indication polarity concern of plant materials. TLC was done to augment the determination of alkaloids components and there in the identification of vascine was located. All these values show that the physic-chemical parameters adopted the values were within the limits and repeated experiments confirmed the verification. HPLC was performed to confirm the quantitative and qualitative presence of vasicine for validation. The present standardization under taken reveal compliance with all the physic-chemical and analytical procedures, therefore it is concluded that Linkus syrup is well standardized product at the base line parameters.

If these analytical profiles compared with the work of Modi *et al.* where Zeal cough syrup employing physico-chemical test and bioassay marker compounds agree with quality and potency [21]. In another study Desai and co worker validated the, manufacturing procedure of Vasu cough syrup with the poly herbal formulation for compliance for their reproducibility [22]. The work done by Khadair and associates validation analysis of hederacoside C, the marker of Ivy plant and percentage recovery was given as 99.6% [23]. In a patent of cough syrup the extract of Adhatoda vasica along with Hedychium and Curcuma cough syrup has been validated in greater details [24]. Therefore the Linkus syrup standardization fall under the specific guide lines of quality herbal medicine and in line with different as mentioned earlier follow the prerequisite for global harmonization.

5. Conclusion

In this study for medicinal plants component, *Glycyrrhiza glabra*, *Hyssopus officinalis*, *Piper longum* and *Alpinia galangal* were formulated for the indication of anti-tussive activity. The physico chemical and organoleptic parameter data so generated were recorded for standardization. TLC was carried out on the aqueous extract and Rf value (0.4) of vasicine as raddish pink spot on exposure to Draggendroff and UV was realized. Quantitative and spectrophotometric estimation of alkaloid was found between the range of 0.035% to 0.07%. Determination of vasicine as biomarker by HPLC in linkus syrup determined as 0.3 mg per 10 mL. The analytical profile of linkus syrup and there in vasicine have been validated to proved that linkus syrup in different batches confirmed the verification. Further study on Linkus syrup is being carried out to determine the efficacy as anti-tussive agent and will be reported elsewhere. The following animal model of cough was used to investigate the anti-tussive potential of Linkus. Healthy Wistar albino rats were treated orally with the recommended doses of Linkus. After 15 minutes, they were individually placed in a closed Plexiglass chamber (20 × 10 × 10 cm) and exposed to citric acid inhalation (0.1 g/ml) for 7 minutes. The cough reflexes were counted for the last 5 minutes and compared with those of the control animals. The results obtained showed good responses.

References

[1] Irwin, R.S., Boulet, L.-P., Cloutier, M.M., *et al.* (1998) Managing Cough as a Defense Mechanism and as a Symptom: A Consensus Panel Report of the American College of Chest Physicians. *Chest*, **114**, 133S-181S. http://dx.doi.org/10.1378/chest.114.2_Supplement.133S

[2] Silva, T.R., Pongravoon, U. and Malmfors, T. (2000) *Adhatoda vasica*: A Critical Review of Ethanopharmacological and Toxicological Data. *Journal of Ethnopharmacology*, **72**, 1-20. http://dx.doi.org/10.1016/S0378-8741(00)00225-7

[3] Bown, D. (1995) Encyclopedia of Herbs and Their Uses. Dorling Kindersley, London.

[4] Numazaki, K., Umetsu, M., Chiba, S. (1994) Effect of Glycyrrhizin in Children with Liver Dysfunction Associated with Cytomegalovirus Infection. *The Tohoku Journal of Experimental Medicine*, **172**, 147-153. http://dx.doi.org/10.1620/tjem.172.147

[5] Tsukiyama, R. (2002) Antibacterial Activity of Licochalcone A against Spore-Forming Bacteria. *Antimicrobial Agents and Chemotherapy*, **46**, 1226-1230. http://dx.doi.org/10.1128/AAC.46.5.1226-1230.2002

[6] Chevalier, A. (1996) The Encyclopedia of Medicinal Plants Dorling Kindersley, London.

[7] Grieve, A. (1984) Modern Herbal. Penguin.

[8] Leung, A.Y. and Foster S. (1996) Encyclopedia of Natural Ingredients. 2nd Edition, John Wiley & Sons, New York.

[9] CSIR (1989) The Wealth of India: A Dictionary o f Indian Raw Materials and Industrial Products. Council of Scientific and Industrial Research, New Delhi, **8**, 96-99.

[10] Kasirajan, B., Maruthamuthu, R., Gopalakrishnan, V., Arumugam, K., Asirvatham, H., Murali, V., *et al.* (2007) A Database for Medicinal Plant Use in Treatment of Asthma. *Bioinformation*, **2**, 105-106. http://dx.doi.org/10.6026/97320630002105

[11] Khare, C.P. (2007) Indian Medicinal Plants—An Illustrated Dictionary. 1st Edition, Springer Science, New York, 9-15.

[12] Blaschek, W., Hager, H., Hänsel, R., Wolf, H.U., Surmann, P., Nyrnberg, E., *et al.* (1990) Hager's Handbuch der Pharmazeutischen Praxis. 5th rev. ed., Springer Verlag, Berlin.

[13] Petkewich, R. and Peter. R. (2006) What's That Stuff Marshmallow. *Chemical & Engineering News*, **84**, 41. http://dx.doi.org/10.1021/cen-v084n016.p041

[14] Hernandez, T., Canales, M., Teran, B., Avila, O., Duran, A., Garcia, A.M., Hernandez, H., Angeles-Lopez, O., Fernandez Ariza, M. and Avila, G. (2007) Antimicrobial Activity of the Essential Oil Extracts of *Cordia curassavica. Journal of Ethnopharmacology*, **111**, 137-141. http://dx.doi.org/10.1016/j.jep.2006.11.002

[15] Sabira, B., Perwaiz, S., Bina, S.S., Khan, S., Fayyaz, S. and Ramzan, M. (2011) Chemical constituents of *Cordia latifolia* and Their Nematicidal Activity. *Chemistry & Biodiversity*, **8**, 850-861. http://dx.doi.org/10.1002/cbdv.201000058

[16] Jiang, J.G., Huang, X.J., Chen, J. and Lin, Q.S. (2007) Comparison of the Sedative and Hypnotic Effects of Flavonoids, Saponins, and Polysaccharides Extracted from Semen *Zizyphus jujuba. Natural Product Research*, **21**, 310-320. http://dx.doi.org/10.1080/14786410701192827

[17] Mahajan, R.T. and Chopda, M.Z. (2009) Phytopharmacology of *Zizyphus jujuba* Mill—A Plant Review. *Pharmacognosy Reviews*, **3**, 320-329.

[18] Kirtikar, K.R. and Basu, B.D. (1999) Indian Medicinal Plants, Vol. 3. 2nd Edition, International Book Distributors, 1699.

[19] Kumar, N., Kumar, R. and Kishore, K. (2013) *Onosma* L.: A Review of Phytochemistry and Ethnopharmacology. *Pharmacognosy Reviews*, **7**, 140-151. http://dx.doi.org/10.4103/0973-7847.120513

[20] Srivastava, S., Verma, R.K., Gupta, M.M., Singh, S.C. and Kumar, S., (2001) HPLC Determination of Vasicine and

Vasicinone in *Adhatoda vasica* with Photo Diode Array Detection. *Journal of Liquid Chromatography & Related Technologies*, **24**, 153-159. http://dx.doi.org/10.1081/JLC-100001478

[21] Modi, J., Soni, H., Pandya, K., Patel, G. and Patel, N. (2014) A Detail Phyto-Chemical Evaluation of Herbo-Mineral Formulation Used in Respiratory Diseases. *Journal of Pharmacognosy and Phytochemistry*, **2**, 36-42.

[22] Desai, L., Oza, J. and Khatri, K. (2012) Prospective Process Validation of Polyherbal Cough Syrup Formulation. *Journal of Advanced Pharmaceutical Technology & Research*, **2**, 225-231.

[23] Khdair, A., Mohammad, M.K., Tawaha, K., Al-Hamarsheh, E., AlKhatib, H.S., Al-khalidi, B., Bustanji, Y., Najjar, S. and Hudaib, M. (2010) A Validated RP HPLC-PAD Method for the Determination of Hederacoside C in Ivy-Thyme Cough Syrup. *International Journal of Analytical Chemistry*, **2010**, Article ID: 478143, 5p.

[24] Herbal Formulation Comprising Extracts of Adhatoda, Hedychium and Curcuma as Cough Syrup, WIPO Patent Application WO/2005/077393 Kind Code: A1.

6

Efficacy of Yiqi Fumai (Freeze-Dried Powder) on Ischemic Diastolic Heart Failure

Dalin Song[1,2*], Mengfen Hu[2], Tongliang Han[1], Hua Zhang[1], Yongjun Mao[2], Tao Tian[3*]

[1]Department of Geriatric Cardiology, Geriatric Institute, Qingdao Municipal Hospital, Qingdao, China
[2]Qingdao University, Qingdao, China
[3]Department of Geriatric Cardiology, Linyi People's Hospital, Linyi, China
Email: [*]dsong55cn@aliyun.com

Abstract

Objective: To evaluate the efficacy of Yiqi Fumai freeze-dry powder (YFP) on ischemic diastolic heart failure. Methods: 100 patients diagnosed with unstable angina accompanying ischemic diastolic heart failure (IDHF) were selected randomly. 52 patients with TCM syndrome of qi-yin deficiency were divided into Chinese and Western combination therapy group. 48 patients have no TCM syndrome of qi-yin deficiency, and were treated with standard western medicine. After treatment, Seattle Angina Questionnaire Evaluation, ECG, conventional and stress echocardiography (SE) index, NT-proBNP were compared between before and after treatment. Results: The differences of PL, TS, DP between before and after treatment by YFP were statistically significant ($P < 0.05$). SE parameters of LVEF, E/A were significantly increase; E/e' decreased. The differences were statistically significant. However, echocardiography parameters showed no significant differences after treatment. After the combination treatment, NT-proBNP level had negative correlation with LVEF, E/A ($r = -0.432, -0.643$, both $P < 0.01$). Conclusion: Yiqi Fumai freeze-dry powder is safe and effective to patients with ischemic diastolic heart failure. Stress echocardiography can improve the diagnostic of ischemic diastolic heart failure, and maybe an effectively predict treatment response.

Keywords

Yiqi Fumai (Freeze-Dried Powder), Diastolic Heart Failure, Seattle Angina Questionnaire (SAQ) Evaluation, Stress Echocardiography

1. Introduction

Cardiovascular events are major fatal disease in China. Acute myocardial infarction (AMI) and ischemic heart

[*]Corresponding authors.

failure (IHF) are the most common and most serious stage in cardiac development. Unstable angina is one type of the acute coronary syndrome and its pathogenesis is unstable coronary plaque that plaque rupture may develop acute myocardial infarction. Myocardial ischemia and wide degeneration, necrosis and fibrosis caused by coronary artery disease can result in myocardial systolic and (or) diastolic dysfunction. Diastolic function occurs prior to systolic function. Diastolic heart failure (DHF) can be further developed to systolic heart failure, which has serious impact on cardiac function and quality of life of patients. Therefore, combination treatment of standardized western medicine joint proprietary Chinese medicine has been increasingly accepted by clinicians.

Coronary heart disease is divided into two categories, thoracic obstruction and angina pectoris, in traditional Chinese medicine (TCM). Both types of coronary disease are severe and require urgent intervention. The pathogenesis of coronary heart disease mainly involves heart vessel blockage or stasis. Delay in the treatment of this chronic disease may cause damage to Yin and Yang as well as Qi and Yin, according to TCM theory. The Yiqi Fumai freeze-dry powder (YFP) was here prepared based on the TCM formula of pulse-activating powder using modern production technology refined for formulation of modern Chinese medicine. The pulse-activating powder formula was taken from a comprehensive TCM book called *Medicine Origin*. It is one of the more famous TCM formulas for pulse activation. It consists of three active ingredients: ginseng, Mai Dong, and Chinese magnoliavine fruit. YFP has a beneficial impact on the replenishment of Qi and pulse activation. It also well nourishes Yin and promotes glandular secretion in TCM theory. Integrative Medicine may bring good results for those patients with Qi and Yin deficiency. However, there is still a lack of reliable clinical studies to prove the efficacy of this treatment. In this study, the Seattle Angina Scale (SAQ), ECG, stress echocardiography (stress echocardiography, SE) and amino-terminal pro-brain natriuretic peptide precursor (NT-proBNP) were used to assess the efficiency of YFP which was based on pulse-activating powder.

2. Materials and Methods

2.1. Ethics

This study was approved by hospital of Qingdao Municipal Hospital and Linyi People's Hospital Committee, and conformed to the guidelines of the National Institutes of Health for the care.

2.2. Study Design

100 patients diagnosed with unstable angina [1] (unstable angina pectoris, UAP) were selected randomly from 2011 to 2012 in both hospitals. Inclusion criteria of UAP cases: >18 years old; diagnosed with coronary heart disease (previous myocardial infarction, or revascularization history, at least one major vascular diameter stenosis > 50% by coronary angiography); or patients with the positive results of stress electrocardiogram test (male), radionuclide or stress echocardiography test; episode of angina; angina (seizure frequency, extent and level of incentives induced angina) has been stable for at least one at entrance; the Canadian Cardiovascular Society angina class I - IV grade. Exclusion criteria of UAP: patients developed acute myocardial infarction in less than three months; postoperative of revascularization (PCI or CABG) in less than three months, so 78 male patients and 22 female patients met these criteria. They were in line with the diagnostic criteria of ischemic diastolic heart failure (IDHF) [2]. Exclusion criteria of IDHF: patients with heart failure caused by non-coronary artery disease; heart failure symptoms aggravated due to digitalis poisoning.

All following patients were excluded: patients with severe hepatic or renal dysfunction (serum ALT levels > 3 times the upper limit of the normal value, serum creatinine level ≥ 442 μmol/L); uncontrolled hypertension (systolic blood pressure ≥ 180 mmHg, diastolic blood pressure ≥ 100 mmHg); Diabetic with glycemic level not controlled satisfactorily; previous history of allergy to ginseng, Ophiopogon japonicus, Schisandra chinensis; pregnant or lactating women.

All subjects signed the informed consent form. Grouping diagrammatic drawing was shown in **Figure 1**. 52 patients with TCM syndrome of qi-yin deficiency were accessed into Chinese and Western combination therapy group (chinese and western medicine treatment group, CWMTG) with 32 male and 20 female, and their ages were from 62 to 74 (average years were 69.5). 48 patients have no TCM syndrome of qi-yin deficiency including 8 females and 40 males with age from 57 to 70 (average years were 65.0 ± 9.0) were treated with standard western medicine (western medicine treatment group, WMTG).

UAP: unstable angina pectoris; TCM: raditional Chinese medicine; MTG: chinese and western medicine

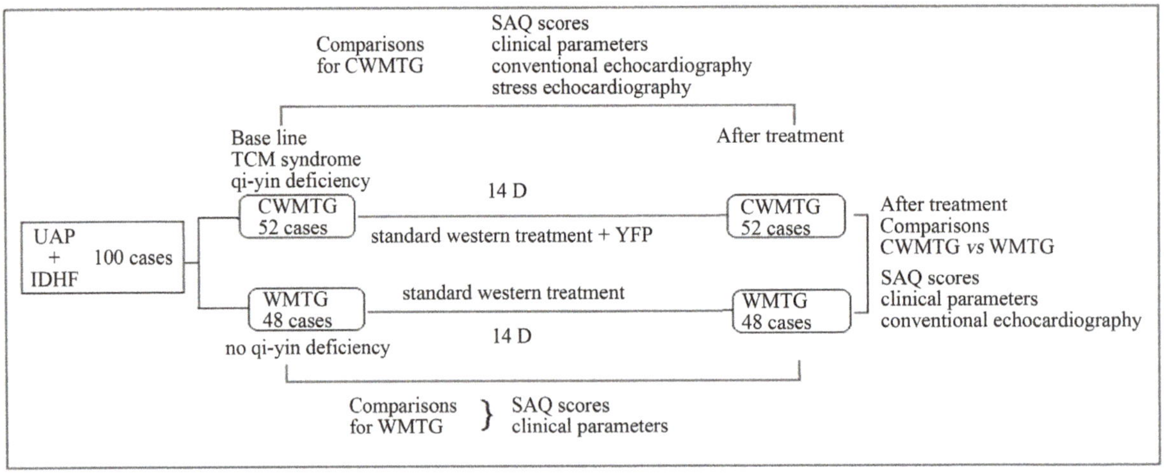

Figure 1. Study design and grouping.

treatment group; WMTG: western medicine treatment group; IDHF: ischemic diastolic heart failure; SAQ: seattle angina questionnaire.

2.3. Treatment

The standard western treatment includes the principles of conventional treatment of IDHF with diuretics, β-blockers, angiotensin-converting enzyme inhibitors (ACEI), angiotensin II receptor blockers (ARB); as well as standard ASC drugs such as aspirin, clopidogrel, isosorbide dinitrate and stantins. Patients in WMTG were given standard western treatment. On the basis of western medicine treatment, patients in CWMTG were given Yiqi Fumai dry powder (Tianjin Tasly Pharmaceutical Co., Ltd. Specification: 0.65 g/bottle. Approval Number: Z20060463). Dosage and Administration: 5.2 g each time, namely 8 bottles at a time, one time per day. The drugs were dissolved in 250 - 500 ml 5% glucose injection or saline intravenous injection and were injected at the rate of about 40 drops per minute for 14 days).

2.4. Seattle Angina Questionnaire (SAQ) Evaluation

With the necessary explanations of SAQ by the doctor before and after treatment, patients independently completed the questionnaire. Seattle Angina scale evaluate the efficiency from following five aspects: physical limitation level (PL, Question 1), angina steady state (AS, Question 2), angina frequency (AF, Questions 3 - 4), treatment satisfaction (TS, Questions 5 - 8), disease perception (DP, Questions 9 - 11), one by one score, the total score is 100 points, the higher the score, the better the patient's quality of life and organism function [3].

2.5. ECG Evaluation

After treatment, disappearance of ischemic manifestation indicated in resting ECG or negative treadmill exercise test were considered markedly effective; that ST segment rebounded 0.05mV, inverted T wave become shallow more than 50% or the inverted, low T wave become upright was effective; ST - T no change was invalid; ST segment descend, or T wave inversion deepens was aggravating.

2.6. Stress Echocardiography

Used Philips IE 33 ultrasonic diagnostic apparatus, X3-1 probe, 1-3MHz frequency, we recorded the left ventricular diastolic diameter (LVDd), interventricular sepal thickness at the end of diastolic (IVSd), left ventricular posterior wall thickness (LVPWd), left atria diameter (LAD). We measured the LVEF, the left ventricular output (CO) and cardiac index (CI) by biplane Simpson on the parasternal long-axis under the resting standard state. Double-blind method was applied. All data measured repeatedly three times. The mean value was reserved. Patients that underwent stress echocardiography were asked to do treadmill exercise until their heart rates were stable at 110/min. After 1 min, the test was terminated, and the indices were recorded at the same site. Indicators of cardiac Doppler echocardiography included cardiac systolic function LVEDV, LVESV, SV, CO, CI, EF, diastolic function E/A etc. All patients completed the test with satisfying results.

2.7. NT-proBNP

N-terminal pro brain natriuretic peptide (NT-proBNP) was detected by euzymelinked immunosorbent assay (biomelieux SA kit).

2.8. Statistical Analysis

SPSS11.5 statistical software was applied. All quantitative data were reported as mean ± S.D. $\left(\bar{x} \pm s\right)$. Indicators between before and after treatment were compared using paired t-test, non-continuous variables between groups were compared using t-test. The continuous variables and rates were compared using X^2 test. Non-parametric continuous variables were represented as the median (minimum - maximum). Paired Wilcoxon test was applied for comparisons before and after treatment; correlation between variables were analyzed using Pearson correlation analysis and independent factors were analyzed using multiple regression. $P < 0.05$ was as statistically significant.

3. Results

3.1. SAQ Scores

There were no significant differences of clinical general characteristics between two groups. Life quality of patients before and after treatment: scores of PL, AS, AF, TS, and DP are shown in **Table 1**. The results showed that the differences of PL, TS, DP between before and after treatment by YFP were statistically significant ($P < 0.05$), indicating that combination of YFP can improve physical limitation extent in patients with unstable angina, and can improve patients' satisfaction and their perception of the disease, making the patient's conditions to be stabilizing. The rate of nitrates use, ECG indicators, SAQ and symptoms were significant different before and after treatment ($P = 0.05$). Patients' satisfaction and disease perception in CWMTG were significantly decreased ($P = 0.05$) and the proportion of ineffectiveness in CWMTG was significantly decreased ($P = 0.02$) (**Figure 2** and **Table 1**).

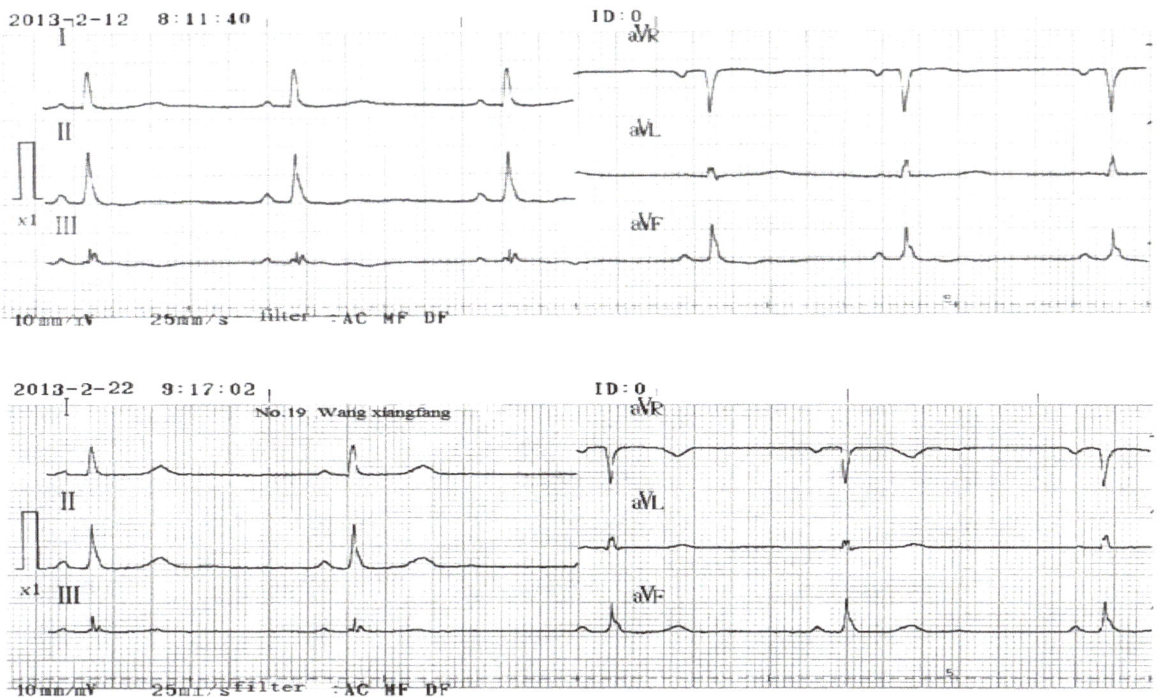

Figure 2. Changes of ECG of patients with IDHF before and after treatment.

Table 1. Seattle angina questionnaire (SAQ) scores of two groups before and after treatment.

	CWMTG (n = 52)			WMTG (n = 48)			P^*
	Before treatment	After treatment	P	Before treatment	After treatment	P	
General clinical characteristics							
Age (years)	65.2 ± 9.7			65.0 ± 9.0			0.55
Male (%)	76.4			78.9			0.21
Diabetes (%)	28.2			29.0			0.89
Hypertension (%)	39.5			38.8			0.66
Hyperlipidemia (%)	60.5			61.2			0.75
Symptoms efficacy							
Markedly	59.2			56.9			0.22
Effective	24.4			20.2			0.21
Ineffectiveness	16.4			22.9			0.02
Treatment							
Anti-platelet (%)	91.2	90.5	0.75	94.2	94	0.66	0.07
β-blockers (%)	65.9	62.2	0.91	64.9	64.2	0.94	0.85
statins (%)	88.4	84	0.45	88.9	86.4	0.28	0.75
ACEI/ARB (%)	57.2	56.9	0.91	61.2	60.5	0.75	0.05
Nitrates (%)	65.6	34.4	0.001	60.5	39.5	0.009	0.05
SAQ							
PL	64 ± 22	54 ± 25	0.02	65 ± 23	60 ± 24	0.05	0.04
AS	40 ± 34	37 ± 31	0.05	39 ± 30	33 ± 20	0.05	0.55
AF	66 ± 27	59 ± 27	0.03	67 ± 26	61 ± 25	0.03	0.75
TS	89 ± 18	96 ± 16	0.001	88 ± 16	90 ± 17	0.004	0.05
DP	42 ± 22	48 ± 23	0.05	44 ± 24	49 ± 22	0.05	0.05

P: Comparisons of each group before and after treatment; P^*: Comparisons of the two groups after treatment.

3.2. Comparisons of Clinical Baseline Data of Patients with IDHF before and after Treatment

Clinical baseline characteristics of patients in CWMTG before and after treatment are shown in **Table 2**. After treatment, plasma NT-proBNP levels and the rate of β-blocker's use were decreased, the exercise tolerance increased. The differences were statistically significant. The rate of diuretics and lipid-lowering drugs use reduced without statistical significance. Plasma NT-proBNP levels of patients in CWMTG decreased significantly after treatment (70.5 (62.0 - 79.0) ng/L vs 74.0 (65.0 - 84.0) ng/L, $P < 0.05$). After treatment, plasma NT-proBNP levels of patients in WMTG were not significantly changed (**Table 2**).

3.3. Changes of Echocardiography of Patients with IDHF before and after Treatment

Comparisons of echocardiography parameters of 52 patients with DHF before and after combination therapy were shown in **Table 3**. The results showed that after treatment, SE parameters of LVEF, E/A were significantly increase; E/e' decreased. The differences were statistically significant. However echocardiography parameters showed no significant differences after treatment (**Figure 3** and **Table 3**).

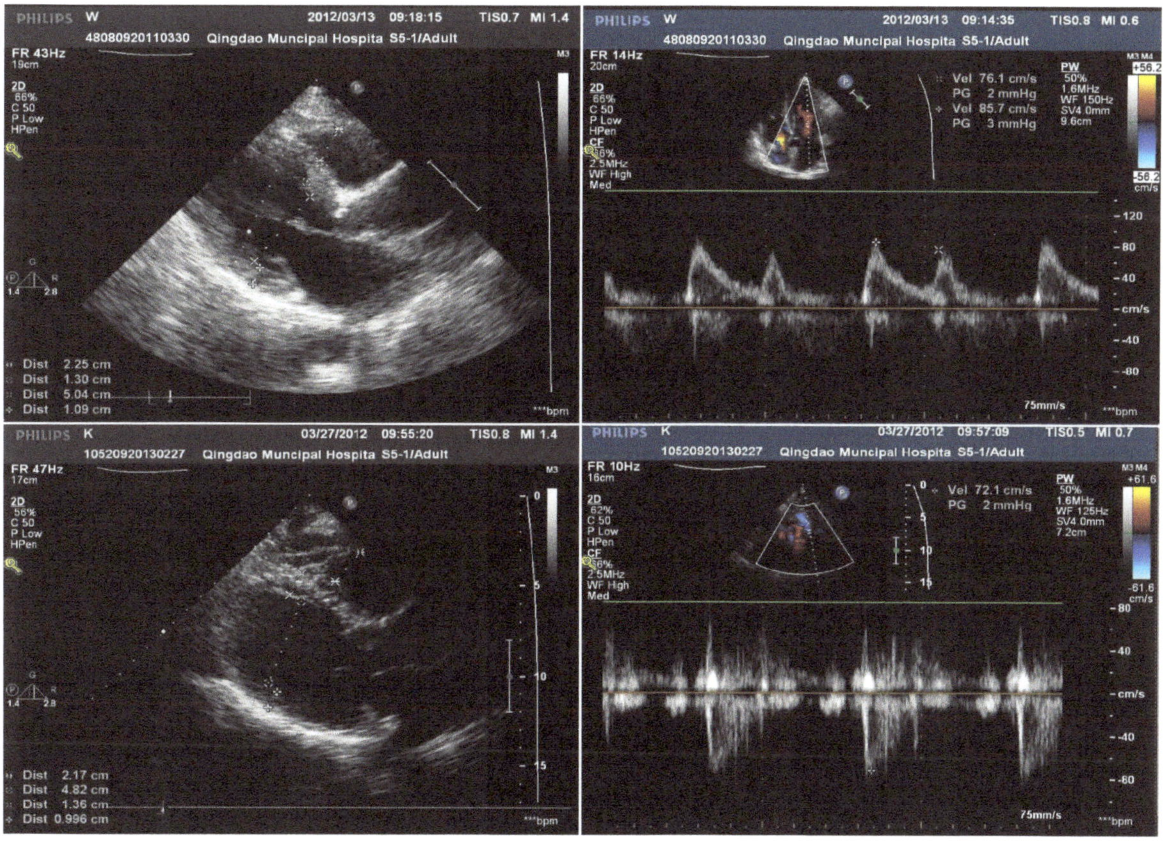

Figure 3. Changes of echocardiography of patients with IDHF before and after treatment.

Table 2. comparisons of clinical parameters of 52 patients with ischemic diastolic heart failure patients before and after treatment.

Clinical parameters	Before treatment	After treatment	P
Demographic characteristics			
Age	69. (62.0 - 74.0)	—	—
Male (%)	32 (61.5%)	—	—
Hypertension (%)	33 (63.5%)	—	—
Diabetes (%)	12 (23.1%)	—	—
Hyperlipidemia (%)	35 (67.3%)	—	—
Fat (%)	19 (36.5%)	—	—
BMI (kg/m^2)	29.5 (26.0 - 33.0)	—	—
Treatment			
Diuretics (%)	27 (52.6%)	20 (38.5%)	0.737
β-blockers (%)	40 (76.3 %)	40 (54.7%)	0.032
Lipid-lowering drugs (%)	33 (63.2%)	27 (52.8%)	0.325
ACEI/ARB (%)	36 (68.4%)	35 (67.9%)	0.960
NT-proBNP (ng/L)	250.7 (167.5 - 544.0)	94.3 (67.0 - 151.5)	<0.001
Hemodynamic			
Heart rate (bpm)	70.5 (62.0 - 79.0)	74.0 (65.0 - 84.0)	0.045
Systolic blood pressure (mmHg)	130.0 (120.0 - 150.0)	130.0 (120.0 - 140.0)	0.042
Diastolic blood pressure (mmHg)	82.5 (80.0 - 95.0)	80.0 (80.0 - 90.0)	0.158
Muscle testing			
Exercise tolerance (s)	387.0 (305.0 - 482.0)	463.0 (382.0 - 527.0)	<0.001

P: Comparisons of before and after treatment.

Table 3. Comparisons of conventional and stress echocardiography index of 52 patients with ischemic diastolic heart failure patients before and after treatment.

The indexes	Before treatment Echo	After treatment Echo	After treatment SE	P
Two-dimensional echocardiography				
EDVI (mL/m^2)	45.0 (39.0 - 54.0)	45.0 (39.9 - 50.0)	45.0 (40.5 - 49.5)	0.717
ESVI (mL/m^2)	16.0 (12.0 - 21.0)	15.2 (12.0 - 18.9)	14.0 (11.0 - 16.5)	0.167
LVEF (%)	54.0 (50.0 - 60.0) a	58.0 (70.0 - 66.0) a	69.5 (66.5 - 73.0) b	0.000
LVMI (g/m^2)	102.5 (88.0 - 123.0) a	101.4 (83.0 - 110.6) a	89.0 (72.0 - 93.5) b	<0.001
LAVI (mL/m^2)	36.0 (29.0 - 41.0) a	34.0 (28.0 - 37.9) a	28.0 (24.0 - 32.0) b	0.001
LVDd	54.7 (50.2 - 55.0)	53.5 (49.7 - 54.1)	51.0 (46.2 - 53.0)	0.03
Left ventricular				
Doppler				
E (cm/s)	77.5 (67.0 - 94.0)	76.0 (65.0 - 96.3)	70.0 (61.5 - 80.0)	0.179
E-exe (cm/s)	107.5 (94.0 - 126.0) a	105.2 (92.3 - 120.2) a	96.0 (83.5 - 102.5) b	0.005
A (cm/s)	92.0 (79.0 - 105.0) a	90.1 (72.2 - 101.4) a	72.0 (65.0 - 79.0) b	<0.001
A-exe (cm/s)	103.0 (92.0 - 121.0) a	101.3 (90.8 - 118.7) a	97.5 (87.0 - 109.5) a,b	0.041
E/A	0.8 (0.7 - 1.0) a	0.8 (0.5 - 1.1) a	1.0 (0.9 - 1.1) b	0.016
E-exe/A-exe	1.0 (0.9 - 1.2)	1.0 (0.8 - 1.2)	0.9 (0.8 - 1.1)	0.826
DT (ms)	189.0 (167.0 - 208.0) a	181.2 (161.2 - 203.0) a	159.5 (149.5 - 189.0) b	0.017
Ard–Ad (ms)	−10.0 (−30.5 - (−1.5))	−11.3 (−30.0 - (−2.2))	−10.5 (−17.0 - (−5.0))	0.640
e' (cm/s)	7.1 (6.3 - 8.4) a	7.9 (6.9 - 9.2) a	9.4 (8.8 - 10.5) b	<0.001
e'-exe (cm/s)	9.3 (8.1 - 10.8) a	9.8 (9.5 - 12.9) a	12.9 (12.0 - 14.3) b	<0.001
a' (cm/s)	9.8 (8.4 - 11.0) a	10.2 (8.9 - 11.7) a	11.2 (9.6 - 12.6) b	0.012
a'-exe (cm/s)	11.1 (9.2 - 13.3) a	12.5 (10.9 - 14.2) a	14.4 (13.0 - 16.5) c	<0.001
s' (cm/s)	7.6 (7.0 - 8.2) a	7.9 (7.8 - 8.6) a	8.8 (8.0 - 9.3) b	<0.001
s'-exe (cm/s)	9.5 (8.8 - 10.3) a	10.5 (8.9 - 13.2) a	13.9 (12.5 - 15.5) c	<0.001
E/e'	10.6 (9.4 - 12.7) a	10.4 (9.0 - 10.9) a	7.0 (6.0 - 8.9) b	<0.001
E-exe/e'-exe	11.0 (9.9 - 12.5) a	10.0 (8.9 - 11.2)	7.2 (6.5 - 7.7) b	<0.001

3.4. Main Echocardiography Parameters of CWMTG Patients and NT-proBNP Correlation Analysis

After the combination treatment, NT-proBNP level had negative correlation with LVEF, E/A, r = −0.432, −0.643, both P < 0.01. After treatment, multiple stepwise regression analysis of NT-proBNP and cardiac function indexes showed that the left ventricular end-diastolic diameter (LVDd), left ventricular ejection fraction (LVEF), early diastolic mitral flow velocity (E), DT, left ventricular isovolumic relaxation time (IVRT), E/A were independent relevant factors of NT-proBNP (**Table 4**).

4. Discussions

In TCM, heart failure is divided into the categories of edema, palpitation, gasp syndrome, phlegm and fluid retention, and blood stasis. Therapy combining Chinese and Western medicine may have pronounced efficacy in the treatment of patients with unstable angina who have been diagnosed with Yin and Qi deficiencies by TCM differentiation. However, there are a few of studies confirming the efficacy of this combination therapy. Studies focusing on objective indicators of improved myocardial function, such as the evaluation index of DHF, regardless of self-reported symptoms of the patients, would be especially useful. In the present work, the SAQ, ECG, stress echocardiography (SE), and the NT-proBNP were all used to assess the efficacy of YFP, which was prepared based on the TCM formula of pulse-activating powder. Assessment of SAQ suggested that treatment with CWMTG brought about significant improvements, including reduced number and severity of angina attacks, and improved the quality of life. In addition, ECG analysis indicated that CWMTG had a more pronounced curative effect than isosorbide denigrate treatment. The results of the SE demonstrated that all patients had symptoms of heart failure and that their LVEF was >50% and the ration of early (E) and late (A) transmittal diastolic velocity

Table 4. Multiple stepwise regression analysis of NT-proBNP and cardiac function indexes of 52 patients after treatment.

Indexes	Non-standardized coefficients	Standardized coefficients	t	P
Two-dimensional echocardiography				
LVEF	1.972°	0.147 b	3.487	0.001
LVDd	8.651	0.131	3.399	0.001
Left ventricular Doppler				
E	6.150°	0.254 a,b	6.260	0.000
E/A	0.104	0.097 b	2.616	0.009
DT	2.296	0.168	3.498	0.001

a: compared with before treatment, $P < 0.05$. b: compared with conventional echocardiography, $P < 0.05$.

(E/A ratio) was <1, suggesting that the patients suffered from DHF. After treatment with CWMTG, the relative number of irregular inter-ventricular sepal (IVS) and LVPW movements was significantly went down. LVEF, CO and CI were significantly increased and the patients showed enhanced diastolic function (E/A ratio). All of these indicated that the LVMI was reduced. Systolic function and diastolic function were improved, and stress echocardiography is more sensitive than conventional echocardiography for evaluating the therapeutic effect of diastolic heart failure.The blood levels of NT-proBNP in the patients of the CWMTG were significantly lower than that in controls. The patients also showed improved exercise tolerance and some of them were able to reduce their doses of diuretics and lipid-lowering drugs.

Clinical symptoms of UAP are chest tightness and pain, chest pain involving the back, back pain involving the chest, shortness of breath, gasping, and restlessness. In severe cases, the disease may lead to death within hours of the initial onset of symptoms. The etiological factors are mainly invasion of pathogenic cold, eating disorders, mental stress and extreme changes in emotional state, disorders of the internal organs caused by fatigue, and old age. The location of the disease is mainly the heart and pathogenesis is heart vessel blockage stasis. In the TCM symptom classification system, patients with the mild form of the disease have hypo function of Yang-Qi in the chest, excessive cold syndrome, and blockage of Qi. Patients with severe form of the disease have accumulation of blood-phlegm, congestion in the chest, and blockage of Qi. Delays in treatment may cause damage to Yin and Yang and deficiencies in Qi and Yin, according to TCM theory. The active ingredients of YFP include *Radix Ginseng Rubra* (Panax ginseng or red ginseng), *Radix Ophiopogonis* (Mai Dong), and *Fructus Schisandrae* (Chinese magnoliavine fruit). Red ginseng reinforces vital energy of body, improves lung function, and promotes glandular secretion. It also provides fixation and hidroschesis. It also provides the principle curative action (sovereign drug). The effects of Mai Dong can nourish Yin and relieve dryness of the body. Combination of this herb with red ginseng may notify both Qi and Yin. Mai Dong is also used as minister drug. Chinese magnoliavine fruit can astringe Yin to stop sweating. Combinations of this herb with red ginseng and Mai Dong may consolidate Qi and glandular secretion to prevent leakage and promote recovery from wastage of Qi and Yin. For this reason, it is also termed an assistant drug, an adjuvant drugs that increases the efficacy or potency of sovereign and minister drugs in TCM. These three herbs are combined: to resolve Qi deficiency using red ginseng as a basis; to prevent Qi leakage using Chinese magnoliavine fruit as a standard; and to replenish Yin using Mai Dong. This eventually allows primordial Qi to be ventilated in the lungs, Yin to be restored, and the pulse to be normalized.

Modern pharmacological research has confirmed that the active ingredients of ginseng extracts (panaxosides or ginsenosides) promote DNA and RNA syntheses, increasing hypoxia tolerance, enhancing myocardial contractility, increasing plasma levels of cyclic adenosine monomphsopate (cAMP) and the synthesis of prostaglandin I_2, or PGI_2, thus inhibiting platelet aggregation and improving myocardial cell metabolism [4]. Mai Dong stabilizes myocardial cell membranes with a positive inotropic effect and eliminates free radicals [5]. Chinese magnoliavine fruit strengthens myocardial contractions, improves microcirculation and inhibits lipid peroxidatiuon. Combinations of these three herbs may enhance myocardial contractility, improve left ventricular function and tolerance of myocardial hypoxia, and protect the injured myocardial ultrastructure [6]. YFP injection can tonify Qi and activate blood circulation; reduce plasma viscosity: promote fibrinolysis; inhibit thrombosis; improve abnormal hemorheology, thereby relieving angina and improving self-reported symptoms [7].

Inhibition of Na^+-K^+-ATPase activity affects Na^+-K^+ and Na^+-Ca^{2+} exchange, thereby increasing Ca^{2+} influx and Ca^{2+} concentration. This promotes the interaction of Ca^{2+} with cardiac troponin, resulting in increases in myocardial contractility and cardiac output [8]. Clinical studies published by Zhong *et al.* demonstrated that pulse-activating injection enhances the capacity of myocardial contraction in patients with ischemic heart disease [9]-[11]. These patients also showed improvement in myocardial compliance and coordination, increased perfusion pressure, and a higher myocardial survival rate and ejection fraction. In the present study, patients' LVEF values were significantly increased and their plasma levels of NT-proBNP were significantly reduced after YFP treatment, suggesting that YFP treatment efficiently improves cardiac function. In addition, these findings are consistent with those of other studies performed using *in vivo* models. In these studies, pulse-activating injection enhanced patients' myocardial contractility and vasodilation but did not increase the heart rate (all regimens either reduced the heart rate or left it unchanged) [12] [13].

It is not subject to the insufficiencies of more commonly used quality of life scales, which do not sufficiently address the specific conditions or psychology of CAD patients, lack internal consistency in some areas, and have poor response to treatment intervention [14]. Repeated assessments involving the SAQ scale has demonstrated its strong reproducibility. In TCM, efficacy is assessed mostly via clinicians' observations of improvements and patient recovery after the examination through TCM's four diagnostic methods of TCM, observation, auscultation and olfaction, interrogation, and assessments of pulse and palpation. However, these assessments do not consider the quality of life of the patients (e.g., patient's comfort, subjective feelings, and degree of life satisfaction). Quality of life does not only represent and integrate personal values with judgment of health status and life satisfaction but also reveals the patient's expectations with respect to the efficacy of the treatment and improvements in function [15].

The SAQ shows that YFP effectively reduces the frequency of clinical attacks of UAP and facilitates significant improvements in UAP self-reported symptoms, quality of life, and patient satisfaction. However, most of the clinical research to date has only focused on adjuvant TCM therapy on the basis of conventional Western medicine. The lack of evidence-based medicine that can be used to assess the clinical efficacy of an individual TCM regimen or TCM regimen used in place of standard UAP drug therapy complicates the assessment of specificity and definite efficacy of TCM treatment. In addition, the standard treatment for UAP has a standardized duration of follow-up after drug administration. However, there are no published reports addressing the long-term use of TCM and duration of TCM administration in this disease. The present work study confirmed that YFP was associated with improvements in patients' self-reported symptoms of UAP and in patients' satisfaction after treatment. It showed efficacy superior to that of a treatment with Western medicine, so it may be possible to use YFP to compensate for some of the insufficiencies of conventional Western medicine.

During myocardial ischemia, abnormalities in cardiac diastolic function occur prior to systolic dysfunction. Left ventricular diastole includes isovolumetric relaxation (early diastole) and ventricular filling phases. The isovolumetric relaxation phase and rapid filling phase involve active energy-consuming processes; but in the slow filling phase and atria systole phase, the ventricle was passively diastole, which was dependent on the stiffness of the left ventricular myocardial muscle. Conventional echocardiography is not sensitive enough to facilitate prognosis or assessment of the efficacy of treatment. This can lead to misdiagnosis and missed diagnoses. In this way, conventional echocardiography has significant limitations. Stress echocardiography (SE) is a new technique that combines a treadmill exercise stress test and an echocardiography analysis. It is a functional test that involves allowing the patient to exercise to increase myocardial oxygen consumption, which induces pronounced homodynamic changes and increases the detection rate of coronary heart disease while maintaining high sensitivity, specificity, and accuracy for the detection of myocardial ischemia. Because of its noninvasiveness, convenience, repeatability, and ability to determine the homodynamic changes in patients, SE can be used to guide treatment and perform prognosis. In this way, it is one of the more reliable and objective tests to have achieved widespread use in clinical settings in recent years. Although all of the patients in this study had DHF with normal systolic function, SE still demonstrated the changes in myocardial systolic function after YFP treatment. LVEF and LVMI changed significantly after YFP treatment, suggesting enhancement of systolic function and further illustrating that SE allows for a comprehensive evaluation of the therapeutic effect. However, evaluation with left ventricular Doppler flow spectrum was affected by heart rate, preload (left atria pressure) and after load (aortic pressure). Exercise increases heart rate, which may affect the results of left ventricular Doppler flow spectrum and may merit further analysis. In this way, SE also has some limitations. The key to improve the sensitivity of SE is correct detection of load-induced segmental wall motion abnormalities (SWMAs). SWMAs occur only during myocardial ischemia. Sometimes, even under circumstances involving severe coronary artery stenosis, SWMAs can remain undetected if myocardial ischemia is not induced by load. In addition, the limitations of traditional tissue Doppler imaging include inability to measure myocardial motions at different sites at the same time and an inability to detect myocardial velocity gradient. These issues should be addressed in future studies.

Modern medicine suggests that heart failure is not only related to homodynamic abnormalities but also associated with the activation of the neuroendocrine system. The NT-proBNP is a cardiac neurohormone. In the human body, it plays a role in diuresis, natriuresis, and vasodilatation. Declined cardiac output, increased tension of the ventricular wall, and overloaded pressure induce the secretion of NT-proBNP, and levels of NT-proBNP can be indicative of the overall situation of circulatory congestion. There is a positive correlation between the NT-proBNP value and the severity of heart failure, indicating that compensatory pathophysiological changes have taken place. The NT-proBNP value is a marker of the state of restoration of the balance of circulation in human body, and it is negatively correlated with the quality of cardiac function [16]. This study suggested that the NT-proBNP is negatively correlated with LVEF and E/A ($r = -0.432$ and -0.643). Left ventricular diastolic dysfunction (LVDd), LVEF, E, diastolic (D wave) flow velocity, isovolumic relax-action time (IVRT), and E/A ratio were found to be independent factors associated with NT-proBNP, suggesting that the increase of left ventricular end-systolic pressure (LVESP) and the diastolic dysfunction may result in increased production of NT-proBNP. The changes in NT-proBNP levels may represent the systolic and diastolic functions of the heart. These results are consistent with the SE evaluation of the severity of heart failure. However, NT-proBNP can distinguish neither the cause of heart failure nor the type of heart failure; whereas SE can compensate this inadequacy, that is to say, SE can distinguish the cause and the type of heart failure. This study examined the comprehensive evaluation of cardiac function using patients' SE and plasma NT-proBNP levels. These methods were found to facilitate diagnosis of chronic heart failure and evaluation of its severity in a more reasonable and accurate manner than other methods. These methods were also used to diagnose the underlying heart conditions of the patients, suggesting that the evaluation in these patients using SE and plasma NT-proBNP index was reliable and sensitive.

This study confirmed that YFP treatment improves self-reported symptoms, increases the degree of satisfaction, and makes up for the drawbacks of standard Western medical regimen. It was here confirmed that SAQ is sensitive and suitable for evaluation of the curative effects of TCM, as been shown in a previous study [17].

Stress echocardiography provides some parameters for evaluation of the changes in IDHF and can serve as a quantitative indicator of the clinical efficacy of YFP treatment. The present study confirmed that YFP treatment is reliable and can improve cardiac function and the exercise tolerance in patients. In this study, we didn't discuss whether YFP is effective to all patients with ischemic diastolic heart failure or just effective to ischemic diastolic heart failure patients with with TCM syndrome of qi-yin deficiency. Besides, the sample cases were too little, we should increase the cases to make the results reliable.Improvements in the SE index, levels of NT-proBNP and clinical symptoms in the patients remained consistent throughout this study, suggesting that the combination of these methods may be helpful for research into integrative therapy involving TCM and Western medicine.

References

[1] Cardiovascular Medicine Branch of Chinese Medical Doctor Association, Evidence-Based Medicine Branch of Chinese Medical Doctor Association Commition (2007) Guidelines and Consensus on Prevention and Treatment of Cardiovascular Diseases 2007[M]. People's Medical Publishing House, Beijing, 37-39.

[2] Young, M.N., Shoemaker, M.B., Kurtz, E.G., *et al.* (2012) Heart Failure with Preserved Left Ventricuiar Function: Diagnosticand Therapeutic Challenges in Patients with Diastolic Heart Failure. *The American Journal of the Medical Sciences.*

[3] Spertus, J.A., Winders, J.A., Dewhurst, T.A., *et al.* (1995) Development and Alidation of the Seattle Angina Questionnaire: *Journal of the American College of Cardiology*, **25**, 333-341. http://dx.doi.org/10.1016/0735-1097(94)00397-9

[4] Yang, W.M. and Zhou, Y.X. (1997) Clinical Observation on Treatment of Chronic Congestive Heart Failure with Shenmai Injection: 62 Cases. *Practical Journal of Integrated Traditional Chinese and Western Medicine*, **10**, 1446.

[5] Wang, J.H. (1994) Handbook of Commonly Used Traditional Chinese Medicine [M]. The Golden Shield Press, Beijing, 112.

[6] Xu, L.H. (2009) Therapeutic Effect of Yiqi Fumai in Patients with Chronic Congestive Heart Faliure. *Clinical Medicine*, **22**, 2418-2419.

[7] Yuan, C.L. and Du, S.L. (2012) Efficacy of Yi Qi Fu Mai Injection on Heart Failure Complicated with Angina Pectoris in Patients with Coronary Heart Disease. *Chinese Journal of New Drugs*, 1774-1777.

[8] Mao, J.Y., Zhang, B.L. and Wang X.L. (2006) Progress in Mechanism of Shenmai Injection in the Treatment of Heart Failure. *Chinese Traditional Patent Medicine*, **28**, 1801-1803.

[9] Dong, Q.Z., Chen, K.Y. and Tu, X.H. (1984) Hemodynamic Effects of Shengmai Injection in the Treatment of Acute Myocardial Infarction. *Chinese Journal of Cardiology*, **12**, 5-6.

[10] Zhong, Y.S. (1998) Effect of Shengmai Injection on Left Ventricular Volume and Function of Patients with Heart Failure after Acute Myocardial Infarction. *Journal of Wuhan Postgraduate Medical College*, **26**, 1-2.

[11] Zhuang, A.L. and Guan, E.J. (1997) Effect of "Sheng Mai" Injection on Cardiac Function of Patients with Ischemic Heart Disease. *Chinese Journal of Integrated Traditional and Western Medicine in Intensive and Critical Care*, **4**, 310-311.

[12] Department of Chest Emergency Coordination Group of the State Administration of Traditional Chinese Medicine Medical Administration. (1995) Clinical and Experimental Studies of Shenmal Injection for Treatment of 219 Cases of Angina Pectoris of CHD. *Journal of Emergency in Traditional Chinese Medicine*, **4**, 152-155.

[13] Meng, Q.Y. (2000) Preliminary Study on Rapid Injection of Shengmai Injection in the Treatment of Hypertensive Emergencies. *Hebei Medicine*, **6**, 133-134.

[14] Xing, W.H. and Chen, X.M. (2004) Feasibility of SF-8 Short Scale for Testing Health Related Quality of Life in Patients with Coronary Heart Disease. *Foreign Medical Sciences* (*Section of cardiovascular*), **5**, 181-184.

[15] Hao, Y.T., Fang, J.Q., Li, C.X., *et al.* (1999) World Health Organization. WHOQOL and Its Chinese Version. *Foreign Medical Sciences* (*Section of Social Medicine*) **16**, 118-122.

[16] Wang, L., Hu, Y.S., Wu, X., *et al.* (2010) Significances of NT-proBNP and hs-CRP in Heart Failure. *National Medical Journal of China*, **90**, 1635-1636.

[17] Liu, T.X., Kong, S.P., Liao, Z.Y., *et al.* (1997) Assessment Study on Physical Function and the Quality of Life for CHD Patients with SAQ. *Chinese Journal of Behavioral Medical Science*, **6**, 127-129.

Abbreviation

IHF: ischemic heart failure
YFP: Yiqi Fumai freeze-dry powder
TCM: traditional Chinese medicine
IDHF: ischemic diastolic heart failure
CWMTG: Chinese and western medicine treatment group
WMTG: western medicine treatment group
SAQ: Seattle Angina Questionnaire
AMI: acute myocardial infarction
DHF: diastolic heart failure
SE: stress echocardiography
UAP: unstable angina pectoris
ACS: acute coronary syndrome
PCI: percutaneous transluminal coronary intervention
CABG: Coronary artery bypass grafting
ACEI: angiotensin-converting enzyme inhibitors
ARB: angiotensin II receptor blockers
LVDd: left ventricular diastolic diameter
IVSd: interventricular sepal thickness at the end of diastolic
LVPWd: left ventricular posterior wall thickness
LAD: left atria diameter
LVEF: left ventricular ejection fraction
CO: left ventricular output

CI: cardiac index
IVS: inter-ventricular sepal
SWMAs: segmental wall motion abnormalities
IVRT: isovolumic relax-action time
LVESP: left ventricular end-systolic pressure
LAVI: left atrial volume index
EDVI: left ventricular end-diastolic volume
ESVI: systolic volume index;
LVMI: left ventricular mass index
E: early diastolic two mitral flow velocity
A: late diastolic mitral flow velocity
E / e ': early diastolic mitral flow velocity and early diastolic mitral annular velocity ratio
DT: mitral E wave deceleration Time
Ard - Ad: aortic root diameter.
Echo: conventional echocardiography
SE: stress echocardiography
ECG: electrocardiogram
NT-proBNP: N-terminal pro brain natriuretic peptide

7

The Origin of Meridians

Li Lei, Ching Wo Tung, Kwai Ching Lo

School of Chinese Medicine, The University of Hong Kong, Hong Kong, China
Email: llie@hku.hk

Abstract

This article explores the origin of meridians. It suggests that the origin of meridians is closely related to the imageries derived by ancient physicians experiencing the circulation of Qi in their bodies during Qigong practice. Based on the cognitive experience from Qigong practice, as well as the symbolic analogy of the flow of rivers and the irrigation system of agriculture, the meridian theory has constructed a model of Qi and blood circulation. Such model is abstract and yet concrete, dialectic and yet intuitive, definite and yet vague, integrated and yet independent, having profound influence on the overall formation of traditional Chinese medicine theories.

Keywords

Meridian, Origin, Circulation of Qi and Blood, Qigong

1. Introduction

Meridian theory is an important component of the basic theories of traditional Chinese medicine.

The time of birth for the meridian concept is not yet clear. There was only a brief description of the eleven-meridians in the silk manuscripts excavated from Mawangdui Han Tombs [1], but later, around the time of the *Yellow Emperor's Canon of Medicine*, the meridian theory had matured in its development. The *Yellow Emperor's Canon of Medicine* established the basic framework of the twelve meridian system, depicting the twelve meridians as an inter-connected system of circulation [2]. The subsequent concepts proposed, such as the concept of "Eight Extraordinary Meridians" by the *Classic on Medical Problems* [3] and the concept of "Fourteen Meridians" combining the twelve meridians with Ren and Du meridians developed by Hua Shou of Yuan dynasty in the *Elucidation of Fourteen Meridians* [4], was no more than supplement and extension of the meridian system in the *Yellow Emperor's Canon of Medicine*.

A meridian is not an anatomical structure. Its morphology has not been in any way traced inside the human body. Even more importantly, theories of traditional Chinese medicine are constructed mainly upon the basis of philosophical thinking, emphasizing macro understanding of the body's functional status as a whole and thus rendering the anatomical description of human structures less important or even dispensable.

The meridian theory has apparently reflected the perceptual characteristics of Chinese culture for its direct image visualization with intuitive logic, which must be a key point when we discuss the origin of meridians.

2. Several Incorrect Viewpoints about the Origin of the Meridians

It has now been widely accepted that the concept of meridians was originated from the propagated sensations produced along a channel during acupuncture or massage treatment. However, such an understanding is not true. While acupuncture stimulation can easily produce propagated sensations, the concept of meridians was conceived much earlier than the invention of acupuncture needles. The Nine-needles made their first appearance during the time of the *Yellow Emperor's Canon of Medicine* when the concept of meridians had already existed. Clearly, the concept of meridians has nothing to do with the propagated sensations of acupuncture needling. In the *Eleven Arms and Feet Meridians for Moxibustion*, it states repeatedly that "for those with symptoms like that, so-and-so meridian should be targeted for moxibustion". It is evident that moxibustion was the only method of treatment applied at that time, while propagated sensation, as produced by the burning of small cones of dried herbs, application of pointed stones, massage or cupping therapies, was a rare clinical phenomenon. Therefore, it is no more than a conjecture to take scattered and indefinite phenomena of propagated sensations as the origin of the circulation pathways of the "Eleven Meridians" and "Twelve Meridians".

Similarly, the concept of meridians did not come from the generalisation and classification of human pathological phenomena, nor the induction of acupoint treatment effects. Systematic classification of human pathological phenomena can be carried out, but it would be difficult to derive the concept of meridians from such classification. As for the acupoints in early times, they form an independent system that was not connected with the meridians. The locating of acupoints was governed by the principle that "acupoint is where the pain is" which clearly reflected the unique feature of an acupoint as the site of pain, pathogen and treatment. The integration of meridians and acupoints took place during the *Yellow Emperor's Canon of Medicine* era. Becoming attached to the meridians, the acupoints hence gained wider practical significance. However, as the concept of meridians was formed long before the compilation of the *Yellow Emperor's Canon of Medicine*, it would only create more confusion about the origin of meridians if the meridians and acupoints were mixed together.

3. The Meridian Concept Stems from the Philosophy Idea

In fact, the concept of meridians was derived merely from a very simple philosophical thinking: human and nature bear resemblance to each other, the human body must therefore have a system of Qi and blood circulation similar to the flow of rivers and lakes in nature.

Ancient China was an agricultural society, the condition of an irrigation system determines the harvest. The legend of Dayu has highlighted the importance of irrigation works to a nation's prospect and people's livelihood. The flow of water over streams and mountains is in itself a natural phenomenon and is a part of the natural environment; it is also closely related to agricultural production. As the way of human beings resembles that of heaven, the human body will certainly have a system of Qi and blood circulation similar to that of rivers and lakes in nature. The *Yellow Emperor's Canon of Medicine* has made it clear that as the Earth has four seas in the east, south, west and north, the human body must also have four "seas", namely, the sea of Shuigu (food digestion), the sea of Twelve Meridians, the sea of Qi and the sea of Marrow, and as there are twelve rivers on earth, so there must be twelve meridians inside the human body.

Drawing analogy between the human body and nature is an evident feature of the philosophy of traditional Chinese medicine.

4. Qigong Practice Laid the Foundation of Meridian Theory

A meridian is a channel of Qi and blood circulation and that is the most basic nature of a meridian. Meridian is the collective name for meridians and collaterals in general, referring to the many blood vessels criss-crossing the human body. The vertical ones are called "meridians" while the horizontal ones are called "collaterals". Originally, "Mai" means blood vessels, but in meridian theory it also means the main channels for Qi circulation.

Undoubtedly, the origin of meridians is closely related to the imageries derived by ancient physicians experiencing the circulation of Qi in their bodies during Qigong practice. As the renowned practitioner of Ming dynasty Li Shizhen said in the *Compendium of Materia Medica*, "the interior channels of the body can only be detected by a self-observing person." [5] In the silk manuscripts excavated from Mawangdui Han Tombs, there was an illustrated guide to physical and breathing exercise with drawings of 44 individuals from different sexes and ages practicing a variety of movements. The bamboo manuscripts excavated from Zhangjiashan Han Tombs in Hubei have documented the theory, key movement guides and practical application of physical and breathing exercise [6]. The 45-word inscription engraved on the ancient jade pendant for promoting Qi circulation, now being kept at the Tianjin History Museum, embodies a complete description of the Qi circulation from the beginning to the end of a Qigong practice [7]. All these historical materials have shown that Qigong had already become very popular long before the *Yellow Emperor's Canon of Medicine* era.

From the experience of Qigong practitioners, it is evident that different Qigong practitioners derive different imageries about the meridians. Comparing the circulation pathways of the twelve meridians as documented by the *Meridians* of the *Spiritual Pivot*, the meridian channels for Qi circulation as perceived during Qigong practice were basically similar to that of the propagated sensations along the meridians. Specifically, the route of Qi circulation along the four limbs in Qigong practice was largely the same as that of the meridian pathways, while that of the chest and abdomen showed certain inconsistencies and that of the head and face showed considerable inconsistencies.

The different imageries perceived by Qigong practitioners have not only explained the existence of two different versions of the meridian pathways as documented by the silk manuscripts of the *Eleven Arms and Feet Meridians for Moxibustion* and the *Eleven Yin and Yang Meridians for Moxibustion* excavated from Mawangdui Han Tombs, but also showed the distribution of the twelve meridians pathways in different parts of the body as described by the *Meridians* of the *Spiritual Pivot*.

Take the pathways of the Gallbladder Meridian as an example, the description by the *Meridians* of the *Spiritual Pivot* is quite clear: there is only one pathway on each lower limb, but is divided into two pathways when it comes to the chest and abdomen, and three on the head and face. In the *Elucidation of the Fourteen Meridians* written by Hua Sou in Yuan Dynasty, the pathway of this meridian on the head has even turned into three divergent folds of lines. For example, the meridian pathway after Wangu (GB12) does not move on to reach the neighbouring Fengchi (GB20), but instead goes up front to Yangbai (GB14) on the forehead before turning down to Fengchi at the back.

The description by the *Elucidation of the Fourteen Meridians* can only be regarded as an illustration of the meridian pathways with meridians and acupoints combined, but it should not be taken as the ultimate version. In spite of this, the multiple meridian pathways on the head have reflected largely the actual Qi circulation in meridian channels as perceived by practitioners during Qigong exercise. The meridian pathways in the four limbs are largely clear while that in the chest and the abdomen are not quite clear, and that on the face and head are mostly not clear. Different Qigong practitioners experience different imageries of Qi circulation and therefore have different documentation of the meridian pathways. The pathways of the twelve meridians described by the *Meridians* of the *Spiritual Pivot* must be the consolidated result of the observations made from a variety of Qigong practice.

5. Conclusions

The concept of meridian should be originated from the observations of human life phenomena by ancient physicians. However, such observations were only vague perceptual understanding. The meridian theory therefore has the typical characteristics of ancient Chinese philosophy. It is constructed upon the perceptual experience gained from Qigong practice as well as the analogical extensions of the flow of rivers in nature and irrigation systems in agriculture. It gives rise to a model of Qi and blood circulation that is abstract and yet concrete, dialectic and yet intuitive, definite and yet vague, integrated and yet independent, hence laying the foundation for the development of acupuncture theories.

In terms of concrete structures, meridians are no more than "blood vessels". However, in macro perspective, the function of Qi and blood circulation represents the basic features of human vitality, and elucidates the intrinsic connections among Yin and Yang, the five elements, viscera, Qi and blood and other traditional Chinese medicine theories, thereby having a profound influence on the overall theoretical construction of traditional Chinese medicine.

References

[1] Collating Group of the Silk Manuscripts Excavated from Mawangdui Han Tombs (1985) The Silk Manuscripts Excavated from Mawangdui Han Tombs (Section Four)[M]. Wenwu Publishing House, Beijing.

[2] Anonymous (1956) Yellow Emperor's Internal Classics: Plain Conversation (Copied Print)[M]. People's Health Publishing House, Beijing.

[3] Anonymous (1956) The Spiritual Pivot (Copied Print)[M]. People's Health Publishing House, Beijing.

[4] Wang, J.-S., Wang, D.-X., Shi, Y.-L., *et al.* (1956) The Variorum of the Classics on Medical Problems. People's Health Publishing House, Beijing.

[5] Wang, L.-Z. and Li, D. (1990) Emendation and Scholiume on "A Study on the Eight Extra-Channels"[M]. Shanghai Scientific and Technical Publishers, Shanghai.

[6] Collating Group of Bamboo Manuscripts Unearthed from 247 Grave in Zhangjiashan (2001) Bamboo Manuscripts Unearthed from a Grave in Zhangjiashan. Cultural Relics Press, Beijing.

[7] Guo, M.-R. (2005) Slavery Era. Chian Renmin University Press, Beijing.

8

Vulvodynia Treated with Acupuncture or Electromyographic Biofeedback

Oroma B. Nwanodi*, Melanie M. Tidman

Department of Interdisciplinary Health Studies, A. T. Still University Arizona School of Health Sciences, Mesa, USA

Email: *o.nwanodi@juno.com

Abstract

First, second, and third line medical treatments of vulvodynia are of limited efficacy. Surgical resection, the fourth line treatment of vulvodynia, may have unforgiving sequela. Therefore, acupuncture and electromyographic (EMG) biofeedback could bridge between medical and surgical treatments of vulvodynia. Of note, EMG biofeedback is more frequently recommended in treatment algorithms for vulvodynia than is acupuncture. Trials of acupuncture for unprovoked vulvodynia demonstrate variable efficacy, whereas trials of EMG biofeedback for provoked vulvodynia demonstrate consistent efficacy. Trials of acupuncture for treatment of provoked and unprovoked vulvodynia using identical acupoints, a vulvar algesiometer for objective pain measurement, and standardized, validated, tools for outcome assessment are needed. Such trials may enable comparison of acupuncture to EMG biofeedback for the treatment of provoked and unprovoked vulvodynia. Similarly, trials of EMG biofeedback for treatment of unprovoked vulvodynia would increase the knowledge base of EMG biofeedback for treatment of vulvodynia.

Keywords

Acupuncture, Biofeedback, Electromyography, Vestibulodynia, Vulvodynia

1. Introduction

This article is a clinical review article on vulvodynia for health care providers including physical therapists, with an interest in alternative, complementary, holistic, or integrated medicine. As the target audience's knowledge base may not focus on gynecology, following the introductory section the relevant anatomy will be reviewed.

The purpose of this review article is to determine whether acupuncture and electromyography (EMG) bio-

*Corresponding author.

feedback have comparable efficacy in the treatment of vulvodynia or vestibulodynia. A secondary goal is to identify why the American guideline for treatment of vulvodynia does not support usage of acupuncture whereas the British guideline supports usage of acupuncture. Additionally, future study options for the treatment of vulvodynia with acupuncture that may use a vulvar algesiometer will be identified. To this end, the pathophysiology, classification, evaluation, and treatments of vulvodynia will be reviewed. Such review should clarify the pathophysiologic basis of vulvodynia, which contributes to the biologic plausibility of both acupuncture and EMG biofeedback for treatment of vulvodynia. Second, the efficacy of acupuncture for treatment of vulvodynia will be presented. Third, the efficacy of EMG biofeedback for treatment of vulvodynia will be reviewed. Fourth, an attempt will be made to determine the comparative treatment efficacy of these two treatment modalities. Such elucidation of comparative efficacy or lack thereof, between acupuncture and EMG biofeedback may reconcile the different recommendations for the treatment of vulvodynia in the American and British guidelines.

1.1. Definition of Terminology

Vulvodynia, a chronic, disabling, burning, discomfort of the vulva was first described in 1976, and given distinction as a discrete clinical entity by the International Society for the Study of Vulval Disease (ISSVD) in 1985 [1]. Initially, vulval vestibulitis was regarded as a distinct disorder from vulvodynia. However, in 2005 the ISSVD reclassified vulval vestibulitis as vestibulodynia, a localized vulvodynia [2].

1.2. Prevalence and Comorbidities

Provoked vestibulodynia has a prevalence of 12% of women [3]. Vestibulodynia is found in 15% of gynecology patients [4]. Immunologic, infectious, inflammatory, neoplastic, and neurologic pathologies should be excluded prior to making a diagnosis of vulvodynia [1] [2] [5]. Anxiety, depression, interstitial cystitis, irritable bowel syndrome, and sexual dysfunction are co-morbidities of vulva pain syndromes [1] [3] [6]. Provoked vestibulodynia is significantly associated with chronic fatigue syndrome (odds ratio [OR] = 2.78), depression (OR = 2.99), fibromyalgia (OR = 2.15), irritable bowel syndrome (OR = 1.86), urinary tract infections (OR = 6.15), and yeast infections (OR = 4.24) [3]. Vulvodynia is known to impair partner intimacy [1] [7], presumably via contribution to the development of dyspareunia [8], hypoactive sexual desire, orgasmic dysfunction, and vaginismus [6].

2. Methods

The PubMed database was searched on August 31, 2013, with the terms "acupuncture treatment vulvodynia", "electromyographic biofeedback vulvodynia", "acupuncture treatment vulvar vestibulitis", and "electromyographic biofeedback vulvar vestibulitis", yielding 10 English language articles. Eight articles were found from the reference lists of the first 10 articles. Three references were sought as original sources of standardized testing instruments. Two references were taken from prior work for neurological background, and one reference for anatomy (**Figure 1**). Of these, three studies on acupuncture and four studies on EMG biofeedback will be reviewed (**Table 1**).

3. Anatomy, Pathophysiology, Classification, Evaluation, and Treatment of Vulvodynia

3.1. Anatomy

The vulva is bounded cephalad by the mons pubis, bilaterally by the lateral margins of the labia majora, and caudad by the anus [9]. Within the vulva, the vestibule is demarcated bilaterally by the labia minora forming Hart's line, cephalad by the clitoris, caudad by the posterior fourchette and fossa navicularis, and in depth by the vaginal introitus [10] [11]. Being contained within the vulva, the vestibule may not be exposed to all the stimuli which the larger vulva is exposed to.

3.2. Pathophysiology

The vulva is primarily innervated by the pudendal nerve plexus from S3 and S4 [12]. Cephalad and lateral portions of the vulva derive innervation from the ilioinguinal, genitofemoral, and posterior femoral cutaneous nerves from L1, L1 and L2, and S1 to S3 respectively [13]. Vulvar pain may be transmitted via rapid, myelin

Table 1. Description of studies included in the review.

Study/ Year	Study Design	Subject Sources/ Diagnosis	Treatment of Interest	Treatment Frequency	Number of Subjects	Outcome Measures	Follow-Up	Results
Reference [1]/1999	Quasi-experimental. No blinding, control group(s), or randomization	Vulval clinic/ vulvodynia	Acupuncture Spleen meridian points 6 & 9, liver meridian point 3, large intestine meridian point 4	Once weekly for 10 weeks	12 women aged 18 - 68 years; all completed treatment	VAS pain score (range not given) and adapted QOL questionnaire scores	5 weeks after last treatment session	Three groups of subject response: good, short-term, and non-responders
Reference [17]/2001	Quasi-experimental. No blinding, control group(s), or randomization	Adolescent health center/ vestibulitis	Acupuncture 4 local and 2 distal points were always used, an additional 2 - 5 points couldalso be used	Once or twice weekly for 10 treatments in total	14 women aged 19 - 26 years; 13 completed treatment	VAS pain score of 0-10, negative/positive QOL questionnaire	11 subjects at 3 months after last treatment session	Statistically significant changes to negative and positive QOL factors p = 0.01 and p = 0.001
Reference [3]/2009	Quasi-experimental No blinding, control group(s), or randomization	Gynecology clinic /provoked vestibulodynia	Acupuncture 10-20 points from the forehead to the knees	Twice weekly for 10 treatments in 5 weeks	8 women aged 21 - 49 years. Mean age 30 years.	FSFI, PCS, PVAQ, and investigator developed pain report	None	Statistically significant improvement in pain with manual genital stimulation on the FSFI, p = 0.05
Reference [12]/1995	Quasi-experimental No blinding, control group(s), or randomization	Vulval clinic/vulvar vestibulitis	EMG biofeedback In-home pelvic floor muscle exercises with vaginal sensor, portable EMG biofeedback instrument, computerized EMG data acquisition	Twice daily for an average of 16 weeks	33women aged 21 - 45 years. Mean age 31.5 years.	Subjective pain scale of 0-10, frequency of coitus, EMG amplitude for contraction, relaxation, and rest periods	6 months	Decreased resting pelvic muscle tension and instability by 68% and 62%. Decreased subjective pain by 83%. Coitus resumed by 78% of abstainers
Reference [8]/2001	Block randomization. Non-blinded. Control groups of group cognitive behavior therapy, vestibulectomy	Media advertisement and referrals/ dyspareunia due to vulvar vestibulitis	EMG biofeedback In-home pelvic floor muscle exercises with vaginal sensor, portable EMG home trainer, computerized EMG data acquisition	Twice daily for 12 weeks	29 per group. Mean age 26.8 years. Total of 9 subjects overall discontinued	PRI and sensory scales of the McGill Pain Questionnaire, frequency of coitus, Derogatis Sexual Functioning Inventory, Brief Symptom Inventory	6 months	Intention-to-treat analysis statistically significant pain reduction in each group, greatest in vestibulectomy group.
Reference [22]/2001	Quasi-experimental No blinding, control group(s), or randomization	Clinic/vulvar vestibulitis	EMG biofeedback In-home pelvic floor muscle exercises with vaginal sensor, portable EMG home trainer, computerized EMG data acquisition	Twice daily for 11 months	29 women aged 25 - 48 years	Subjective pain scale of 0 - 10 for assessment of dyspareunia. EMG amplitude for contraction and relaxation	None	Significant decrease in pain for 84.7% of subjects. Coitus resumed by 69% of subjects
Reference [23]/2006	Joint computer generated randomization, control group given 2% topical lidocaine gel and 5% lidocaine ointment	Two vulvar clinics/vulvar vestibulitis	EMG biofeedback In-home pelvic floor muscle exercises with vaginal sensor, portable EMG home trainer, computerized EMG data acquisition	Twice daily for 4 months	23 women per group	Negative/positive QOL questionnaire, PRIME MD, Short Form 36, VAS 0 - 100 pain scale, Vulvar pressure pain threshold measured by vulvar algesiometer calibrated for 3 - 1000 grams force	6 and 12 months	Equivalent improvement in vestibular pressure pain thresholds, QOL, and coitus were achieved by each treatment group.

EMG, Electromyography; FSFI, Female Sexual Function Index; PCS, Pain Catastrophizing Scale; PRI, Pain Rating Index; PVAQ, Pain Vigilance and Awareness Questionnaire; PRIME MD, Primary Care Evaluation of Mental Disorders; QOL, Quality of Life; VAS, Visual analogue scale.

ated, A-δelta fibers with encephalin mediated spinal cord synapses between inhibitory communication cells and Waldeyer cells connected with the spinothalamic tract and serotonin mediated descending pain inhibitory channels [1]. An initial painful stimulus to the vulva can cause central pain sensitization.

In central pain sensitization the dorsal horn neurons are hypersensitized to any subsequent vulval stimulus [14]. Meaning that, after the initial provocation to the vulva, nociceptor thresholds are lowered and hyperalgesia occurs [7]. Now, progressively reduced stimuli can generate an increasingly greater pain response [7]. Distal-

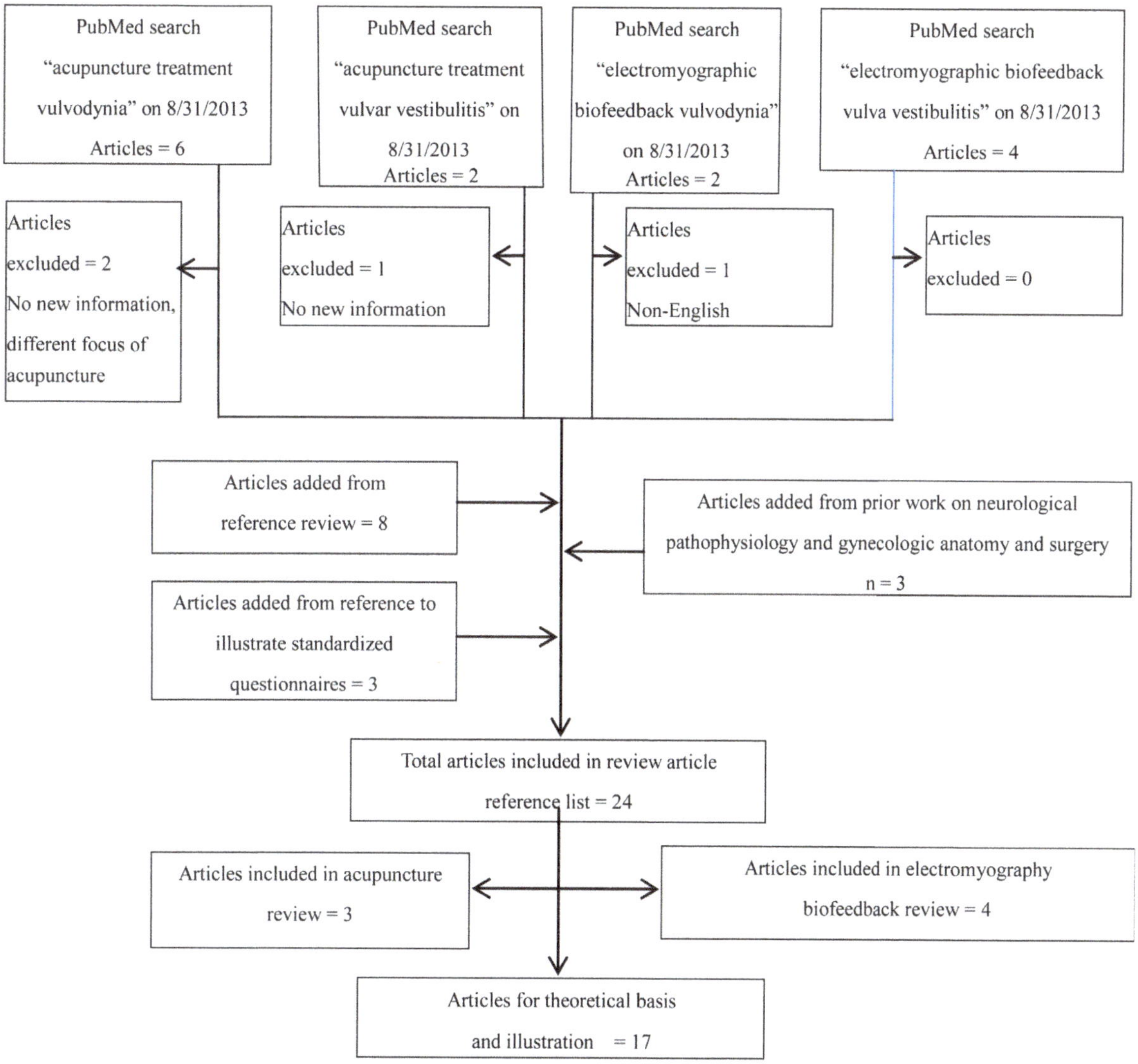

Figure 1. Article selection flow chart.

stimuli may elicit a response previously derived from local stimuli. The nociceptor field of reception increases with central sensitization and hyperalgesia [7]. Allodynia follows when nociceptors respond to what would ordinarily be non-noxious stimuli [7]. Persistent pelvic floor muscle stimulation may progress into contracture of the pubovaginalis and puborectalis portions of the pubococcygeus muscle [7] which receive innervation from S3 and S4 via the pudendal nerve [12]. Unprovoked myofascial pain ensues [7]. Baseline vulval electromyography (EMG) of healthy female controls averages 1 - 2 μV RMS [12]. Women with provoked vulvodynia have baseline EMG of 2.5 μV RMS, whereas women with unprovoked vulvodynia demonstrate further increased voltage of 3 - 5 μV RMS [12]. The progressive increase in vulva EMG voltage from healthy controls with normal pain sensation may reflect disease progression from central sensitization with hyperalgesia in provoked vulvodynia, to allodynia in unprovoked vulvodynia.

Alternatively, the concept of cross-talk pain from visceral inflammation postulates that normally inactive mucosal afferents of the bladder, urethra, and vagina are activated when sympathetic nervous system synapses are shared with afferents from viscera including the distal large intestines and rectum [14]. The pudendal dorsal root ganglia of S2 through S4 are shared with parasympathetic pelvic splanchnic nerves innervating the vagina and cervix, the inferior hypogastric plexus (from which the pelvic nerves derives) innervating the uterus and cervix, sympathetic sacral splanchnic nerves, and the vagal nerve which innervates the vagina, cervix, and uterus.

The ilioinguinal, genitofemoral, and posterior femoral cutaneous nerves share the inferior mesenteric ganglia with the lumbar splanchnic nerve from T12. In turn, the least splanchnic nerve from T12 shares the celiac and superior mesenteric ganglia with the greater and lesser splanchnic nerves. Therefore, innervation deriving from T12 can expose vulva innervation to stimuli from the ascending and transverse colon, kidney, liver, small and large intestines, spleen, stomach, and pancreas [15].

Up to 15% of afferents combine somatic and para-sympathetic motor activity permitting neurogenic sensitization, upregulation, and neurogenic inflammation in organs distant from the original inciting event, resulting in cross-talk pain [14] [16]. The anatomic location and etiologic pathophysiology of vulvodynia described above are important determinants of classification of vulvodynia and extent to which surgical treatment may eventually be recommended.

3.3. Classification of Vulvodynia

The ISSVD distinguishes between generalized vulvodynia of the entire vulva and localized vulvodynia pertaining to specific parts of the vulva [2]. Vestibulodynia is a localized vulvodynia of the vestibule anatomically described above [10] [11]. Generalized and localized vulvodynia may be provoked by nonsexual stimuli, sexual stimuli, or a combination thereof. Alternatively, generalized and localized vulvodynia may be unprovoked, or may result from a combination of provocation and non-provocation based on the described theories of central sensitization, allodynia, and cross-talk.

According to Friedrich's criteria, vestibulodynia involves six months of vestibular erythema, elicitation of pain upon application of pressure to the vestibulum, and extreme pain upon vulva penetration [17]. The classifications of provoked or unprovoked vulvodynia and vestibulodynia may affect treatment of refractory cases.

3.4. Evaluation of Vulvodynia

On physical exam, pain is elicited by the poorly reproducible operator dependent application of a cotton swab to the vulva [10] [11]. Therefore, a vulvar algesiometer (**Figure 2**) that measures pressure pain was developed [18]. Using four vulvar locations (**Figure 3**) for the vulvar algesiometer a correlation was found between 25 patients' subjective reports of pain and objective vulvar algesiometer scores. Post-treatment patients were able to tolerate increased force setting of the vulvar algesiometer force probe [18].

3.5. Treatment of Vulvodynia

Initially, vulvodynia and vestibulodynia are treated identically. Acute vulvodynia of less than three months du-

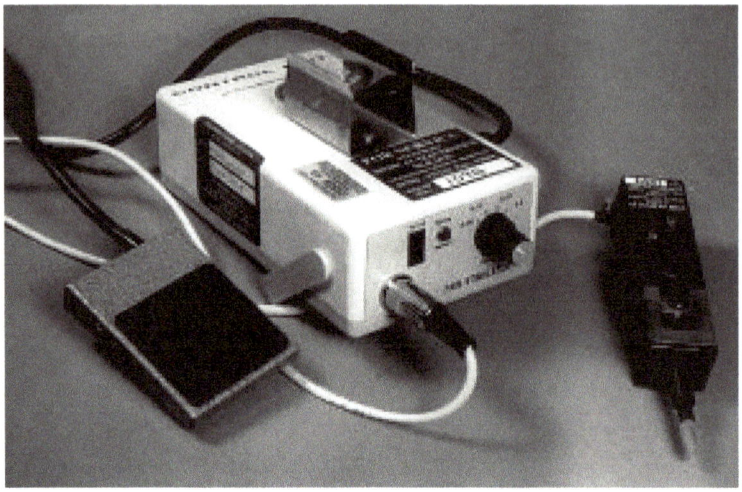

Figure 2. V ulvar algesiometer. Reproduced with permission from Eva, L.J., Reid, W.M.N., MacLean, A.B., & Morrison, G.D. (1999) Assessment of response to treatment in vulvar vestibulitis syndrome by means of the vulvar algesiometer. American Journal of Obstetrics and Gynecology, 181 (1), 99 - 102 (**Figure 1**).

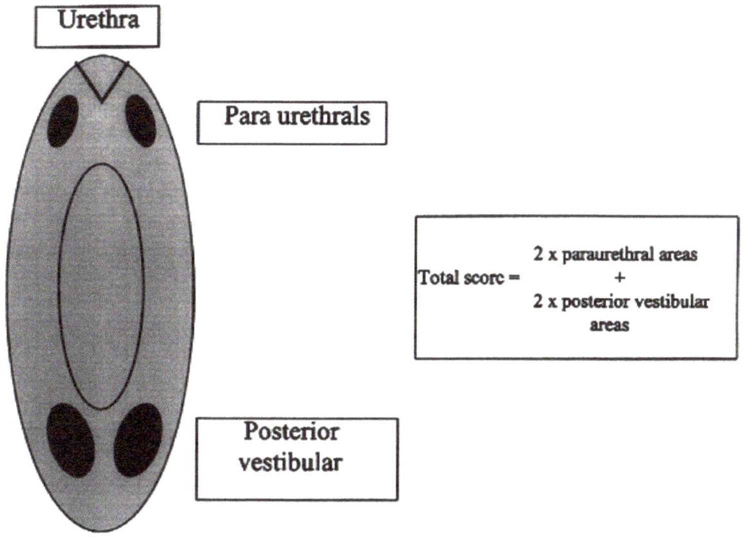

Figure 3. Positions of Application of Vulvar Algesiometer Probe. Reproduced with permission from Eva, L.J., Reid, W.M.N., MacLean, A.B., & Morrison, G.D. (1999) Assessment of response to treatment in vulvar vestibulitis syndrome by means of the vulvar algesiometer. American Journal of Obstetrics and Gynecology, 181(1), 99-102 (**Figure 2**).

ration may be treated by lifestyle changes such as the removal of irritant stimuli, suppression of inflammation and neuropathic pain [1] [5]. Bacterial and viral sexually-transmitted diseases, candidiasis, and urinary incontinence should be treated if identified. Usage of douches, harsh soaps, perfumed feminine hygiene products, propylene glycol or polyethylene glycol containing lubricants and spermicide, and tampons may provide irritant stimulus and should be discontinued [1] [5]. Underlying chronic conditions including interstitial cystitis and lichen sclerosis should be identified and treated if present. Topical steroids may be over-used by patients and are not recommended [5] [9] [12]. However, emollients and non-irritative lubricants may be used [1] [5]. These are all first line treatments.

Oral antidepressants and anticonvulsants form second line treatment [5]. Injectable anesthetic and steroid combinations are used as third line treatment when topical treatments provide inadequate relief [5]. Refractory vestibulodynia with dyspareunia achieving partial response to topical anesthetics may be more successfully treated with vestibulectomy than is unprovoked vestibulodynia [2]. Vulvectomy is the surgical alternative for refractory vulvodynia. Vestibulectomy involves the excision of painful tissue within the vestibule. Vestibulectomy is less extensive than a perineoplasty which additionally excises perineal tissue close to the anus [5]. Anatomically more extensive, vulvectomy is preferably reserved for patients with vulvar cancer. A complete or almost complete resolution of refractory vestibulodynia was achieved by 68% of participants in a randomized controlled trial (RCT) of vestibulectomy [3]. However, by six months post-procedure success rates start to decline to as low as 40 percent [10].Vulvectomy and vestibulectomy are major surgeries with the possibility of intractable post-operative adhesion formation and pudendal neuralgia [13]. Given the irreversible invasiveness of fourth line treatments of vulvodynia and vestibulodynia: vulvectomy, vestibulectomy, and perineoplasty; there is need for less invasive, reversible, alternative treatments of vulvodynia and vestibulodynia. Acupuncture and EMG biofeedback may be alternative treatments of vulvodynia and vestibulodynia.

For refractory vulvodynia, the American vulvodynia guideline recommends biofeedback and physical therapy, including electromyographic (EMG) biofeedback [5]. Acupuncture is absent from the American vulvodynia guideline [5]. Yet, the British Society for the Study of Vulval Diseases Guideline Group includes acupuncture as a possible treatment for unprovoked vulvodynia [2]. Acupuncture is efficacious as treatment of pain in dysmenorrhea, fibromyalgia, headache, lumbago, myofascial pain, and osteoarthritis [3]. Of note, while the efficacy of acupuncture for the above ailments is comparable to that of mainstream medical treatments, much fewer adverse events are encountered with usage of acupuncture than with mainstream medical treatments [3] [17]. Therefore, it is biologically plausible that acupuncture may be a safe, efficacious treatment of vulvodynia, including vestibulodynia, a local vulvodynia.

Given that currently available medical treatments do not adequately treat vulvodynia, there is room for additional effective treatment modalities of vulvodynia absent the systemic adverse events frequently associated with oral medications. Moreover, the vulvar algesiometer provides for objective, noninvasive assessment of vulvar pain that may be more highly regarded than subjective visual analogue scales (VAS) for determining efficacy of different treatment modalities for vulvodynia [18]. Clinical trials may specifically select cases of either provoked or unprovoked vulvodynia or vestibulodynia for study. Now that the vulvar algesiometer is available, an objective pain measurement may be used in clinical studies.

4. Efficacy of Acupuncture for Treatment of Vulvodynia

Penetration of acupuncture needles at acupoints by rotation or thrusting triggers numbness or fullness in the patient, referred to as "de chi" which in turn activates the release of opioid peptides[3] [17]. Acupuncture increases the concentration of β endorphins [1]. Acupuncture mediated opioid peptide β endorphin release is confirmed by opioid antagonist naloxone reversal of analgesia following acupuncture [1]. Therefore, acupuncture could alter the response of spinal cord synapses to afferent sensation of rapid, myelinated, A-δelta fibers in vulvodynia and vular vestibulitis [1].

Increased localization of analgesics or healing promoting substances at the target site facilitated by acupuncture in turn, increase rates of transmission of electromagnetic signaling from the brain [3]. Additionally, acupuncture may promote immune and central nervous system functioning [3]. Like longitude and latitude which traverse the entire globe, acupuncture meridians traverse the entire body. Meridians are energy pathways through the body, used by both acupuncture and bioenergy medicine. The acupuncture meridians of the liver, kidney, and spleen pass through the genitalia, permitting distant acupoints on the liver, kidney, and spleen meridians to elicit a therapeutic response at the vulva [3]. These acupuncture meridians echo the described interrelations between the ilioinguinal, genitofemoral, posterior femoral, and pudendal nerves that innervate the vulva, and the splanchnic nerves that innervate the liver, kidney, and spleen via sharing of the inferior mesenteric ganglia with the lumbar splanchnic nerve from T12. Thus, based on cross-talk, it is biologically plausible that acupuncture for treatment of vulvodynia and vestibulodynia need not be performed directly on the vulva or vulval vestibule.

Reference [1] performed a case series of 12 patients with unprovoked vulvodynia. Four acupoints were used weekly for 10 weeks. Two of 12 patients achieved good response, three of 12 patients achieved short-term response; seven of 12 patients were non-responders [1]. Standardized questionnaires for outcome determination were not used [1]. A pilot study of 14 women with vestibulodynia treated with acupuncture used ten treatments performed by a physiotherapist with more than 10 years of experience [17]. Each treatment done at one to two week intervals used at least six acupoints (**Table 1**), with 1 - 3 mechanical rotations for a total of 30-45 minutes [17]. Again, standardized questionnaires for outcome determination were not used [17]. Before treatment, after treatment, and three months post treatment VAS vulvar pain scores for patient-provoked vulvar pain were recorded for negative outcomes: the three major disabling effects of vestibulodynia as determined by each participant, and for positive outcomes such as "desire" and "joy of living" [17]. Statistically significant improvement of median VAS for both negative and positive outcomes occurred immediately after treatment with $p = 0.004$ and $p = 0.04$ respectively [17]. Three months post treatment a continued statistically significant but slightly changed improvement persisted with $p = 0.01$ for negative outcomes and $p = 0.001$ for positive outcomes [17].

Subsequently, reference [3] performed a pilot trial of acupuncture for treatment of provoked vestibulodynia with eight patients. Two traditional Chinese medicine practitioners (TCMs) performed 10 one-hour long acupuncture sessions utilizing 10 - 20 needles inserted from the forehead to the knees within five weeks. Reference [3] used standardized questionnaires for outcome determination. The Female Sexual Function Index (FSFI) [19], the Pain Catastrophizing Scale (PCS) [20], and the Pain and Vigilance Awareness Questionnaire (PVAQ) [21] were administered prior to initial treatment, then after the fifth and tenth treatments [3]. Following each treatment session, the investigators administered an investigator-selected questionnaire with 10 point Likert scale ranking. Analysis of reference 3 yielded a single statistically significant finding attributable to small sample size: pain reduction with manual genital stimulation ($p = 0.05$) [3].

5. Efficacy of Electromyographic Biofeedback of Pelvic Floor Musculature for Treatment of Vulvodynia

Physiotherapy with biofeedback has efficacy of up to 83% pain reduction in the treatment of provoked vulvodynia due to hypertonicity of the pelvic floor [3] [12]. Reference [12] performed an initial assessment in office, then studied 33 women using a surface EMG single user vaginal sensor with a separate portable EMG biofeedback machine at home on a twice daily basis with six intermittent in-office surveillance visits over 16 weeks. If necessary EMG biofeedback from accessory muscles of the abdomen, buttocks, and legs, as well as videotaped demonstration of pelvic floor muscle contractions were used to elicit correct pelvic floor muscle contraction. Patients learned to hold pelvic floor muscle contractions for one, ten, and 60 seconds. Each twice daily at-home cycle comprised of 10 second contractions alternated with 10 second rests for 60 repetitions, totaling 20 minutes. At each clinic session, patients reported pain on a Likert scale with 0 representing no pain and 10 representing the worst pain. By the 16-week clinic session, pain had decreased by 83%. Patients continued twice-daily pelvic floor contraction cycles without biofeedback for at least three months. A final evaluation was performed three months thereafter. Statistically significant decrease in pain, increase in number of patients able to have sexual intercourse, increase in pelvic floor muscle strength, and decreases in EMG amplitude during relaxation periods were achieved, with $p < 0.0001$ for each variable [12].

Reference [12] was retested with a study of 29 women, five of whom had undergone vestibular surgery [22]. The investigatory team performing the retest included the lead author of the original study as a co-investigator [22]. At 11 months from treatment initiation, reduction of pain to mild or negligible ratings was achieved in 84.7% of study subjects [22]. Moreover, 75% of study subjects were sexually active 11 months from study initiation [22].

The first RCT of treatment of provoked vestibulodynia was a comparative efficacy trial of 12 weeks of group cognitive-behavioral therapy (CBT), 12 weeks of EMG bio-feedback, and vestibulectomy involving 78 initial subjects assigned to trial arms by block randomization [8]. A subject recruitment, selection, and trial completion diagram is not provided [8]. In addition to assessing nonsexual vulvar pain via a Likert scale, perceived treatment efficacy and dyspareunia per se were also assessed [8]. Additionally, the Pain Rating Index (PRI), the Sensory scale of the McGill Pain Questionnaire (MPQ, the Global Sexual Functioning score of the Sexual History Form, the Sexual Information scale of the Derogatis Functioning Inventory, and the Global Severity Index of the Brief Symptom Inventory (BSI-GSI) [8]. Intent-to-treat analysis showed that at six months post vestibulectomy, subjects had statistically significant lower pain score than EMG biofeedback subjects ($p < 0.05$). Each treatment arm had identical improvement in pain from pretreatment to six months post treatment, MPQ-PRI pain, Sensory scale of the MPQ, sexual function, sexual history, and sexual frequency, ($p < 0.01$ for each treatment arm and variable). However, the vestibulectomy arm contained seven drop-outs, whereas the CBT group did not have any drop-outs [8].

Reference [23] performed a computer randomized comparative efficacy clinical trial of EMG biofeedback versus topical lidocaine gel with 23 subjects in each arm, of which 18 subjects completed EMG biofeedback and 19 subjects completed topical lidocaine treatment. EMG biofeedback used an identical vaginal sensor as in reference [8]. EMG biofeedback, comprised of three 10-minute sessions daily comprising of ten 5-second contractions and 5-second relaxations, followed by a 60-second rest, then fifteen 10-second contractions and 10-second relaxations, ending with a 60-second contraction [23]. Vulvar algesiometers measured vestibular pressure pain thresholds, while a 0 to 100 VAS was used to record subjective pain, sexual functioning, and dyspareunia [23]. The Short form 36 (SF 36), Primary Care Evaluation of Mental Disorders (PRIME MD, and a quality-of-life (QOL) instrument were also used. Vulvar algesiometer data at four months yielded greater improvement in pressure pain thresholds for the topical lidocaine group (site A, $p = 0.008$; site B, $p = 0.007$) than the EMG biofeedback group (Site A, $p = 0.002$; Site B $p = 0.02$), but at twelve months both groups and sites have statistically identical outcomes with p = non-significant for any difference. Reduction in frequency of non-coital vestibular pain was greatest for EMG biofeedback given $p = 0.003$, and was the only VAS variable with a statistically significant difference when both treatment arms were compared, $p = 0.009$ [23].

6. Comparative Efficacy of Acupuncture and Electromyographic Biofeedback of Pelvic Floor Musculature

The studies on acupuncture for treatment of unprovoked vulvodynia lacked placebo controls [1] [3] [17]. Therefore, assessment of a placebo effect when treating vulvodynia with acupuncture cannot be performed. As is commonly a difficulty in comparing trials on acupuncture, each study used different acupuncture protocols in terms of duration of individual treatments, frequency and total number of treatments, and number of acupoints [1] [3] [17]. Furthermore, different outcome assessment methods were used in each study [1] [3] [17]. A direct comparison of these three studies cannot be made.

Similarly, the studies on EMG biofeedback for provoked vulvodynia have protocol differences. References [12] and [22] used different EMG biofeedback equipment, assessment protocol software, and durations of initial treatment. Reference [8] used different EMG biofeedback equipment and treatment repetition pattern than references [12] and [22], but the same assessment software asreference [22]. Reference [23] used a different treatment repetition pattern than references [8], [12], and [22]. As references [12] and [22] did not present study data in the same format a direct comparison of results between these two studies, of which the former was ostensibly to ascertain reproducibility of the latter is not facilitated. Furthermore, references [8] and [23] used numerous assessment questionnaires. Despite this, all four trials individually support the efficacy of EMG with biofeedback in treatment of vestibulodynia whereas none of the trials on acupuncture resoundingly demonstrate efficacy of acupuncture for treatment of vulvodynia [8] [12] [22] [23]. Yet, given that women with unprovoked vulvodynia have higher resting EMG of 3 - 5 μV RMS than an average 2.5 μV RMS in women with provoked vulvodynia [12], it is unclear why none of the trials of EMG with biofeedback in vulvodynia studied women with unprovoked vulvodynia.

7. Conclusions

Consistent with the 1997 NIH finding that evidence in support of medical applications of acupuncture was weak, at present, there is insufficient data to argue for the efficacy of acupuncture for treatment of unprovoked vulvodynia, and no data on the efficacy of acupuncture for treatment of provoked vulvodynia [24]. Therefore, it is understandable that American guidelines for the treatment of vulvodynia exclude acupuncture [5]. However, the absence of adverse events from acupuncture, and suggestion of response were sufficient for the British guidelines to include acupuncture as a treatment for unprovoked vulvodynia [2]. As acupuncture and EMG biofeedback have been used to treat different forms of vulvodynia a direct comparison of the two treatment modalities cannot be made.

Vulvectomy and vestibulectomy, the treatments of last resort for provoked vulvodynia or provoked vestibulodynia have only a culminative 68% almost cured or cured rate. Therefore, additional treatments for provoked vulvodynia including provoked vestibulodynia are needed. Given the favorable adverse event profile of acupuncture, it is reasonable to thoroughly evaluate acupuncture as a mode of treatment for provoked vulvodynia. Therefore, randomized controlled trials (RCTs) of acupuncture for treatment of provoked vulvodynia are needed. Such RCTs of acupuncture for treatment of provoked vulvodynia should use clearly delineated acupoints [1] [17], a vulvar algesiometer for reproducibility of pressure pain [23], and standardized, validated, tools for outcome assessment [3]. Designed in this fashion, RCTs of acupuncture for treatment of vulvodynia could facilitate comparison of acupuncture and EMG with biofeedback for the treatment of provoked vulvodynia. Similarly, well-designed and performed trials of acupuncture for treatment of unprovoked vulvodynia would increase the body of evidence for the use of acupuncture in the treatment of vulvodynia.

Trials of EMG biofeedback demonstrate efficacy. EMG biofeedback may be less efficacious than vestibulectomy. EMG biofeedback is also less invasive than vestibulectomy, therefore, it may be prudent to recommend a trial of EMG biofeedback prior to proceeding with vulvectomy or vestibulectomy for refractory provoked vulvodynia or refractory provoked vestibulodynia.

Acknowledgements

This paper is based on coursework previously submitted to the Arizona School of Health Sciences in partial fulfillment of the requirements for the Doctor of Health Sciences Degree, A. T. Still University.

References

[1] Powell, J. and Wojnarowska, F. (1999) Acupuncture for Vulvodynia. *Journal of the Royal Society of Medicine*, **9**, 579-581.

[2] Mandal, D., Nunns, D., Byrne, M., Mclelland, J., Rani, R., Cullimore, J., *et al.* (2010) Guidelines for the Management of Vulvodynia. *British Journal of Dermatology*, **162**, 1180-1185. http://dx.doi.org/10.1111/j.1365-2133.2010.09684.x

[3] Curran, S., Brotto, L.A., Fisher, H., Knudson, G. and Cohen, T. (2009) The ACTIV Study: Acupuncture Treatment in Provoked Vestibulodynia. *The Journal of Sexual Medicine*, **7**, 981-995. http://dx.doi.org/10.1111/j.1743-6109.2009.01582.x

[4] Goetsch, M.F. (1991) Vulvar Vestibulitis: Prevalence and Historic Features in a General Gynecologic Practice Population. *American Journal of Obstetrics and Gynecology*, **164**, 1609-1614; discussion, 1614-1616. http://dx.doi.org/10.1016/0002-9378(91)91444-2

[5] Haefner, H., Collins, M.E., Davis, G.D., Edwards, L., Foster, D.C., Hartmann, E.H., *et al.* (2005) The Vulvodynia Guideline. *Journal of Lower Genital Tract Disease*, **9**, 40-51.http://dx.doi.org/10.1097/00128360-200501000-00009

[6] Nunns, D. and Mandal, D. (1997). Psychological and Psychosexual Aspects of Vulvar Vestibulitis. *Genitourinary Medicine*, **73**, 541-544.

[7] Jantos, M. (2008) Vulvodynia: A Psychophysiological Profile Based on Electromyographic Assessment. *Applied Psychophysiology and Biofeedback*, **33**, 29-38. http://dx.doi.org/10.1007/s10484-008-9049-y

[8] Bergeron, S., Binik, Y.M., Khalifé, S., Pagidas, K., Glazer, H.I., Meana, M. and Amsel, R. (2001) A Randomized Comparison of Group Cognitive-Behavioral Therapy, Surface Electromyographic Biofeedback, and Vestibulectomy in the Treatment of Dyspareunia Resulting from Vulvar Vestibulitis. *Pain*, **91**, 297-306. http://dx.doi.org/10.1016/S0304-3959(00)00449-8

[9] McKay, M. (1992) Vulvodynia Diagnostic Patterns. *Dermatology Clinics*, **10**, 423-433.

[10] Baggish, M.S. and Miklos, J.R. (1995) Vulvar Pain Syndrome: A Review. *Obstetrical & Gynecological Survey*, **50**, 618-627. http://dx.doi.org/10.1097/00006254-199508000-00023

[11] Haefner, H. (2000) Critique of New Gynecological Surgical Procedures: Surgery for Vulvar Vestibulitis. *Clinical Obstetrics & Gynecology*, **43**, 689-700. http://dx.doi.org/10.1097/00003081-200009000-00028

[12] Glazer, H.I., Rodke, G., Swencionis, C., Hertz, R. and Young, A.W. (1995) Treatment of Vulvar Vestibulitis Syndrome with Electromyographic Biofeedback of Pelvic Floor Musculature. *The Journal of Reproductive Medicine*, **40**, 283-290.

[13] Baggish, M.S. and Karram, M.M. (2011) Atlas of Pelvic Anatomy and Gynecologic surgery. 3rd Edition, Elsevier Saunders, Saint Louis.

[14] Bergeron, S., Binik, Y.M., Khalifé, S. and Pagidas, K. (1997) Vulvar Vestibulitis Syndrome: A Critical Review. *The Clinical Journal of Pain*, **13**, 27-42.http://dx.doi.org/10.1097/00002508-199703000-00006

[15] What-When-How. (n.d.) The Autonomic Nervous System (Integrative Systems) Part 1. The Crankshaft Publishing. http://what-when-how.com/neuroscience/the-autonomic-nervous-system-integrative-systems-part-1/

[16] Ustinova, E.E., Fraser, M.O. and Pezzone, M.A. (2010) Cross-Talk and Sensitization of Bladder Afferent Nerves. *Neurourology and Urodynamics*, **29**, 77-81.http://dx.doi.org/10.1002/nau.20817

[17] Danielsson, I., Sjöberg, I. and Östman, C. (2001) Acupuncture for the Treatment of Vulvar Vestibulitis: A Pilot Study. *Acta Obstetricia et Gynecologica Scandinavica*, **80**, 437-441. http://dx.doi.org/10.1034/j.1600-0412.2001.080005437.x

[18] Eva, L.J., Reid, W.M.N., MacLean, A.B. and Morrison, G.D. (1999) Assessment of Response to Treatment in Vulvar Vestibulitis Syndrome by Means of the Vulvar Algesiometer. *American Journal of Obstetrics and Gynecology*, **181**, 99-102. http://dx.doi.org/10.1016/S0002-9378(99)70442-4

[19] Rosen, R., Brown, C., Heiman, J., Leiblum, S., Meston, C., Shabsigh, R., *et al.* (2000) The Female Sexual Function Index (FSFI): Multidimensional Self-report Instrument for the Assessment of Female Sexual Function. *Journal of Sex & Marital Therapy*, **26**, 191-208.http://dx.doi.org/10.1080/009262300278597

[20] Sullivan, M.J.L., Bishop, S. and Pivik, J. (1995) The Pain Catastrophizing Scale: Development and Validation. *Psychological Assessment*, **7**, 524-532.http://dx.doi.org/10.1037/1040-3590.7.4.524

[21] McCracken, L. M. (1997) "Attention" to Pain in Persons with Chronic Pain: A Behavioral Approach. *Behavior Therapy*, **28**, 271-284. http://dx.doi.org/10.1016/S0005-7894(97)80047-0

[22] McKay, E., Kaufman, R. H., Doctor, U., Berkova, Z., Glazer, H. and Redko, V. (2001) Treating Vulvar Vestibulitis with Electromyographic Biofeedback of Pelvic Floor Musculature. *The Journal of Reproductive Medicine*, **46**, 337-342.

[23] Danielsson, I., Torstensson, T., Brodda-Jansen, G. and Bohm-Starke, N. (2006) EMG Biofeedback versus Topical Lidocaine Gel: A Randomized Study for the Treatment of Women with Vulvar Vestibulitis. *Acta Obstetricia et Gynecologica*, **85**, 1360-1367. http://dx.doi.org/10.1080/00016340600883401

[24] Schnyer, R., Lao, L., Hammerschiag, R., Wayne, P., Langevin, H.M., Napadow, V., *et al.* (2008) Society for Acupuncture Research: 2007 Conference Report; The Status and Future of Acupuncture Research: 10 Years Post-NIH Consensus Conference. *The Journal of Alternative and Complementary Medicine*. **14**, 859-860. http://dx.doi.org/10.1089/acm.2008.SAR-2

9

Effects of Rivastigmine Combined with Reinhartdt and Sea Cucumber Capsule in Patients with Mild-to-Moderate Parkinson's Disease Dementia: A Pilot Study

Yongxing Yan[1], Lizhen Liang[1*], Tao Xie[2], Yonghui Shen[1], Yanjing Cao[1]

[1]Department of Neurology, The Third People's Hospital of Hangzhou, Hangzhou, China
[2]Department of Neurology, University of Chicago Medicine, Chicago, USA
Email: [*]yuanyr@sohu.com

Abstract

Many patients with Parkinson's disease suffer cognitive impairment or dementia. Cholinesterase inhibitors (ChEIs) have positive effects on patients with Parkinson's Disease Dementia (PDD). But it is only improve symptoms. There is no etiological cure for PDD. So, In order to achieve the best outcomes, the combination of ChEIs and other therapeutic strategies is needed to study. In the present study, we investigate the efficacy and safety of rivastigmine combined with Reinhartdt and Sea Cucumber Capsule (RSC) in patients with mild-to-moderate PDD, and its effect on thyroid function. There were 52 patients were randomly assigned to receive either rivastigmine (3 mg/day) or rivastigmine plus RSC (2.7 g/day) treatment for 24 weeks. Efficacy was investigated by the change of the scores of Alzheimer's Disease Assessment Scale cognitive subscale (ADAS-Cog), Activities of Daily Life (ADL) and Unified Parkinson's Disease Rating Scale (UPDRS) part III (motor scale). Meanwhile, thyroid hormone levels were detected before and after 12 weeks, 24 weeks treatment in all patients. Results showed that the patients treated with rivastigmine plus RSC showed more improvement in the cognition and the daily life activities compared to those treated with rivastigmine alone. Significant difference was present after being treated for 12 weeks or more. However, no group difference was found on UPDRS part III, thyroid hormone level change and the incidence of adverse events (11.1% vs 16.0%) between the two groups of treatment. Adverse effects were nausea and vomiting which were the main reasons for the dropout. The finding suggests that Rivastigmine plus RSC may improves the treatment effects in cognition and the ADL of the patients with mild-to-moderate PDD, compared with the rivastigmine treatment alone. However, no effect was observed on the motor symptoms and thyroid hormone levels. In addition, this joint treatment is safe.

[*]Corresponding author.

Keywords

Parkinson's Disease, Cognitive Function, Rivastigmine, Reinhartdt and Sea Cucumber

1. Introduction

Parkinson's disease characterized by bradykinesia, tremor, rigidity, and postural instability is one of common neurodegenerative disease, its incidence of 14 per 100,000 [1] [2]. In China, the incidence rate is about 2% in the population of age ≥ 65-year old [3]. In addition to the typical motor symptoms of Parkinson's disease, it also have cognitive impairment or dementia [4]. Some studies have shown that about 30% of patients suffer dementia in Parkinson's disease [5] [6]. Parkinson's Disease Dementia (PDD) greatly affects functioning and quality of life. It can also increase caregiver burden, health-related costs, and duration of hospital stays etc [7]-[9].

In patients with PDD, cognitive changes are linked to disease-related disturbances of cholinergic activity [10]. Bohnen NI *et al.* found cholinergic deficits in PDD are more obvious in Alzheimer's disease, compared with similar levels of cognitive impairment [11]. Studies of cholinergic deficits in patients with PDD suggested that treatment of cholinesterase inhibitors (ChEIs) may effectively improve the impact of the disease on the cholinergic circuits. A Cochrane analysis supports the use of ChEIs in patients with PDD and shows that ChEIs have positive effects on cognitive function [12].

Although ChEIs have effects on PDD, up to date, many treatments all were symptomatic therapy. there is no etiological cure for PDD. In order to achieve the best treatment outcomes, the combination of ChEIs and other therapeutic strategies is widely studied. In China, some traditional herbs have been reported to improve cognitive function in dementia patients [13]-[15]. The combination of traditional herb and ChEIs suggested an obvious effect in treating the patients with Alzheimer's disease and vascular dementia [16] [17].

Reinhartdt and Sea Cucumber Capsule (RSC) has been used for many years in China to improve the cognition of Alzheimer's disease and vascular dementia [18] [19]. Here we hypothesize that RSC combined with a ChEIs rivastigmine may improve the treatment of mild-to-moderate PDD. the efficacy and tolerance of rivastigmine combined with RSC will be examined on the Alzheimer's Disease Assessment Scale cognitive subscale (ADAS-Cog), Activities of Daily Life (ADL) and Unified Parkinson's Disease Rating Scale (UPDRS) part III (motor scale) of the patients with mild-to-moderate PDD, and its effect on thyroid function axis.

2. Materials and Methods

2.1. Participants

Patients received a diagnosis of Parkinson's disease according to the clinical diagnostic criteria of the United Kingdom Parkinson's Disease Society Brain Bank [20] and a diagnosis of dementia due to Parkinson's disease based on criteria established by a Movement Disorders Society taskforce [21]. Patients had mild-to-moderately dementia as defined by a Mini-Mental State Examination (MMSE) score of 10 to 26. The vision, hearing and mental states of all patients were allowed cooperation to complete neuropsychological testing. All cases were in good nutritional status and had normal range of liver and kidney function in the blood. There was no history of thyroid disease, or drugs which can affect thyroid metabolism nearly a month.

Exclusion criteria included any causes of dementia other than Parkinson's disease; a history of a major depressive disorder; a history of hypersensitivity to ChEIs; the use of a cholinesterase inhibitor or other traditional herbal medicine which can interfere with the evaluation during the four weeks before randomization; serious abnormal heart, liver, kidney function; history of allergies and seafood allergy; a known or suspected history of alcoholism or drug abuse.

2.2. Study Design

In this 24-week, randomized, open-label and evaluator-blinded controlled study, all patients were informed and agreed to be consecutively enrolled in the study by their physicians. The random number table was used for randomized controlled trial design in the study. Basically, we randomly picked one number in the random number table for the first patient who was enrolled in the study. And the numbers following the first picked number in the random number table were consecutively assigned to other subjects according to the order of treatment. The subjects with singular number were treated with rivastigmine (Brand name: Exelon, Novartis Pharmaceutical Co., Switzerland) and the subjects with plural number were treated with rivastigmine plus Reinhartdt and Sea Cucumber Capsule (Brand name: Fufanghaishe, Hangkang Ocean Biological Pharmaceutical Co. Ltd., China).

During the treatment, all participants in rivasigmine group took rivastigmine orally at the doses of 3 mg/day, divided twice a day. In the combination treatment group, RSC was given at the dose of 0.9 g/time, three times a day orally. No other ChEIs or nootropics was taken by the patients in both groups during the treatment.

Patients were required to attend a regular interview every 4 weeks for the following evaluations. The following evaluations were routine physical and mental examination, psychometric tests (ADAS-Cog, ADL and UPDRS-III), and adverse events monitoring. Blood, urine, stool routine, liver and kidney function and Electrocardiography (ECG) were detected before and after 12 weeks and 24 weeks treatment in all patients. Thyroid hormone levels were also checked by immune chemiluminescence detection at the same time. Test box was provided by Bayer Co. Each normal reference values were: TT_3: 0.8 - 2.2 μg/L; TT_4: 42 - 135 μg/L; FT_3: 2.5 - 9.82 pmol/L; FT_4: 10 - 25 pmol/L; TSH: 0.2 - 7.0 mIU/L).

This study was conducted in accordance with the ethical standards of the responsible committee on human experimentation and with the Helsinki Declaration as revised in 1983.

2.3. Assessing Measurements

ADAS-Cog was used to measure the cognitive domains of PDD. The cognitive portion of the ADAS assesses orientation, memory, language, visuospatial, and praxis functions. Total scores ranged from 0 to 70, the higher the score, the greater the cognitive impairment. ADL was assessed with a standardized 20-item ADL scale. The scores ranged from 0 to 80 and a higher score, the greater less functional ability.

Changes in symptoms of Parkinson's disease were assessed by means of the motor section of the UPDRS (part III), for which scores can range from 0 to 108 points, with higher scores indicating more severe motor symptoms.

During the whole study, blinded and well trained evaluators performed the experiments to test MMSE, ADAS-Cog, ADL, UPDRS-III. All evaluators analyzed the data without any information about the patient group.

2.4. Statistical Analysis

Analyses were done on data from all patients who underwent randomization and who received at least one dose of study drug, applying the principle of intention-to-treat (ITT). We used the last-observation-carried-forward (LOCF) method to impute values if no follow-up information was available.

Statistical analyses were performed with the use of SPSS software, version 10.0. The basal comparison of characteristics in patients with two treatments was analyzed by a chi square test and student's t test. Changes from baseline in the ADAS-cog, ADL and UPRDS-III scores were assessed by means of analysis of covariance. Thyroid hormone levels data were expressed as mean ± standard deviation. Variance analysis (one-way ANOVA) was used in group while the Q test (post-hoc multiple comparisons between groups were made with Least-significant difference) was used between groups. A p-value < 0.05 was considered statistically significant.

3. Results

3.1. Patient Disposition

A total of 58 eligible patients were enrolled to attend the study. During the study, 3 patients previously took cholinesterase inhibitors, 2 patients quitted the study and 1 patient had severe renal dysfunction. Those 6 patients were excluded from our randomized study for treatment. The Consolidated Standards of Reporting Trias (CONSORT)-like flowchart was showed in **Figure 1**. The rest of 52 subjects were randomly divided into two treatment group. One group of 25 patients (11 males and 14 females) of aged 69.7 ± 4.2 years old (from 60 to 76

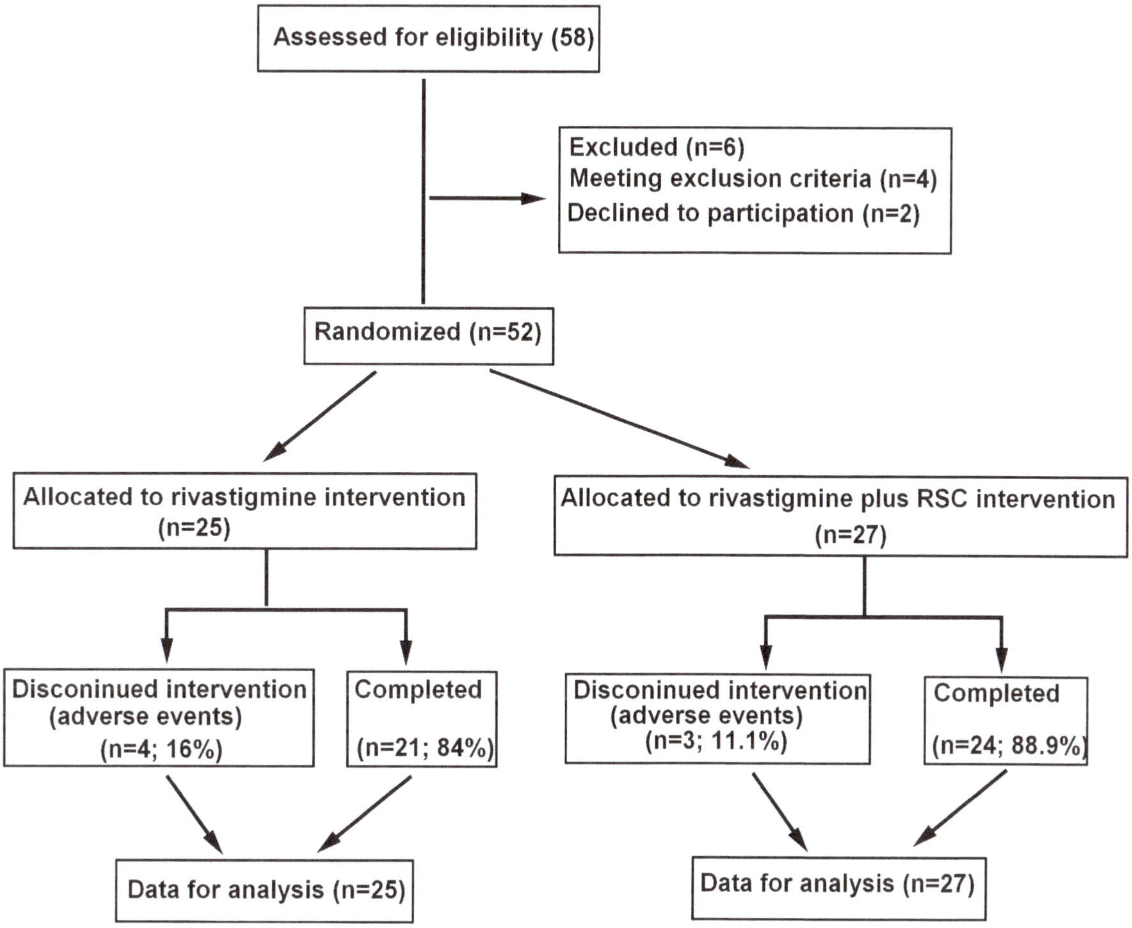

Figure 1. The CONSORT-like flowchart of patients.

years old) were treated with rivastigmine alone. The average duration of PDD for those patients was 1.6 ± 0.9 years. Another group of 27 patients (16 males and 11 females) of aged 70.6 ± 6.9 years (from 58 to 82 years old) were treated with rivastigmine plus RSC. The average duration of PDD was 1.6 ± 0.8 years. The results did not show any significant difference between the two groups in baseline data, the characteristics of two groups were shown in **Table 1**.

All patients with PDD from the two groups were also administered the following concomitant medications (single rivastigmine treatment vs rivastigmine plus RSC): levodopa agents (96.0% vs 92.6%), dopamine agonists agents (76.0% vs 81.5%), Amantadine (36.0% vs 25.9%), Comtan (catechol-O-methyltransferase inhibitor; Entacapone) (16.0% vs 11.1%), antidepressants (28.0% vs 22.2%), antianxiety agents (32.0% vs 37.0%),and antipsychotic agents (32.0% vs 33.3%). There were no significant differences between two groups ($p > 0.05$) in most common concomitant medications.

3.2. Efficacy

The ADAS-Cog scores declined at the beginning of the treatment in both groups. This meant the cognition of the patients improved after the treatments. Compared to the rivastigmine treatment alone group, rivastigmine plus RSC group had significantly more reduction in ADAS-Cog scores and ADL scores. The ADAS-Cog scores in the combined group had an obvious decrease ($p < 0.05$ at 12weeks, $p < 0.01$ after 16 weeks) and the patients displayed much better cognition since the 12th week (**Figure 2**). The ADL scores also significantly decreased in rivastigmine plus RSC treatment group from the 12th week to the end of the study as compared with rivastigmine treatment alone (**Figure 3**). There is no difference was observed in the UPDRS part III score between two groups at each time (**Figure 4**).

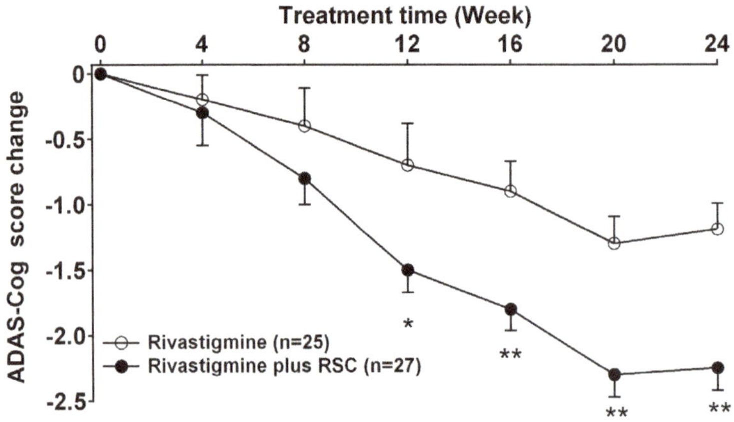

Figure 2. The change of the scores of ADAS-Cog in each group (mean ± SD). *: $p < 0.05$, **: $p < 0.01$ between the rivastigmine treatment and the rivastigmine plus RSC treatment.

Table 1. The characteristics of the patients in each group.

Parameter	Rivastigmine, N = 25	Rivastigmine plus RSC, N = 27	Statistic values
Sex (male/female)-no.	11/14	16/11	$x^2 = 1.211$; $p = 0.271$
Age (mean ± SD)	69.7 ± 4.2	70.6 ± 6.9	t = 0.571; p = 0.570
Education (mean ± SD)	9.1 ± 2.1	8.9 ± 3.1	t = 0.316; p = 0.753
Duration of PD (mean ± SD)	7.9 ± 1.9	7.8 ± 2.4	t = 0.292; p = 0.771
Duration of PDD (mean ± SD)	1.6 ± 0.9	1.6 ± 0.8	t = 0.044; p = 0.965
MMSE score (mean ± SD)	20.8 ± 3.9	19.8 ± 3.8	t = 0.283; p = 0.778
ADAS-cog score (mean ± SD)	25.4 ± 9.4	26.2 ± 9.1	t = 0.320; p = 0.750
ADL score (mean ± SD)	42.6 ± 9.3	42.1 ± 11.0	t = 0.173; p = 0.863
UPDRS part III score (mean ± SD)	33.6 ± 11.1	33.3 ± 12.5	t = 0.092; p = 0.927
Medications used-no. (%)			
Levodopa	24 (96%)	25 (92.6%)	$x^2 = 0.277$; $p = 0.599$
Dopamine agonists	19 (76.0%)	22 (81.5%)	$x^2 = 0.234$; $p = 0.629$
Amantadine	9 (36.0%)	7 (25.9%)	$x^2 = 0.618$; $p = 0.432$
Comtan	4 (16.0%)	3 (11.1%)	$x^2 = 0.266$; $p = 0.606$
Antidepressants	7 (28.0%)	6 (22.2%)	$x^2 = 0.231$; $p = 0.631$
Antianxiety agents	8 (32.0%)	10 (37.0%)	$x^2 = 0.146$; $p = 0.703$
Antipsychotic agents	8 (32.0%)	9 (33.3%)	$x^2 = 0.010$; $p = 0.918$

Thyroid hormone levels of the two groups of patients were evaluated before and after 12 weeks, 24 weeks treatment, but no statistical difference was found between the each time period ($p > 0.05$, **Table 2**).

3.3. Safety

The main treatment-related adverse events were nausea and vomiting in this study. Three participants (2 patients vomiting, 1 patient nausea) in the rivastigmine plus RSC and four subjects (1 patient vomiting, 3 patients nausea) in the single rivastigmine group experienced mild-to-moderate adverse events related to nausea and vomiting. They all failed to complete the study due to the adverse events. No serious adverse events were occurred during the study. The statistical results found no significant difference in the laboratory and auxiliary examination (blood, urine, stool routine, liver and kidney function, ECG). The discontinuation rate was similar in two groups

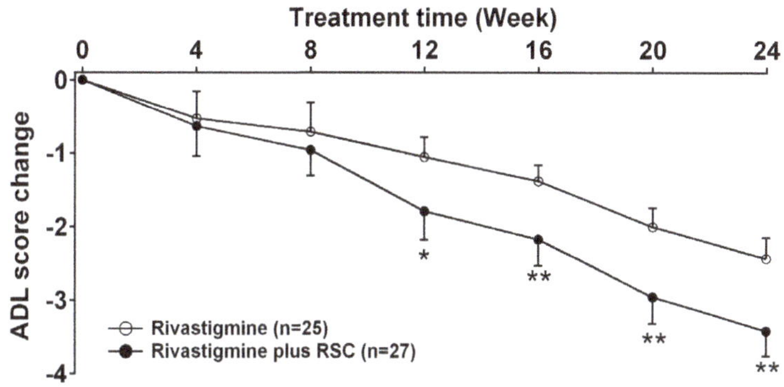

Figure 3. The change of the scores of ADL in each group (mean ± SD). *p < 0.05, **p < 0.01 between the rivastigmine treatment and the rivastigmine plus RSC treatment.

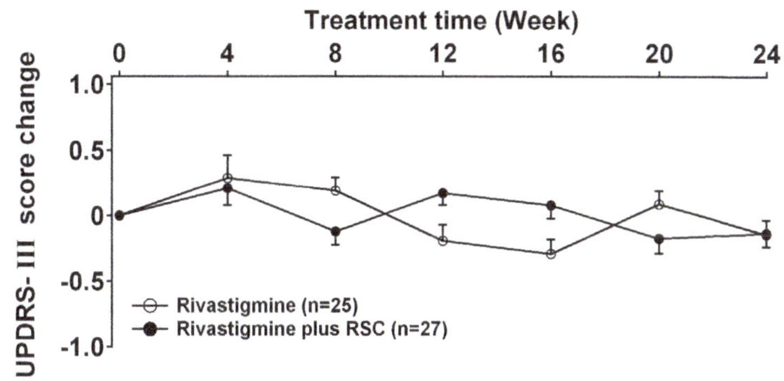

Figure 4. The change of the scores of UPDRS-III in each group (mean ± SD). There is no difference between two groups at each time.

Table 2. Thyroid hormone levels before and after treatment in each group (mean ± SD).

Groups	No.	Period	TSH (mIU/L)	TT_3 (μg/L)	TT_4 (μg/L)	FT_3 (pmol/L)	FT_4 (pmol/L)
Rivastigmine	25	Before treatment	4.0 ± 0.9	1.6 ± 0.3	76.1 ± 10.7	5.8 ± 2.1	18.0 ± 3.5
	25	After 12 weeks	4.0 ± 0.9	1.7 ± 0.2	74.6 ± 9.3	5.7 ± 1.7	17.7 ± 2.9
	25	After 24 weeks	4.2 ± 0.8	1.7 ± 0.3	76.6 ± 8.1	5.6 ± 1.8	17.9 ± 2.9
Rivastigmine plus RSC	27	Before treatment	4.1 ± 0.9	1.7 ± 0.3	78.2 ± 10.7	6.0 ± 1.3	17.8 ± 3.7
	27	After 12 weeks	4.1 ± 1.0	1.7 ± 0.3	79.2 ± 9.6	5.7 ± 1.3	18.1 ± 3.2
	27	After 24 weeks	4.2 ± 0.9	1.6 ± 0.2	78.0 ± 9.7	6.1 ± 1.3	16.9 ± 3.3

(11.1% in rivastigmine plus RSC group; 16.0% in rivastigmine alone group). No difference was observed between two groups in reasons for discontinuation ($p > 0.05$).

4. Discussion

Dementia in Parkinson's disease is linked to disease-related disturbances of cholinergic activity [10]. Cholinergic neuron loss as the main feature of non-dopaminergic neurons dysfunction was an important pathophysiological mechanism in Parkinson's disease dementia [10] [11]. The main neuropathological change was that the Lewy bodies widely appear in the basal ganglia and the limbic system [22]-[24]. Thus, base on the pathophysiological mechanism, many scholar think that mechanism-based treatments can improve cognition in Parkinson's disease. The first study about ChEIs treatment PDD in 1996, it showed the cognition of patients with PDD improved after treated with tacrine [25]. Although only seven patients with PDD in the study, the result of this study provided the rationale for large randomized controlled trials of ChEIs in PDD. EXPRESS study which a

24-week randomized placebo-controlled trial, showed that rivastigmine significantly improved cognition and clinical outcomes compared with placebo [26]. Meanwhile ,The results of extension phase also showed that rivastigmine might provide sustained benefits for up to 48 weeks [27].when the patients with PDD were treated with rivastigmine, amplified brain perfusion on Single-photon Emission Computed Tomography and increased α-activity on quantitative EEG in frontal regions were found [28] [29]. Now, rivastigmine is widely approved for clinical use in the treatment of PDD [30]. In this study, we observed obvious improvement in cognition and the daily activities of patients with mild-to-moderate PDD after taking rivastigmine 3 mg/d for 24 weeks. In China, some traditional herbal medicine can improve cognitive function in dementia patients [13]-[15]. RSC is one of traditional Chinese medicine which improves the cognition of Alzheimer's disease and vascular dementia and has been used for many years in China [18] [19]. RSC is a natural product which is made of Hainan semirings sea snakes, Yuzu sea cucumber and polygala tenuifolia by biological engineering technology. The main ingredients were sea snakes, sea cucumbers, Polygala and stone calamus. Researches about RSC in cell and molecular level indicated that it could significantly increase the content of acetylcholine and superoxide dismutase in the brain, and reduce the glutamic acid and lipid peroxide levels. The mechanism for improving cognitive and memory function is changing a variety of brain neurotransmitters and biochemical factors [31]-[33]. ChEIs was also reported to treat the patients with Alzheimer's disease and vascular dementia with a certain effect [17] [34]. In the present study, we observed more improvement in cognition and the daily activities of patients after 24-weeks treatment with rivastigmine plus RSC group compared with rivastigmine alone treatment group. Significant difference was found in ADAC-cog, ADL scores at the 12-weeks. Patients showed better cognitive and behavior abilities with rivastigmine plus RSC treatment. These results suggest that rivastigmine plus RSC treatment has a better effect on improving the cognitive deficit in PDD patients than rivastigmine alone treatment. It also indicated the potency of RSC in delaying the cognitive decline in PDD when treated with rivastigmine simultaneously. In our study, the improvement of the cognition and the daily function of the patients in the combined treated group may be due to the improvement of acetylcholine content in the brain. The improvement of daily living function may be due to the improvement in cognition, as the motor function remains unchanged after the treatment.

Thyroid hormone plays an important role in the central nervous system development and normal function [35] [36]. Slight change in thyroid hormone level even in the normal range may be associated with the elderly emotional and cognitive function change. Previous studies have shown that thyroid hormone levels were closely linked with Alzheimer's disease. Thyroid hormone levels were reported to be changed in Alzheimer's disease patients after cholinesterase inhibitor therapy [37] [38]. Our previous study also found that the RSC combined with donepezil therapy in patients with Alzheimer's disease and vascular dementia raised its T_3, T_4 level, synergistically improving cognitive function [17] [34]. However, in present study, no change about thyroid hormone levels was found before and after 12 weeks and 24 weeks in either single rivastigmine treatment or rivastigmine plus RSC treatment. It is consistent with previous researches that thyroid hormone levels were not correlated to the severity of Parkinson's disease [39] [40].

The predominant adverse events caused by cholinergic disorder are nausea,vomiting, tremor, diarrhea, anorexia, etc. Most of these adverse events were reversible, and were mild to moderate. Although tremor may occurred during the initial treatment period, the analysis about rivastigmine effect on motor effects showed that Parkinson's disease did not get worse during 48 weeks in the EXPRESS study [41]. Adverse events were not observed to be different in UPDRS motor scores including tremor-related items between the control groups and treatment group [24]. Compared to the treatment in previous studies, the combination treatment in our study indicated a lower incidence of side effects (13.5%, 7 cases). The side effect is the reason for withdrawing from the study. It mainly showed nausea (3 cases), vomiting (4 cases), and symptoms improved after withdraw. No tremor and other movement disorders aggravation were observed. There was no difference in UPDRS motor scores. It may be related to rivastigmine used in small dosage (3 mg/day) in our study.

Of cause, some limitations are still present in our study. First, these results may partly reflect a normal clinical treatment, not a double-blind, randomized, controlled trial. Second, the sample size is still small, due to the strict inclusion and exclusion criteria. A better rigorous research with more patients needs to be performed in the future.

5. Conclusion

In conclusion, our results show that rivastigmine plus RSC treatment has a better effect in improving the symptoms of the patients with mild-to-moderate PDD than rivastigmine treatment alone. The formula was safe and it had no effect on thyroid hormone levels in PDD patients.

Competing Interests

The authors have declared that no competing interest exists.

References

[1] Jankovic, J. (2008) Parkinson's Disease: Clinical Features and Diagnosis. *Journal of Neurology, Neurosurgery & Psychiatry*, **79**, 368-376. http://dx.doi.org/10.1136/jnnp.2007.131045

[2] Hirtz, D., Thurman, D.J., Gwinn-Hardy, K., Mohamed, M., Chaudhuri, A.R. and Zalutsky, R. (2007) How Common Are the "Common" Neurologic Disorders? *Neurology*, **68**, 326-337. http://dx.doi.org/10.1212/01.wnl.0000252807.38124.a3

[3] Zhang, Z.X., Roman, G.C., Hong, Z., Wu, C.B., Qu, Q.M., Huang, J.B., Zhou, B., Geng, Z.P., Wu, J.X., Wen, H.B., Zhao, H. and Zahner, G.E. (2005) Parkinson's Disease in China: Prevalence in Beijing, Xian, and Shanghai. *Lancet*, **365**, 595-597. http://dx.doi.org/10.1016/S0140-6736(05)17909-4

[4] Galvin, J.E., Pollack, J. and Morris, J.C. (2006) Clinical Phenotype of Parkinson Disease Dementia. *Neurology*, **67**, 1605-1611. http://dx.doi.org/10.1212/01.wnl.0000242630.52203.8f

[5] Aarsland, D., Zaccai, J. and Brayne, C. (2005) A Systematic Review of Prevalence Studies of Dementia in Parkinson's Disease. *Movement Disorders*, **20**, 1255-1263. http://dx.doi.org/10.1002/mds.20527

[6] Riedel, O., Klotsche, J., Spottke, A., Deuschl, G., Förstl, H., Henn, F., Heuser, I., Oertel, W., Reichmann, H., Riederer, P., Trenkwalder, C., Dodel, R. and Wittchen, H.U. (2010) Frequency of Dementia, Depression, and Other Neuropsychiatric Symptoms in 1449 Outpatients with Parkinson's Disease. *Journal of Neurology*, **257**, 1073-1082. http://dx.doi.org/10.1007/s00415-010-5465-z

[7] Winter, Y., von Campenhausen, S., Arend, M., Longo, K., Boetzel, K., Eggert, K., Oertel, W.H., Dodel, R. and Barone, P. (2011) Health-Related Quality of Life and Its Determinants in Parkinson's Disease: Results of an Italian Cohort study. *Parkinsonism & Related Disorders*, **17**, 265-269. http://dx.doi.org/10.1016/j.parkreldis.2011.01.003

[8] Vossius, C., Larsen, J.P., Janvin, C. and Aarsland, D. (2011) The Economic Impact of Cognitive Impairment in Parkinson's Disease. *Movement Disorders*, **26**, 1541-1544. http://dx.doi.org/10.1002/mds.23661

[9] Fletcher, P., Leake, A. and Marion, M.H. (2011) Patients with Parkinson's Disease Dementia Stay in the Hospital Twice as Long as Those without Dementia. *Movement Disorders*, **26**, 919. http://dx.doi.org/10.1002/mds.23573

[10] Klein, J.C., Eggers, C., Kalbe, E., Weisenbach, S., Hohmann, C., Vollmar, S., Baudrexel, S., Diederich, N.J., Heiss, W.D. and Hilker, R. (2010) Neurotransmitter Changes in Dementia with Lewy Bodies and Parkinson Disease Dementia *in Vivo*. *Neurology*, **74**, 885-892. http://dx.doi.org/10.1212/WNL.0b013e3181d55f61

[11] Bohnen, N.I., Kaufer, D.I., Ivanco, L.S., Lopresti, B., Koeppe, R.A., Davis, J.G., Mathis, C.A., Moore, R.Y. and DeKosky, S.T. (2003) Cortical Cholinergic Function Is More Severely Affected in Parkinsonian Dementia Than in Alzheimer Disease: An *in Vivo* Positron Emission Tomographic Study. *Arch Neurol*, **60**, 1745-1748. http://dx.doi.org/10.1001/archneur.60.12.1745

[12] Rolinski, M., Fox, C., Maidment, I. and McShane, R. (2012) Cholinesterase Inhibitors for Dementia with Lewy Bodies, Parkinson's Disease Dementia and Cognitive Impairment in Parkinson's Disease. *Cochrane Database of Systematic Reviews*, **3**, CD006504. http://dx.doi.org/10.1002/14651858.CD006504.pub2

[13] Wu, T.Y., Chen, C.P. and Jinn, T.R. (2011) Traditional Chinese Medicines and Alzheimer's Disease. *Taiwanese Journal of Obstetrics and Gynecology*, **50**, 131-135. http://dx.doi.org/10.1016/j.tjog.2011.04.004

[14] Lin, H.Q., Ho, M.T., Lau, L.S., Wong, K.K., Shaw, P.C. and Wan, D.C. (2008) Anti-Acetylcholinesterase Activities of Traditional Chinese Medicine for Treating Alzheimer's Disease. *Chemico-Biological Interactions*, **175**, 352-354. http://dx.doi.org/10.1016/j.cbi.2008.05.030

[15] Kim, H.G. and Oh, M.S. (2012) Herbal Medicines for the Prevention and Treatment of Alzheimer's Disease. *Current Pharmaceutical Design*, **18**, 57-75. http://dx.doi.org/10.2174/138161212798919002

[16] Li, D.Q., Zhou, Y.P. and Yang, H. (2012) Donepezil Combined with Natural Hirudin Improves the Clinical Symptoms of Patients with Mild-to-Moderate Alzheimer's Disease: A 20-Week Open-Label Pilot Study. *International Journal of Medical Sciences*, **9**, 248-255. http://dx.doi.org/10.7150/ijms.4363

[17] Yan, Y.X., Liang, L.Z. and Zhou, Z.L. (2007) Clinical Study of Combined Treatment with Compound Reinhartdt and Sea Cumber Capsule and Donepezil for Vascular Dementia. *Chinese Journal of Integrated Traditional and Western Medicine*, **27**, 887-890.

[18] Wang, C.F., Ma, Y.X., Gu, Y.D., Xie, S.Z., Yu, Z.Y. and Yang, J.Y. (2000) A Double-Blind Clinical Study on the Reinhardt and Sea Cucumber Capsule in Treating Dementia in the Aged. *Geriatrics & Health Care*, **6**, 11-15.

[19] Kang, J. (2009) Research of Compound Reinhartdt and Sea Cumber Capsule Treating Encephalopathy. *World Chinese Medicine*, **4**, 58-59.

[20] Gibb, W.R. and Lees, A.J. (1988) The Relevance of the Lewy Body to the Pathogenesis of Idiopathic Parkinson's Disease. *Journal of Neurology, Neurosurgery & Psychiatry*, **51**, 745-752. http://dx.doi.org/10.1136/jnnp.51.6.745

[21] Emre, M., Aarsland, D., Brown, R., Burn, D.J., Duyckaerts, C., Mizuno, Y., Broe, G.A., Cummings, J., Dickson, D.W., Gauthier, S., Goldman, J., Goetz, C., Korczyn, A., Lees, A., Levy, R., Litvan, I., McKeith, I., Olanow, W., Poewe, W., Quinn, N., Sampaio, C., Tolosa, E. and Dubois, B. (2007) Clinical Diagnostic Criteria for Dementia Associated with Parkinson's Disease. *Movement Disorders*, **22**, 1689-1707. http://dx.doi.org/10.1002/mds.21507

[22] Hurtig, H.I., Trojanowski, J.Q., Galvin, J., Ewbank, D., Schmidt, M.L., Lee, V.M., Clark, C.M., Glosser, G., Stern, M.B., Gollomp, S.M. and Arnold, S.E. (2000) Alpha-Synuclein Cortical Lewy Bodies Correlate with Dementia in Parkinson's Disease. *Neurology*, **54**, 1916-1921. http://dx.doi.org/10.1212/WNL.54.10.1916

[23] Aarsland, D., Perry, R., Brown, A., Larsen, J.P. and Ballard, C. (2005) Neuropathology of Dementia in Parkinson's Disease: A Prospective, Community-Based Study. *Annals of Neurology*, **58**, 773-776. http://dx.doi.org/10.1002/ana.20635

[24] Braak, H., Rüb, U., Jansen Steur, E.N., Del Tredici, K. and de Vos, R.A. (2005) Cognitive Status Correlates with Neuropathologic Stage in Parkinson Disease. *Neurology*, **64**, 1404-1410. http://dx.doi.org/10.1212/01.WNL.0000158422.41380.82

[25] Hutchinson, M. and Fazzini, E. (1996) Cholinesterase Inhibition in Parkinson's Disease. *Journal of Neurology, Neurosurgery & Psychiatry*, **61**, 324-325. http://dx.doi.org/10.1136/jnnp.61.3.324-a

[26] Emre, M., Aarsland, D., Albanese, A., Byrne, E.J., Deuschl, G., De Deyn, P.P., Durif, F., Kulisevsky, J., van Laar, T., Lees, A., Poewe, W., Robillard, A., Rosa, M.M., Wolters, E., Quarg, P., Tekin, S. and Lane, R. (2004) Rivastigmine for Dementia Associated with Parkinson's Disease. *The New England Journal of Medicine*, **351**, 2509-2518. http://dx.doi.org/10.1056/NEJMoa041470

[27] Poewe, W., Wolters, E., Emre, M., Onofrj, M., Hsu, C., Tekin, S. and Lane, R., EXPRESS Investigators (2006) Long-Term Benefits of Rivastigmine in Dementia Associated with Parkinson's Disease: An Active Treatment Extension Study. *Movement Disorders*, **21**, 456-461. http://dx.doi.org/10.1002/mds.20700

[28] Ceravolo, R., Volterrani, D., Frosini, D., Bernardini, S., Rossi, C., Logi, C., Manca, G., Kiferle, L., Mariani, G., Murri, L. and Bonuccelli, U. (2006) Brain Perfusion Effects of Cholinesterase Inhibitors in Parkinson's Disease with Dementia. *Journal of Neural Transmission*, **113**, 1787-1790. http://dx.doi.org/10.1007/s00702-006-0478-6

[29] Fogelson, N., Kogan, E., Korczyn, A.D., Giladi, N., Shabtai, H. and Neufeld, M.Y. (2003) Effects of Rivastigmine on the Quantitative EEG in Demented Parkinsonian Patients. *Acta Neurologica Scandinavica*, **107**, 252-255. http://dx.doi.org/10.1034/j.1600-0404.2003.00081.x

[30] van Laar, T., De Deyn, P.P., Aarsland, D., Barone, P. and Galvin, J.E. (2011) Effects of Cholinesterase Inhibitors in Parkinson's Disease Dementia: A Review of Clinical Data. *CNS Neuroscience & Therapeutics*, **17**, 428-441. http://dx.doi.org/10.1111/j.1755-5949.2010.00166.x

[31] Wang, C.F., Ma, Y.X., Xie, S.Z., Li, W.B., Zhang, B.L. and Tao, G.S. (1999) The Study of Reinhartdt and Sea Cucumber Capsule on the Efficacy and Mechanism of Action in the Dementia Model. In: Ma, Y.X., Wang, C.F. and Shi, F,Y., Eds., *New Progress of Aging and Geriatrics*, 1st Edition, FU Dan University Press, Shanghai, 477-487.

[32] Lv, J., Jia, H., Jiang, Y., Ruan, Y., Liu, Z., Yue, W., Beyreuther, K., Tu, P. and Zhang, D. (2009) Tenuifolin, an Extract Derived from Tenuigenin, Inhibits Amyloid-Beta Secretion *in Vitro*. *Acta Physiologica*, **196**, 419-425. http://dx.doi.org/10.1111/j.1748-1716.2009.01961.x

[33] Jia, H., Jiang, Y., Ruan, Y., Zhang, Y., Ma, X., Zhang, J., Beyreuther, K., Tu, P. and Zhang, D. (2004) Tenuigenin Treatment Decreases Secretion of the Alzheimer's Disease Amyloid Betaprotein in Cultured Cells. *Neuroscience Letters*, **367**, 123-128. http://dx.doi.org/10.1016/j.neulet.2004.05.093

[34] Zhou, Z.L., Liang, L.Z. and Yan, Y.X. (2007) Clinical Study of Reinhartdt and Sea Cucumber Capsule Combined with Donepezil in Treating Alzheimer's Disease. *Chinese Journal of Integrated Traditional and Western Medicine*, **27**, 110-113.

[35] Jahagirdar, V. and McNay, E.C. (2012) Thyroid Hormone's Role in Regulating Brain Glucose Metabolism and Potentially Modulating Hippocampal Cognitive Processes. *Metabolic Brain Disease*, **27**, 101-111. http://dx.doi.org/10.1007/s11011-012-9291-0

[36] Carreón-Rodríguez, A. and Pérez-Martínez, L. (2012) Clinical Implications of Thyroid Hormones Effects on Nervous System Development. *Pediatric Endocrinology Reviews*, **9**, 644-649.

[37] Bauer, M., Goetz, T., Glenn, T. and Whybrow, P.C. (2008) The Thyroid-Brain Interaction in Thyroid Disorders and

Mood Disorders. *Journal of Neuroendocrinology*, **20**, 1101-1114. http://dx.doi.org/10.1111/j.1365-2826.2008.01774.x

[38] Bunevicius, R. (2009) Thyroid Disorders in Mental Patients. *Current Opinion in Psychiatry*, **22**, 391-395. http://dx.doi.org/10.1097/YCO.0b013e328329e1ae

[39] Schaefer, S., Vogt, T., Nowak, T. and Kann, P.H., German KIMS board (2008) Pituitary Function and the Somatotmphie System in Patients with Idiopathic Parkinson's Disease under Chronic Dopaminersic Therapy. *Journal of Neuroendocrinology*, **20**, 104-109. http://dx.doi.org/10.1111/j.1365-2826.2007.01622.x

[40] Bonuccelli, U., D'Avino, C., Caraccio, N., Del Guerra, P., Casolaro, A., Pavese, N., Del Dotto, P. and Monzani, F. (1999) Thyroid Function and Autoimmunity in Parkinson's Disease: A Study of 101 Patients. *Parkinsonism & Related Disorders*, **5**, 49-53. http://dx.doi.org/10.1016/S1353-8020(99)00010-3

[41] Oertel, W., Poewe, W., Wolters, E., De Deyn, P.P., Emre, M., Kirsch, C., Hsu, C., Tekin, S. and Lane, R. (2008) Effects of Rivastigmine on Tremor and Other Motor Symptoms in Patients with Parkinson's Disease Dementia: A Retrospective Analysis of a Double-Blind Trial and an Open-Label Extension. *Drug Safety*, **31**, 79-94. http://dx.doi.org/10.2165/00002018-200831010-00007

10

Anticancer Effect of Ginseng Leaves Crude Polysaccharides on Human Hepatoma Cell SMMC-7721

Xiaozhen Fu[1], Dan Shi[1], Chao Qu[1], Guangying Zhong[1], Wei Zou[1,2*#], Jing Liu[3#]

[1]College of Life Sciences, Liaoning Normal University, Dalian, China
[2]Liaoning Key Laboratories of Biotechnology and Molecular Drug Research and Development, Dalian, China
[3]The First Affiliated Hospital, Dalian Medical University, Dalian, China
Email: [*]weizou60@126.com

Abstract

Background: Polysaccharides extracted from the medicinal herbs are known to possess antitumor effects. Although there is a significant number of evidences implicated on the beneficial effects of the ginseng leaves ginsenoside with diverse associated mechanisms, reports on the anticancer by the ginseng leaves crude polysaccharides (GLCP) are not sufficient. Experiments were carried out to unravel the anticancer effects of GLCP. Methods: Cells were treated with GLCP (0.5 - 2 mg/ml) for 48h. MTT method was used to detect the cell viability. Western blot and flow cytometry were used to detect apoptotic rate. Western blot and acridine orange staining were used to detect the cell autophagy. Results: Compared with the normal human liver cell (Chang liver), GLCP (1.5 - 2 mg/ml) significantly reduction cell viability, promote apoptosis-related proteins expression, promote cell apoptosis and autophagy in SMMC-7721 cells. But *caveolin-1* gene silencing could inhibit the anticancer effect of GLCP. Conclusions: These data suggest that GLCP promote autophagy and apoptosis in human hepatoma cell SMMC-7721. We speculate that its mechanism may be associated with the *caveolin-1* which is an essential structural molecule of caveolae. Although the effect of GLCP inhibited of liver cancer is not very strong, we are more interested in the GLCP which plays a tumor suppressor role in health care.

Keywords

Anticancer, Ginseng Leaves Crude Polysaccharides (GLCP), *Caveolin-1*, Autophagy, Apoptosis

[*]Corresponding author.
[#]Jing Liu and Wei Zou contributed equally to this work.

1. Introduction

Hepatoma is currently the sixth most common type of cancer and the third leading cause of cancer-related death in the world [1]. In China, more than 401,000 new patients are diagnosed with hepatoma and more than 371,000 patients are killed by the terrible disease annually [2]. Although recent advances in chemotherapeutic agents in hepatoma have been achieved, treatment options are still limited and are associated with significant morbidity and mortality.

Ginseng is a kind of traditional Chinese medicine, ginseng polysaccharides which because of its anti-tumor, anti-oxidation, hypoglycemic, and many other activities was widespread concern in recent years [3] [4]. The ginseng root requires 6 - 7 years to harvest, while ginseng leaves can be harvested annually; recent studies have shown that there was the same active ingredient in the ginseng and ginseng leaves, such as fatty acids, alkaloids, polysaccharides, sesquiterpenes, ginsenosides and so on [5] [6]. But the ginseng leaves activities especially the anticancer activity have not been reported.

In the present study, we have investigated the anticancer effects of ginseng leaves crude polysaccharides (GLCP) in human hepatoma cell SMMC-7721. Herein, we show that GLCP promote cell apoptosis and autophagy in SMMC-7721 cells. Furthermore, we demonstrated that *caveolin-1* gene silencing inhibits the anticancer effect of GLCP. So its mechanism may be associated with the *caveolin-1* which is an essential structural molecule of caveolae.

2. Materials and Methods

2.1. Materials

RPMI-1640 medium, Opti-MEM® reduced serum media and newborn bovine serum (NBCs) were purchased from Gibco Laboratories (Grand Island, NE, USA). Penicillin and streptomycin were purchased from Invitrogen (Carlsbad, CA, USA). The primary antibodies were purchased from Cell Signaling Technology (Boston, MA, USA).

2.2. Cell Lines and Culture Condition

The human hepatoma cell (SMMC-7721) and normal human liver cell (Chang liver) were obtained from the Cell Bank of the Institute of Biochemistry and Cell Biology, China Academy of Sciences (Shanghai, China). Cav-1 knockdown hepatoma SMMC-7721 cells using RNA interference technology to build early in our laboratory. The cells were grown in RPMI-1640 medium containing 15% newborn bovine serum (NBCs), penicillin (100 μg/ml), and streptomycin (100 μg/ml). Cultures were maintained at 37°C in a humidified 5% CO_2 atmosphere. Ginseng leaves crude polysaccharides (GLCP) was dissolved in the complete medium and adjusted to the indicated final concentrations with culture medium before use.

2.3. Cell Viability Measurement Assay

The effect of GLCP on the growth of human hepatoma cell SMMC-7721 was evaluated using 5×10^3 cells seeded onto 96-well plates, which were treated with GLCP after 24h at the time of cell plated. To evaluate the effect of GLCP at concentrations 0.5, 1, 1.5, and 2 mg/ml, cells were maintained in media with various concentrations of GLCP for 48 h and cell numbers were determined by 3-[4,5-dimethylthiazol-2-yl]-2,5-diphenyltetrazolium bromide (MTT) assay, and absorbance was read at 570 nm.

2.4. Western Blot Analysis

Cells were plated in 6-well plates and were treated with GLCP for 48 h. After treatment, the cells were harvested and resuspended in ice-cold cell lysis buffer, and the homogenate was centrifuged at 10,000 g for 15 min at 4°C. The total supernatant protein concentration was measured using a bicinchoninic acid (BCA) protein assay kit (Kangchen Biotech, Shanghai, China). An equal volume of sodium dodecyl sulfate (SDS) gel loading buffer [100 mM Tris-HCl (pH 6.8), 200 mM dithiothreitol (DTT), 4% SDS, 0.1% bromophenol blue and 20% glycerol] was added to samples, which were subsequently boiled for 7 min. The total proteins from each sample were separated by 15% sodium dodecylsulfate-polyacrylamide gel electrophoresis (SDS-PAGE) and were transferred to a polyvinylidene difluoride (PVDF) membrane. The membrane was blocked with 5% fat-free dry milk in PBS-T for 1 h at room temperature followed by incubation with primary antibodies to *caveolin-1* (1:1000), LC3B (1:1000), Bcl-2 (1:1000), P53 (1:1000) and β-actin (1:2000) overnight at 4°C. The next day, the membranes were washed and subsequently incubated with HRP-conjugated secondary antibodies for 2 h at room temperature. Following three washes with PBS-T, the membranes were developed using an enhanced chemiluminescence (ECL) kit and exposed to X-ray films. Gel-Pro analyzer 4 software was used to quantify the protein expression levels.

2.5. Acridine Orange Staining

Cells were plated in 24-well plates and were treated with GLCP for 48 h. After washed twice with phosphate buffered saline (PBS), the cells were fixed with 95% ethanol for 10 min. Acridine orange was added at a final concentration of 0.1 mg/ml for 25 min at 4°C, after washed twice with PBS, added 0.1 mol $CaCl_2$ in the cells for colour separation. Finally, cells were washed with phosphate buffered saline. Pictures were obtained with a fluorescence microscope.

2.6. Flow Cytometry

Cell apoptosis was quantified by flow cytometry using PI and Annexin V double staining, and it was performed as previously described using FACScalibur (Becton Dickinson, Franklin Lakes, NJ).

2.7. Statistical Analysis

All of the experiments were performed at least three times. The values were expressed as the means ± S.E.M. Statistical analysis was performed between groups by *ANOVA* using SPSS 16.0 software (SPSS Inc, Chicago, IL, USA). A probability value of $p < 0.05$ was considered significant.

3. Results

3.1. Ginseng Leaves Crude Polysaccharides Promote Apoptosis in Human Hepatoma Cell SMMC-7721

MTT analysis showed that compared with the control group, the relative viability of SMMC-7721 cell decreased significantly after adding different concentrations (0.5, 1, 1.5, and 2 mg/ml) of GLCP, at the same time, GLCP activity of normal liver cells in some role in promoting (**Figure 1(a)**). Using flow cytometry detection after adding the 1.5 mg/ml polysaccharide on apoptosis in SMMC-7721 cells, the results showed that, adding polysaccharide treatment significantly increased apoptosis rate (**Figure 1(b)**). Western blot to detect the apoptosis associated protein expression changes after adding the GLCP in human hepatoma cell SMMC-7721. We can see from the quantitative, GLCP inhibits the expression of BCL-2 proteins in human hepatoma cell SMMC-7721 and promotes the expression of NF-κ b (**Figure 1(c)**).

3.2. GLCP Promote Human Hepatoma Cell SMMC-7721 Autophagy

To determine if GLCP induced autophagy in SMMC-7721 cells, acridine orange staining for autolysosome was performed. Results showed that the GLCP at the concentration of 1.5 mg/ml drastically increased the formation of autolysosome in SMMC-7721 cells (**Figure 2(a)**).Western blot showed the marker protein levels of autophagy, compared with control group the LC3-II/LC3- Ⅰ level was increased significantly after adding 1.5 mg/ml GLCP (**Figure 2(b)**).

3.3. *Caveolin-1* Gene Silencing Inhibits the Anticancer Effect of GLCP

MTT method and flow cytometry were used to detect the anticancer effect of GLCP in *caveolin-1* gene silencing SMMC-7721 cells. Compared with the SMMC-7721 cells, the relative viability of *caveolin-1* gene silencing SMMC-7721 cells basically unchanged after adding different concentrations (0.5, 1, 1.5, and 2 mg/ml) of GLCP (**Figure 3(a)**). Using flow cytometry detection after adding the 1.5 mg/ml polysaccharide on apoptosis in SMMC-7721 cells and the *caveolin-1* gene silencing SMMC-7721 cells, the results showed that, adding polysaccharide treatment the apoptosis rate of the *caveolin-1* gene silencing SMMC-7721 cells was unchanged

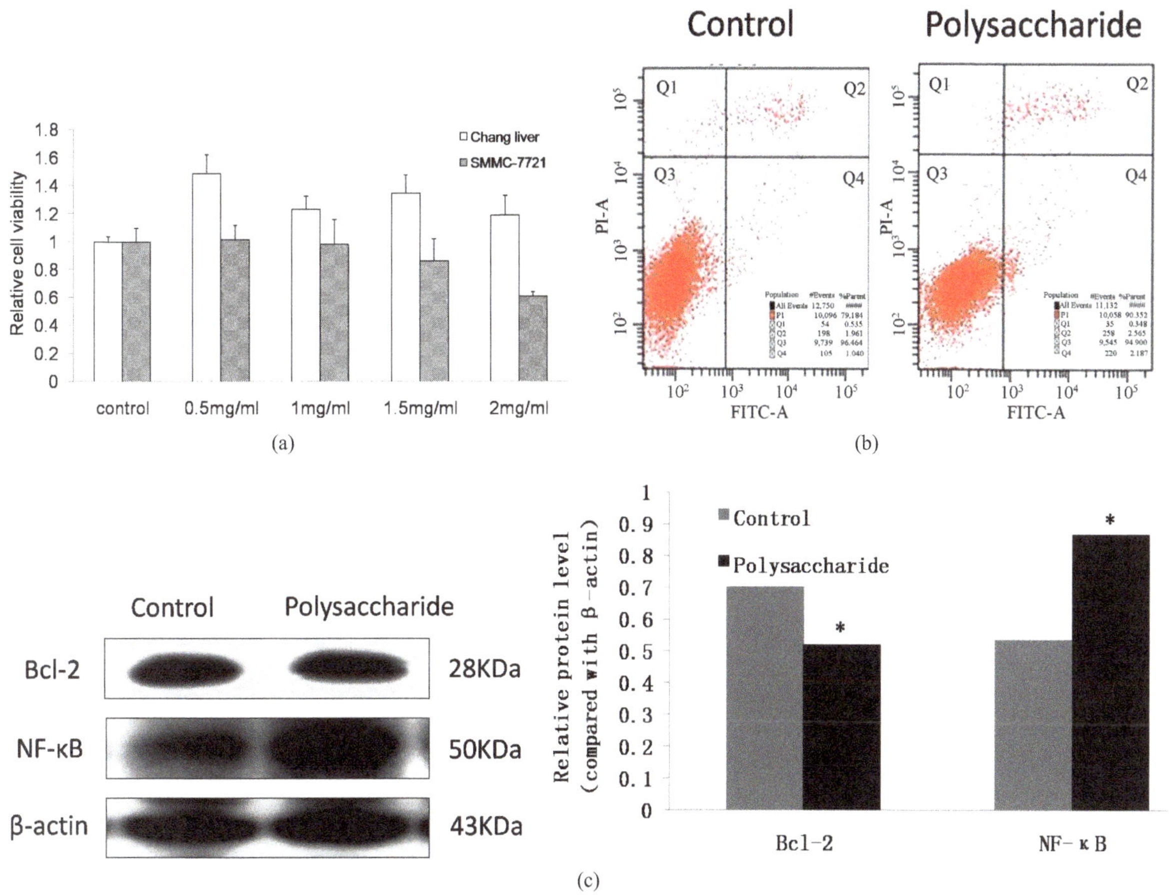

Figure 1. Compared with the normal human liver cell (Chang liver), GLCP promote cell apoptosis in human hepatoma cell SMMC-7721. (a) The cells were treated with 0.5 - 2 mg/ml GLCP for 48 h. Cell viability was measured by the MTT assay as described in methods. (b) The SMMC-7721 cell was treated with 1.5 mg/ml GLCP for 48 h. The cell apoptosis level was examined by flow cytometry. (c) The SMMC-7721 cell was treated with 1.5 mg/ml GLCP for 48 h. Western blot was used to examine the relative protein expression of Bcl-2 and NF-κB, the protein level was compaerd with the β-actin. The data represent the mean of three independent experiments ± SD. $^{*}p < 0.05$; $^{**}p < 0.01$ versus control.

(**Figure 3(b)**). Western blot to detect the apoptosis associated protein expression changes after adding the GLCP in human hepatoma cell SMMC-7721 and the *caveolin-1* gene silencing SMMC-7721 cells. The results showed that, *caveolin-1* gene silencing inhibits the anticancer effect of GLCP.

4. Discussion

Hepatocellular carcinoma (HCC) is widespread primary malignant tumor of the liver. It is the third and ninth most common cause of cancer associated deaths in men and women, respectively [7]. Current anti-tumor treatments, such as radiotherapy, chemotherapy, immunotherapy, and suicide gene therapy, act on tumor by inducing tumor cell apoptosis [8]. Chemotherapy is the most common treatment option for hepatoma [9]. However, its effectiveness is often compromised because of inherent or acquired drug resistance, with major impediment being frequent appearance of multi-drug resistant cancer cells during drug treatment [10]. So looking for non-toxic or low toxic anti-cancer drugs from natural products become a new hotspot in recent years [11] [12].

A variety of active polysaccharide extracted from plants can influence the humoral immunity, innate and adaptive immunity. Now, the lentinan and polysaccharides of ganoderma lucidum, bidentata, polyporus, huangqi and etc are commonly used in clinical [13]. However, the activity of plant polysaccharides not only in strengthening the immune system as concerned, the same has anti-cancer effect [14] [15]. Use of plant polysaccharides as anticancer health food has long been applied in our country, but due to its mechanism of action is not clear, this treatment still cannot be received by the international community.

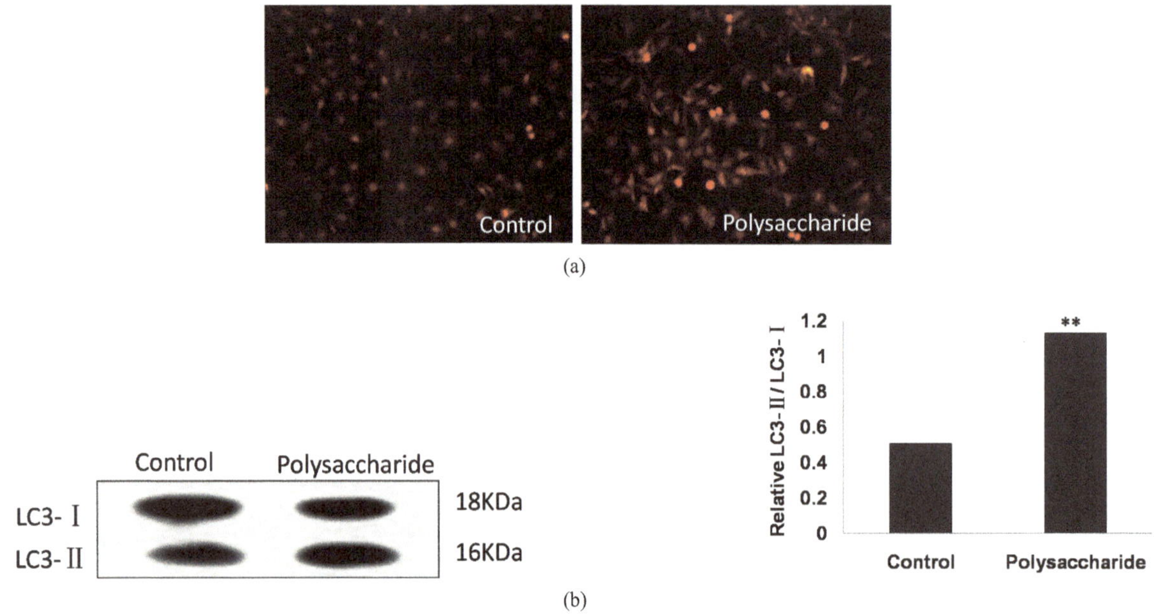

Figure 2. Induction of autophagy in human hepatoma cell SMMC-7721 after treatment with GLCP. SMMC-7721 cells were treated with 1.5 mg/ml GLCP for 48 h. (a) The accumulation of acidic vesicular organelles (AVOs), which emitted bright red fluorescence, was visualized by acridine orange staining; (b) Western blot was used to examine the protein expression of LC3, using LC3-II/ LC3-I to represent the level of the autophagy.

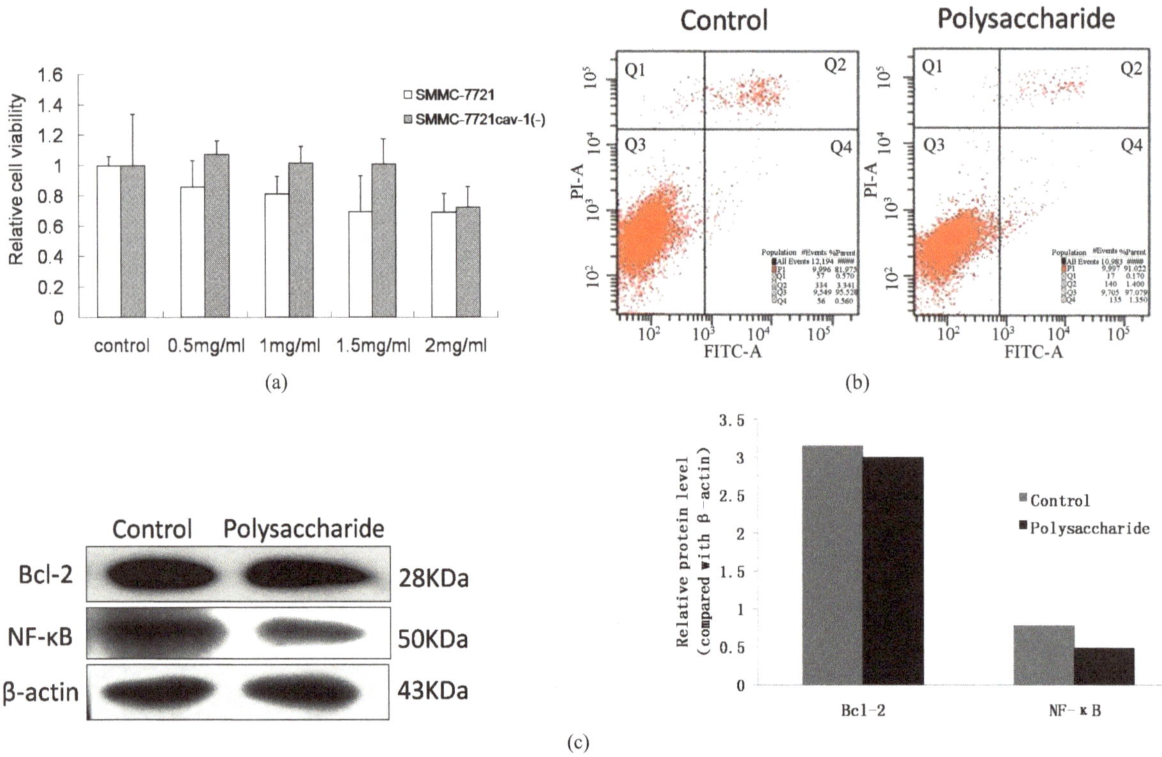

Figure 3. Compared with human hepatoma cell SMMC-7721, *caveolin-1* gene silent resisted GLCP promote the cell apoptosis. (a) The cells were treated with 0.5 - 2 mg/ml GLCP for 48 h. Cell viability was measured by the MTT assay as described in methods. (b) The SMMC-7721$^{cav-1(-)}$ cell was treated with 1.5 mg/ml GLCP for 48 h. The cell apoptosis level was examined by flow cytometry. (c) The SMMC-7721$^{cav-1(-)}$ cell was treated with 1.5 mg/ml GLCP for 48 h. Western blot was used to examine the relative protein expression of Bcl-2 and NF-κB, the protein level was compaerd with the β-actin. The data represent the mean of three independent experiments ± SD. $^{*}p < 0.05$; $^{**}p < 0.01$ versus control.

Caveolin-1 is a kind of 21 - 24 KD membrane protein, and it is an essential structural molecule of caveolae [16]. Its function are quite diverse, ranging from cellular cholesterol transport, cell membrane composing, cellular signal transduction, cell cycle regulation and control, cell transformation to tumorigenesis [17] [18]. Previously studies in our lab have demonstrated that *caveolin-1* gene silencing activates estrogen receptor alpha expression and leads to 17 beta-estradiol-stimulated mammary tumorigenesis [19]. Recent studies have showed that *caveolin-1* has close relation with breast epithelial cell transformation and breast tumor formation [20]. Downregulation of *caveolin-1* could increase cell apoptosis *in vitro* [21] [22]. In this paper, *caveolin-1* has been shown to participate in the mechanism of GLCP-induced hepatoma cell apoptosis.

In this study we used the traditional extracted method of oriental medicines to obtain the ginseng leaves crude polysaccharides (GLCP) [23]. Ginseng leaves (50 g) was extracted with 1L of boiling water for 4 h, after filtered it was precipitated with ethanol and deproteinized by the Sevag method and then lyophilized, producing an average yield of 28.53%. The powdered extract (GLCP) was dissolved in complete medium and then filtered through a 0.22 μm syringe filter. Then observe its biological effect on normal liver cells and liver cancer cells.

Our experiments show that GLCP promote apoptosis and autophagy in human hepatoma cell SMMC-7721, at the same time it had no effect on the activity of normal liver cell Chang liver. And its mechanism may be associated with the *caveolin-1*, because when *caveolin-1* gene silencing the anticancer effect of GLCP had been disappeared. Although the results show that the effect of GLCP inhibited of liver cancer is not very strong, here we study primary focus the mechanism of the anticancer effect, and to provide a dietary health reference. In the future studies, we will separate the active ingredients from the GLCP, to looking for the non-toxic or low toxic natural anti-cancer drugs.

5. Conclusion

The result shows that GLCP promote autophagy and apoptosis in human hepatoma cell SMMC-7721, and the mechanism may be associated with the *caveolin-1* which is an essential structural molecule of caveolae.

Acknowledgements

This work was supported by a grant from the National Natural Science Foundation of China (No. 30970353), the National Natural Science Foundation of China (No.30570225) and the National Science and Technology Cooperation Project of Ministry of Science and Technology (2010DFR30850).

References

[1] Gu, W., Fang, F.F., Li, B., *et al.* (2012) Characterization and Resistance Mechanisms of a 5-Fluorouracil-Resistant Hepatocellular Carcinoma Cell Line. *Asian Pacific Journal of Cancer Prevention*, **13**, 4807-4814. http://dx.doi.org/10.7314/APJCP.2012.13.9.4807

[2] Ferlay, J., Shin, H.R., Bray, F., *et al.* (2010) Estimates of Worldwide Burden of Cancer in 2008: GLOBOCAN 2008. *International Journal of Cancer*, **127**, 2893-2917.

[3] Kim, J. (2008) Protective Effects of Asian Dietary Items on Cancers—Soy and Ginseng. *Asian Pacific Journal of Cancer Prevention*, **9**, 543-548.

[4] Wee, J.J., Mee Park, K. and Chung, A.S. (2010) Biological Activities of Ginseng and Its Application to Human Health. Source Herbal Medicine: Biomolecular and Clinical Aspects. 2nd Edition. CRC Press, Boca Raton; 2011. Chapter 8.

[5] Yang, S.O., Lee, S.W., Kim, Y.O., *et al.* (2013) HPLC-Based Metabolic Profiling and Quality Control of Leaves of Different Panax Species. *Journal of Ginseng Research*, **37**, 248-253.

[6] Choi, S.Y., Cho, C.W., Lee, Y., *et al.* (2012) Comparison of Ginsenoside and Phenolic Ingredient Contents in Hydroponically-Cultivated Ginseng Leaves, Fruits, and Roots. *Journal of Ginseng Research*, **36**, 425-429. http://dx.doi.org/10.5142/jgr.2012.36.4.425

[7] Semela, D. and Heim, M. (2011) Hepatocellular Carcinoma. *Therapeutische Umschau*, **68**, 213-217. http://dx.doi.org/10.1024/0040-5930/a000153

[8] Fulda, S. and Debatin, K.M. (2006) Extrinsic versus Intrinsic Apoptosis Pathways in Anticancer Chemotherapy. *Oncogene*, **25**, 4798-4811. http://dx.doi.org/10.1038/sj.onc.1209608

[9] Wong, R. and Frenette, C. (2011) Updates in the Management of Hepatocellular Carcinoma. *Journal of Gastroenterology and Hepatology* (N Y), **7**, 16-24.

[10] Mellor, H.R. and Callaghan, R. (2008) Resistance to Chemotherapy in Cancer: A Complex and Integrated Cellular Response. *Pharmacology*, **81**, 275-300. http://dx.doi.org/10.1159/000115967

[11] Boh, B. (2013) Ganoderma Lucidum: A Potential for Biotechnological Production of Anti-Cancer and Immunomodulatory Drugs. *Recent Patents on Anti-Cancer Drug Discovery*, **8**, 255-287. http://dx.doi.org/10.2174/1574891X113089990036

[12] Zong, A., Cao, H. and Wang, F. (2012) Anticancer Polysaccharides from Natural Resources: A Review of Recent Research. *Carbohydrate Polymers*, **90**, 1395-410.

[13] He, X.J., Niu, X.Y., Li, J., *et al.* (2012) Immunomodulatory Activities of Five Clinically Used Chinese Herbal Polysaccharides. *Journal of Experimental and Integrative Medicine*, **2**, 15-27.

[14] Liu, L.N., Guo, Z.W., Zhang, Y., *et al.* (2012) Polysaccharide Extracted from Rheum Tanguticum Prevents Irradiation-Induced Immune Damage in Mice. *Asian Pacific Journal of Cancer Prevention*, **13**, 1401-145. http://dx.doi.org/10.7314/APJCP.2012.13.4.1401

[15] Song, K.S., Li, G., Kim, J.S., *et al.* (2011) Protein-Bound Polysaccharide from Phellinus Linteus Inhibits Tumor Growth, Invasion, and Angiogenesis and Alters Wnt/β-Catenin in SW480 Human Colon Cancer Cells. *BMC Cancer*, **11**, 307. http://dx.doi.org/10.1186/1471-2407-11-307

[16] Lajoie, P. and Nabi, I.R. (2012) Lipid Rafts, Caveolae, and Their Endocytosis. *International Review of Cell and Molecular Biology*, **282**, 135-163. http://dx.doi.org/10.1016/S1937-6448(10)82003-9

[17] Boscher, C. and Nabi, I.R. (2012) *Caveolin-1*: Role in Cell Signaling. *Advances in Experimental Medicine and Biology*, **729**, 29-50. http://dx.doi.org/10.1007/978-1-4614-1222-9_3

[18] Fang, K., Fu, W., Beardsley, A.R., *et al.* (2007) Overexpression of *Caveolin-1* Inhibits Endothelial Cell Proliferation by Arresting the Cell Cycle at G0/G1 Phase. *Cell Cycle*, **6**, 199-204.

[19] Zhang, X., Shen, P., Coleman, M., *et al.* (2005) *Caveolin-1* Gene Silencing Activates Estrogen Receptor Alpha Expression and Leads to 17 Beta-Estradiol-Stimulated Mammary Tumorigenesis. *Anticancer Research*, **1**, 369-375.

[20] Syeed, N., Husain, S.A., Abdullah, S., *et al.* (2010) *Caveolin-1* Promotes Mammary Tumorigenesis: Mutational Profile of the Kashmiri Population. *Asian Pacific journal of Cancer Prevention*, **11**, 689-696.

[21] Zhao, X.N., Ma, C., Cai, X.L., Lei, D.P., Liu, D.Y., *et al.* (2011) RNA Interference of *Caveolin-1* via Lentiviral Vector Inhibits Growth of Hypopharyngeal Squamous Cell Carcinoma Fadu Cells *in Vitro* and *in Vivo*. *Asian Pacific journal of Cancer Prevention*, **12**, 397-401.

[22] Feng, S., Wang, Y., Wang, X., *et al.* (2010) *Caveolin-1* Gene Silencing Promotes the Activation of PI3K/AKT Dependent on Eralpha36 and the Transformation of MCF10ACE. *Science China Life Sciences*, **53**, 598-605.

[23] Yang, L., Qu, H., Mao, G., *et al.* (2013) Optimization of Subcritical Water Extraction of Polysaccharides from Grifola Frondosa Using Response Surface Methodology. *Pharmacognosy Magazine*, **9**, 120-129.

11

Long-Term Treatment with an Herbal Formula MCC Ameliorates Obesity-Associated Metabolic Dysfunction in High Fat Diet-Induced Obese Mice: A Comparative Study among MCC and Various Combinations of Its Constituents

Pou Kuan Leong[1], Hoi Yan Leung[1], Hoi Shan Wong[1], Ji Hang Chen[1], Wing Man Chan[1], Chung Wah Ma[2], Yi Ting Yang[2], Kam Ming Ko[1*]

[1]Division of Life Science, Hong Kong University of Science and Technology, Hong Kong, China
[2]Infinitus (China) Company Ltd., Guangzhou, China
Email: [*]bcrko@ust.hk

Abstract

Obesity has been found to be associated with increased incidence of various metabolic disorders. Anti-obesity interventions are therefore urgently needed. An earlier study has demonstrated that treatment with an herbal formula MCC, which comprises the fruit of *Momordica charantia* (MC), the pericarpium of *Citri reticulate* (CR) and L-carnitine (CA), reduced the weight gain in high fat diet (HFD)-fed mice. In the present study, we investigated the effect of long-term treatment with MCC (6 g/kg/day × 40 doses) and various combinations of its constituents in HFD-fed female ICR mice. Body weight change was monitored during the course of the experiment. Total and differential adiposity, plasma lipid contents, metabolic enzyme activities and mitochondrial coupling efficiency in skeletal muscle were measured. Glucose homeostasis was also assessed. Results showed that HFD increased the body weight, total and differential adiposity, and plasma lipid contents as well as impaired metabolic status in skeletal muscle and glucose homeostasis. MCC and all combinations of its constituents reduced the weight gain in HFD-fed mice, which was accompanied with an improvement on glucose homeostasis. While MC, CA and CR independently suppressed the HFD-induced weight gain in mice, MC seems to be the most effective in weight reduction, all of which correlated with the induction of mitochondrial uncoupling in skeletal muscle. Only CA and

[*]Corresponding author.

CR, but not MC, significantly reduced the total adiposity and visceral adiposity as well as plasma cholesterol level. However, the two component combinations, MC + CR and MC + CA, decreased the degree of visceral adiposity and plasma cholesterol level, respectively. MCC treatment at 1.5 g/kg (but not a higher dose of 6 g/kg) suppressed visceral adiposity and induced mitochondrial uncoupling in skeletal muscle in HFD-fed mice. The finding suggests that MCC may offer a promising prospect for ameliorating the diet-induced obesity and metabolic disorders in humans.

Keywords

High Fat Diet; Obesity; Weight Control; Momordica Charantia; Citri Reticulata; L-Carnitine

1. Introduction

The worldwide epidemic of obesity has been found to be associated with increased incidence of cardiovascular diseases, type 2 diabetes as well as the metabolic syndrome, leading to severe economic burden on healthcare system in modern society. Body mass index (BMI), which indicates the ratio of body weight to height, is a conventional metrics for assessing the health risk arising from obesity. Recent studies have demonstrated an inverse relationship of obesity and mortality in cardiovascular diseases and diabetes, suggesting that BMI may be not a reliable benchmark of healthy individual [1]. Alternatively, the mass of visceral fat pad, which is the fat pad of intra-abdominal cavity, is causally related to metabolic diseases, presumably by virtue of its secretion of pro-inflammatory adipokines [2]. In addition to visceral fat mass, a high ratio of low-density lipoprotein cholesterol (LDL-C) to high-density lipoprotein cholesterol (HDL-C) in combination with hypertriglyceridemia correlates well with a high risk of coronary heart disease [3]. In this regard, anti-obesity interventions, which aimed at controlling not only body weight but also plasma lipids as well as visceral fat mass, are urgently needed.

Regular physical exercise combined with low calorie diet is a commonly used intervention for the treatment of obesity. However, only a small portion of obese individuals with intervention on lifestyle can maintain a prolonged and sustained weight control [4]. Therapeutic interventions, including the use of pancreatic lipase inhibitor and stimulator of central noradrenaline release, are alternative approach to treating obesity. Despite their efficacy of weight reduction, adverse effects, such as steatorrhoea and liver injury, were observed in some obese individuals [5]. Recently, Tseng *et al.* have proposed a novel target of obesity therapy by increasing cellular bioenergetics [6]. As such, the dissipation of proton gradient across the mitochondrial inner membrane (*i.e.* mitochondrial uncoupling) can cause an inefficient generation of cellular ATP, with a resultant increase in energy expenditure. In this connection, the induction of mitochondrial uncoupling, particularly in skeletal muscle, offers a potential treatment of obesity [7].

In an effort to develop safe interventions for obesity, herbal medicine, which has a long history of use in weight reduction, has attracted a lot of interest. An herbal formula MCC, which is comprised of the fruit of *Momordica charantia* (MC, also called bitter melon), the pericarpium of *Citri reticulata* (CR) and L-carnitine (CA), was found to reduce the weight gain, visceral fat mass and hyperlipidemia in high fat diet (HFD)-induced obese mice [8]. However, the role of the three constituents of MCC formula in producing the pharmacological action remains to be investigated.

In the present study, we endeavored to define the role of the three constituents of MCC formula by comparing the weight reduction effect of MCC and various combinations of its constituents (*i.e.*, 1- and 2-component combinations), using a mouse model of HFD-induced obesity. The body weight gain was monitored during the course of 8-week experiment. To examine the degree of adiposity and plasma lipid levels, the mass of gonadal fat, mesenteric fat and subcutaneous fat as well as various plasma lipid contents [triglyceride (TG), LDL-C and HDL-C] were measured after the 8-week HFD feeding. To investigate the glucose homeostasis of HFD-fed mice, plasma glucose levels after 24-h fasting as well as glucose intolerance and insulin sensitivity index in oral glucose tolerance test (OGTT) were measured. To assess the metabolic status of skeletal muscle, activities of myocellular phosphofructokinase (PFK), β-hydroxyacyl-Co A dehydrogenase (β-HAD), carnitine palmitoyl CoA transferase (CPT) and citrate synthase (CS), as well as state 3 and state 4 respiratory rates of isolated mitochondria of skeletal muscle were assayed. The mitochondrial coupling efficiency was then estimated by computing the ratio of state 3 to state 4 mitochondrial respiratory rate.

2. Materials and Methods

2.1. Chemicals

PicoLab® Rodent diet 20 (normal diet) was purchased from LabDiet® (City, State, USA). The "Original" High Fat Diet (Diet-induced Obesity Formula D12492, 60% energy from fat) was purchased from Research Diets, Inc. (New Brunswick, NJ, USA). TG and cholesterol assay kits were purchased from Wako Pure Chemical Industries, Ltd (Okasa, Japan). HDL-C test kit was purchased from Wako Diagnostics (Richmond, VA, USA). Glucose assay reagent was obtained from Sigma Chemical Co. (St. Louis, MO, USA). ELISA kit for measuring mouse insulin was purchased from Crystal Chem Inc. (Downers Grove, USA). The water extracts of MC and CR as well as CA were manufactured and supplied by Infinitus (China) Company Ltd., Guangzhou, China. The MCC formula is comprised of MC, CR and CA with the mass ratio of MC:CR:CA being 1:3.5:10. All other chemicals were of analytical grade.

2.2. Animal Care

Female ICR mice (8 - 10 weeks old, 20 - 25 g) were maintained under a 12-hour dark/light cycle at about 22°C, and allowed food and water *ad libitum* in the Animal and Plant Care Facilities at the Hong Kong University of Science and Technology (HKUST). All experimental protocols were approved by the University Committee on Research Practice at HKUST

2.3. Animal Treatment

In a preliminary study, MCC treatment was found to reduce the high fat diet-induced weight gain in both male and female ICR mice, with similar changes in the tested biochemical parameters. In the present study, only female ICR mice were used, which were randomly assigned to 10 groups, with 10 - 15 mice in each group: 1) Normal diet (ND, 13% energy from fat, PicoLab) control; 2) High fat diet (HFD, 60% energy from fat, Test Diet) control; 3) HFD, MC 0.17 g/kg; 4) HFD, CR, 0.6 g/kg; 5) HFD, CA, 1.71 g/kg; 6) HFD, MC + CR, 0.17 + 0.6 g/kg; 7) HFD, MC + CA, 0.17 + 1.71 g/kg; 8) HFD, CR + CA, 0.6 + 1.71 g/kg; 9) HFD, MCC, 1.5 g/kg; 10) HFD, MCC, 6.0 g/kg; 11) Emodin, 40 mg/kg. Doses of various combinations were equivalent to 6.0 g/kg of MCC. Mice were administered intragastrically at the indicated dose 5 days per week for 8 weeks. Control mice received water (vehicle) only. Twenty-four hours after the last dosing, blood samples were drawn from overnight fasted, phenobarbital-anesthetized mice by cardiac excision using syringes rinsed with 0.5% heparin in saline (w/v), and the mice were then sacrificed by cervical dislocation. Samples of gastrocnemius muscle and fat pads (gonadal, mesenteric and subcutaneous fat) were excised, and they were subjected to further analysis.

2.4. Preparation of Samples

Plasma samples were obtained by centrifuging whole blood samples at 1500 × g for 10 minutes at 4°C. Plasma samples were then subjected to biochemical analysis.

Minced gastrocnemius muscle tissues were digested by collagenase solution [0.075% (w/v) in buffer] at 4°C for 20 min. After removing the collagenase solution by centrifugation, the digested tissues were mixed with 20 mL of ice-cold homogenizing buffer (100 mM KCl, 50 mM MOPS, 10 mM EGTA, pH 7.2) and subjected to homogenization with a Teflon-glass homogenizer at 4000 rpm for 25 - 30 complete strokes. Then the homogenates were centrifuged at 600 × g for 10 min at 4°C. The resultant supernatant was nucleus-free fraction. For measurements of β-HAD, CS and CPT activities, nucleus-free fraction was diluted with 0.2% Triton X-100 (w/v, in K_2HPO_4 buffer) [8].

Mitochondrial pellets were prepared from nucleus-free fractions of muscle homogenates by centrifugation at 9200 × g at 4°C for 30 min. The mitochondrial pellets were then resuspended in a buffer containing 250 mM sucrose, 50 mM Tris, pH 7.5 and constituted the mitochondrial fractions [8].

2.5. Measurement of Body Weight and Fat Pad Weight

Body weight of mice was measured once a week during the 8-week course of experiment. Gonadal, mesenteric, and subcutaneous fat pads were weighed. The ratio of a particular fat pad weight to body weight was estimated and expressed as fat pad index [8].

2.6. Biochemical Analysis

Plasma glucose levels were measured using an assay kit basing on coupled hexokinase-catalyzed and glucose-6-phosphate dehydrogenase-catalyzed reactions, with a resultant NAD reduction. Absorbance changes at 340 nm were monitored spectrophotometrically by Victor[3] Multi-label Counter (Perkin Elmer, Turku, Finland). Plasma levels of TG, HDL-C, and TC levels were measured using assay kits. LDL-C level was estimated by Friedewald's formula: $\mathrm{LDL} = \mathrm{TC} - (\mathrm{HDC} - \mathrm{C} + \mathrm{TG}/5)$ [9]. Plasma insulin level was measured using an ELISA kit. PFK, *β*-HAD, CS and CPT activities in skeletal muscle were measured using enzymatic methods, as described as Leong *et al.* and Colberg *et al.* [8] [10].

2.7. Oral Glucose Tolerance Test

After 8 weeks of experiment, oral glucose tolerance test (OGTT) was performed. Six hour post-fasting, blood samples were collected as initial levels of plasma glucose and insulin (*i.e.* time = 0). Then, glucose (2 g/kg) was orally administered to the mice. Blood samples were collected at 15, 30, 60 and 120 min post-dosing of glucose. Plasma glucose and insulin levels were measured. Glucose intolerance was estimated by computing the area under the curve (AUC) plotting plasma glucose level against time and expressed in arbitrary unit. Insulin sensitivity index (ISI) was estimated by following equation:

$$1000 \Big/ \left\{ \text{Square root of} \left[(\mathrm{FPG} \times \mathrm{FPI}) \right] \times (\text{Mean OGTT glucose}) \times (\text{mean OGTT insulin}) \right\},$$

where FPG = fasting plasma glucose; FPI = fasting plasma insulin [10].

2.8. Measurement of Mitochondrial Respiration

Mitochondrial respiratory was measured polarographically by a Clark-type oxygen electrode (Hansatech Instruments Ltd., Norfolk, UK) at 30˚C. Mitochondrial fraction (~0.5 mg protein/mL) was incubated in a buffer containing 30 mM KCl, 6 mM $MgCl_2$, 75 mM sucrose, 1 mM EDTA, 20 mM KH_2PO_4 and 0.1% (w/v) fatty acid-free BSA, pH 7.0. Substrate solution containing 10 mM glutamate and 2.5 mM malate was added, and after a stable state 2 respiration had been established, state 3 respiration (coupling) was initiated by the addition of ADP (final concentration 0.6 mM). When all of the added ADP was used up for ATP generation, oligomycin (ATP synthase inhibitor) was added to induce the state 4 respiration (uncoupling). The respiratory control ratio (RCR) was estimated by calculating the ratio of state 3 to state 4 respirations [11].

2.9. Statistical Analysis

The time dependent changes in the body weight during the course of 8 week experiment was analyzed by mixed Analysis of Variance (mixed ANOVA). Other data were analyzed by one-way Analysis of Variance (ANOVA). Post-hoc multiple comparisons were performed using Least Significant Difference (LSD). P values < 0.05 were regarded as statistically significant.

3. Results

3.1. Effects of MCC and Various Combinations of Its Constituents on Body Weight Gain in HFD-Fed Mice

ND slightly but not significantly increased the body weight during the course of 8-week experiment in mice. HFD accelerated the body weight increase during the course of experiment in mice, with the degree of stimulation being 24%, when compared with that of ND (**Figure 1**). MCC and all combinations of its constituents were found to inhibit the HFD-induced body weight gain (**Table 1**). While MC (0.17 g/kg) completely abrogated the HFD-induced body weight gain, MC + CR (0.17 and 0.6 g/kg) caused the largest degree of suppression (91.6%) among the 2-component combinations (**Table 1**). The 3-component combination MCC (6.0 g/kg) also suppressed the HFD-induced body weight gain, with the extent of inhibition being 76% (**Figure 1** and **Table 1**).

3.2. Effects of MCC and Various Combinations of Its Constituents on Various Fat Pad Indices in HFD-Fed Mice

The HFD-induced body weight gain was associated with an increase in total fat pad index (162%), as well as

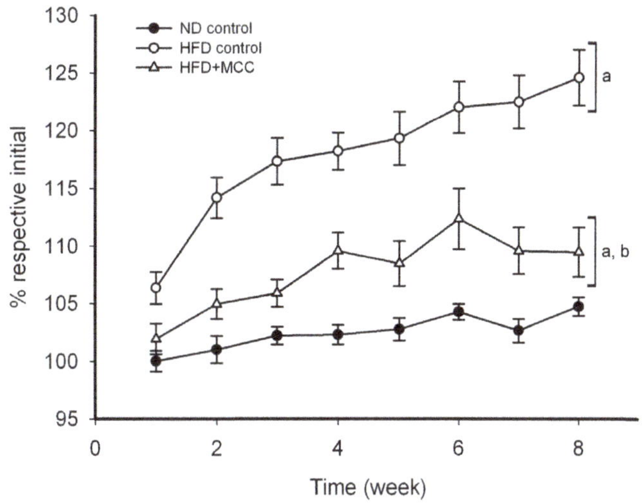

Figure 1. Effect of MCC on body weight gain during the course of 8-week experiment in HFD-fed mice. Mice were allowed food [ND (13% energy from fat) or HFD (60% energy from fat)] and water *ad libitum*, during the course of 8-week experiment. In the drug treatment groups, mice were intragastrically administered with MCC (6 g/kg/day) 5 days per week for 8 weeks (*i.e.* 40 doses), while control mice received water (vehicle) only. Body weights of mice were monitored by measuring the body weight of mice every week during the 8-week period. Data were expressed as % initial, by normalizing with initial body weight (*i.e.* time = week 0) of the respective mouse. Value given are means ± SEM, with n = 10 - 15. The initial values of body weight of each group were given as follows: 1) ND control = 33.1 ± 0.5 g; 2) HFD control = 33.2 ± 1.0 g; 3) HFD + 6 g/kg MCC = 36.1 ± 0.7 g. [a]Significantly different from time-matched ND-fed control; [b]significantly different from time-matched HFD-fed control.

Table 1. Effects of MCC and various combinations of its constituents on body weight in HFD-fed mice.

Treatment	Body weight (% control)	% Suppression of weight gain
ND		
Control	104.8 ± 0.8	
HFD		
Control	124.6 ± 2.4[a]	
MC	103.5 ± 2.9[b]	106.3
CR	108.6 ± 2.4[b]	80.6
CA	112.2 ± 2.2[b]	62.4
MC + CR	106.4 ± 2.8[b]	91.6
MC + CA	106.7 ± 3.1[b]	90.5
CR + CA	109.3 ± 2.6[b]	77.0
MCC	109.5 ± 2.1[b]	76.2

[a]Significantly different from ND-fed control; [b]significantly different from HFD-fed control.

differential increases in gonadal fat pad (184%), mesenteric fat pad (93%) and subcutaneous fat pad (162%) indices, when compared with the ND control (**Table 2**). Among the single-component treatments, MC and CR suppressed the HFD-induced increases in total fat pad index (39% and 36%, respectively) as well as gonadal fat pad index (47% and 38%), whereas CA reduced the gonadal fat pad index (46%) and mesenteric fat pad index

(103%) in HFD-fed mice (**Table 2**). CR further suppressed the subcutaneous fat by 23%. Among the 2-component treatments, MC + CR and MC + CA decreased the total fat pad index (41% and 74%, respectively) and gonadal fat pad index (57% and 87%) in HFD-fed mice. In addition, MC + CA also suppressed increases in fat pad indices of total fat pad (64%) and subcutaneous fat pad (50%) of HFD-fed mice. CR + CA reduced the subcutaneous fat index (27%) in HFD-fed mice (**Table 2**). MCC (6.0 g/kg) did not produce detectable changes the total and differential fat pad indices.

3.3. Effects of MCC and Various Combinations of Its Constituents on Plasma Lipid Levels in HFD-Fed Mice

The HFD-induced increases in total and differential fat pad indices were paralleled by increases in plasma levels of TG and TC and (36% and 79%, respectively), as well as the ratio of LDL-C to HDL-C (27%) in HFD-fed mice (**Figure 2**). MCC (6.0 g/kg) and various combinations of its constituents differentially modulated the plasma lipid level in HFD-fed mice (**Figure 2**). The HFD-induced elevation in plasma TG level was decreased by MCC and all tested combinations (except CA), with complete suppression produced by MC + CA, CR + CA and MCC. MCC and all tested combinations reduced the plasma TC level in HFD-fed mice, with the extent of suppression afforded by CR + CA (77%) being most prominent, followed by MCC (71%). The HFD-induced increase in LDL-C/HDL-C ratio was suppressed by MCC and all tested combinations (except MC and MC + CA), with the complete inhibition produced by MCC.

3.4. Effects of MCC and Various Combinations of Its Constituents on Glucose Homeostasis in HFD-Fed Mice

In addition to increases in plasma lipid levels, HFD also impaired the glucose homeostasis, as indicated by increases in fasting plasma glucose level (28%) and oral glucose intolerance (25%) as well as the decrease in insulin sensitivity (65%) (**Figures 3(A)-(C)**). MCC and all tested combinations caused reversal changes on fasting plasma glucose level, oral glucose intolerance and insulin sensitivity in HFD-fed mice. Treatment with CR, MC + CR or CA + CR caused complete normalization of fasting plasma glucose level in HFD-fed mice (**Figure 3(A)**). In the oral glucose tolerance test, MC, MC + CR, MC + CA, CR + CA and MCC completely reversed the glucose intolerance, while CA, MC + CR, MC + CA and MCC completely restored the insulin sensitivity in HFD-fed mice.

3.5. Effects of MCC and Various Combinations of Its Constituents on Various Metabolic Enzyme Activities of Skeletal Muscle in HFD-Fed Mice

The HFD-induced impairment of glucose homeostasis was associated with the reduced PFK activity (20%) of

Table 2. Effects of MCC and various combinations of its constituents on various fat pad indices in HFD-fed mice.

Treatment	Total	Differential		
	Fat pad index	Subcutaneous fat pad index	Gonadal fat pad index	Mesenteric fat pad index
ND				
Control	0.044 ± 0.004	0.017 ± 0.001	0.021 ± 0.002	0.0064 ± 0.0005
HFD				
Control	0.115 ± 0.010[a]	0.043 ± 0.004[a]	0.059 ± 0.006[a]	0.0124 ± 0.0009[a]
MC	0.082 ± 0.11[b]	0.033 ± 0.005	0.038 ± 0.005[b]	0.0112 ± 0.0014
CR	0.079 ± 0.09[b]	0.032 ± 0.004[b]	0.037 ± 0.005[b]	0.0104 ± 0.0012
CA	0.087 ± 0.008	0.039 ± 0.004	0.039 ± 0.004[b]	0.0087 ± 0.0009[b]
MC+CR	0.092 ± 0.014	0.043 ± 0.008	0.038 ± 0.006[b]	0.0103 ± 0.0011
MC+CA	0.073 ± 0.017[b]	0.031 ± 0.007[b]	0.033 ± 0.010[b]	0.0084 ± 0.0014[b]
CR+CA	0.097 ± 0.020	0.029 ± 0.006[b]	0.057 ± 0.013	0.0102 ± 0.0015
MCC	0.101 ± 0.008	0.035 ± 0.003	0.056 ± 0.005	0.0109 ± 0.0008

[a]Significantly different from ND-fed control; [b]significantly different from HFD-fed control.

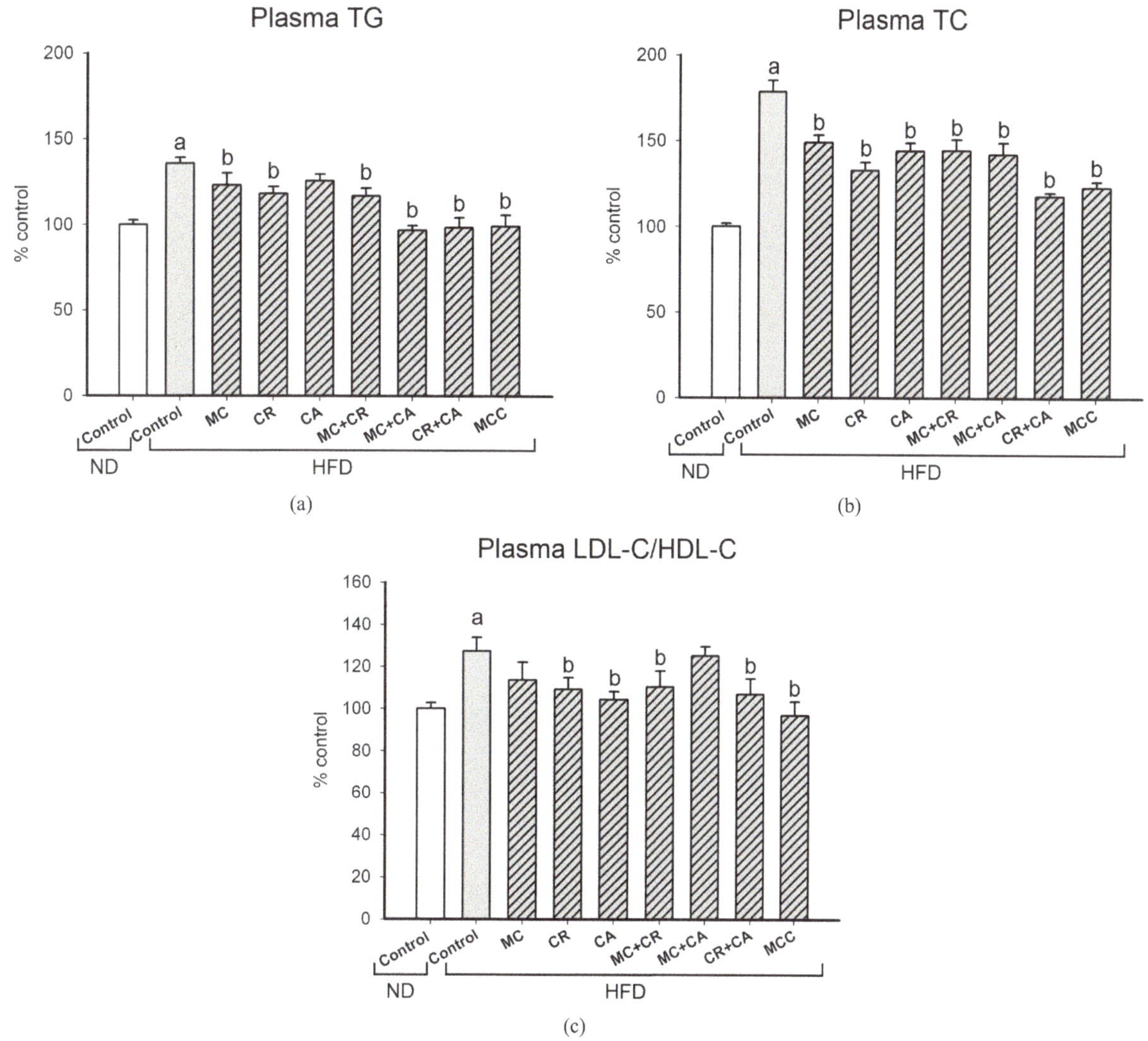

Figure 2. Effects of MCC and various combinations of its constituents on plasma lipid levels in HFD-fed mice. Mice were sacrificed at 24 h after the last dosing of MCC as described in Materials and Methods. Plasma triglyceride (TG) level (ND control = 59.0 ± 2.5 mg/dL), total lipoprotein cholesterol (TC) level (ND control = 146.3 ± 5.2 mg/dL) and ratio of low density lipoprotein cholesterol (LDL-C) to high density lipoprotein cholesterol (HDL-C) (ND control = 1.4 ± 0.11) were measured, as described in Materials and methods. Data were expressed as % control by normalizing with ND control. Value given are means ± SEM, with n = 10 - 15. [a]Significantly different from ND control; [b]Significantly different from HFD control.

skeletal muscle (**Table 3**). In addition, HFD increased the β-HAD activity (24%) and CPT activity (18%) of skeletal muscle in HFD-fed mice (**Table 3**). No detectable changes in CS activity of skeletal muscle in HFD-fed mice were observed. While MC, CR, CA and MC + CA partially reversed the HFD-induced reduction in PFK activity, CR, CA, MC + CR and MC + CA suppressed the CPT activity in HFD-fed mice.

3.6. Effects of MCC and Various Combinations of Its Constituents on Mitochondrial Coupling Efficiency of Skeletal Muscle in HFD-Fed Mice

HFD did not cause detectable change in mitochondrial coupling efficiency of skeletal muscle in HFD-fed mice. All single-component (MC, CR and CA) treatments decreased the coupling efficiency (36%, 19% and 31%, respectively), with the extent of reduction afforded by MC being most prominent (**Figure 4**). Among the 2-component combinations, only MC + CR and MC + CA decreased the mitochondrial coupling efficiency (28% and 20%, respectively) of skeletal muscle in HFD-fed mice. MCC did not affect the mitochondrial coupling effi-

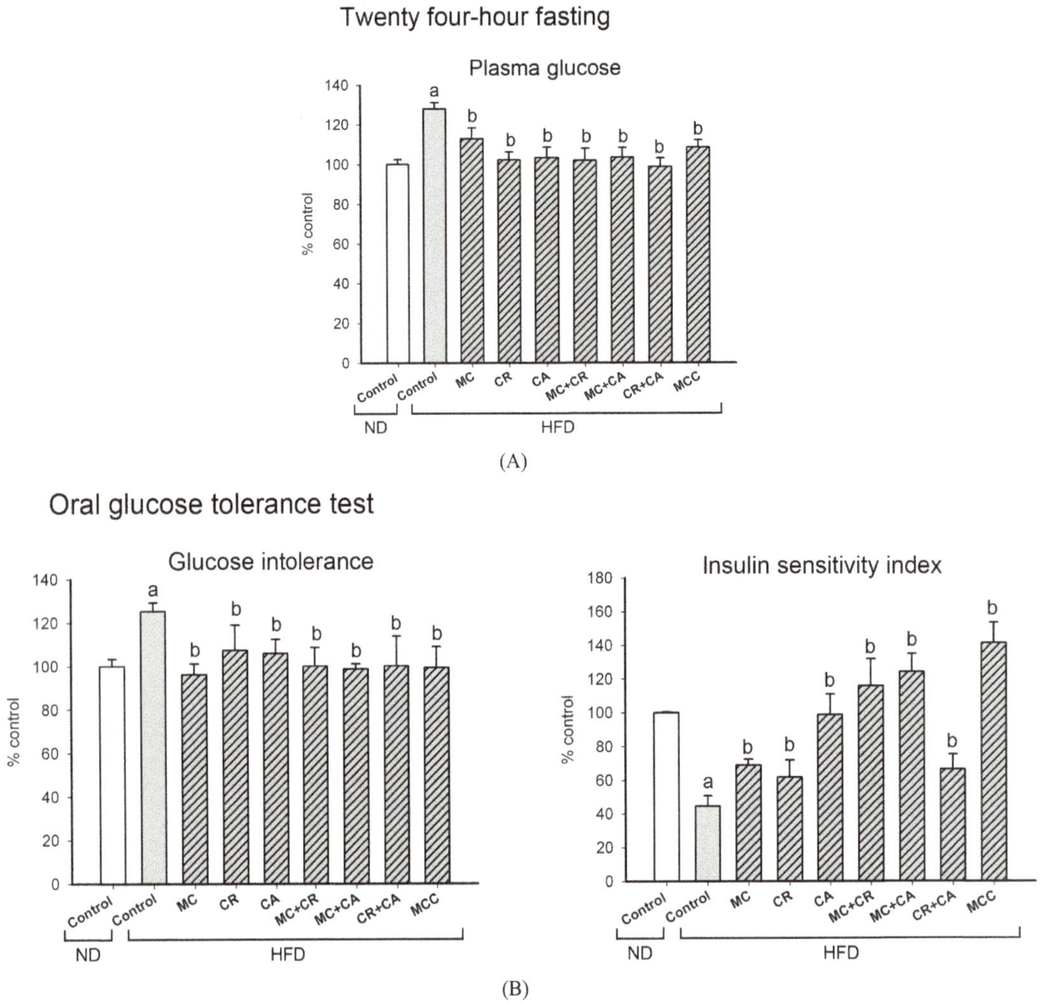

Figure 3. Effects of MCC and various combinations of its constituents on glucose homeostasis in HFD- fed mice. (A) Mice were sacrificed at 24 h after the last dosing of MCC as described in Materials and Methods. Plasma glucose level (ND control = 80.7 ± 4.2 mg/dL) was measured. (B) Mice were objected to oral glucose tolerance test at 24 h after the last dosing of MCC as described in Materials and Methods. Blood samples were collected at 15, 30, 60 and 120 min post-dosing of glucose. Plasma glucose and insulin levels were measured. Glucose intolerance was estimated by computing the area under the curve (AUC) plotting plasma glucose level against time and expressed in arbitrary unit (ND control = 1030 ± 40). Insulin sensitivity index (ISI) was estimated (ND control = 2623 ± 14), as described in Materials and Methods. Data were expressed as % control, by normalizing with ND control. Value given are means ± SEM, with n = 10 - 15. [a]Significantly different from ND control; [b]significantly different from HFD control.

ciency of skeletal muscle.

3.7. Effects of a Low Dose of MCC on Various Parameters in HFD-Fed Mice

The effects of MCC treatment at a low dose of 1.5 g/kg were also investigated in HFD-fed mice (**Table 4**). MCC (1.5 g/kg) reduced the HFD-induced body weight gain, with the degree of suppression being 64%. In contrast to the that of high dose of 6.0 g/kg, the weight reduction caused by the low dose of MCC was associated with decreases in total fat pad index (22%) as well as subcutaneous and mesenteric fat pad indices (36% and 66%, respectively) in HFD-fed mice. Consistent with this, MCC treatment also reduced the HFD-induced elevations of plasma TG and TC levels (by 65% and 72%, respectively) as well as plasma LDL-C to HDL-C ratio (127%). MCC also improved the glucose homeostasis in HFD-fed mice, as evidenced by the reversal of changes in fasting plasma glucose level (83%), glucose intolerance (100%) and insulin sensitivity (29%). Despite the fact

Table 3. Effects of MCC and various combinations of its constituents on various metabolic enzymes of skeletal muscle in HFD-fed mice.

Treatment	PFK	*β*-HAD	CS	CPT
ND				
Control	100 ± 2.6	100.0 ± 1.6	100.0 ± 1.3	100.0 ± 1.9
HFD				
Control	79.7 ± 1.6[a]	124.3 ± 3.5[a]	102.9 ± 3.0	117.9 ± 1.5[a]
MC	95.1 ± 3.5[b]	125.9 ± 1.8	101.1 ± 3.5	115.2 ± 2.8
CR	89.5 ± 4.8[b]	119.7 ± 6.1	102.7 ± 2.7	103.9 ± 2.6[b]
CA	91.4 ± 3.8[b]	122.5 ± 5.3	108.8 ± 1.7	104.2 ± 3.7[b]
MC + CR	88.1 ± 3.0	120.9 ± 4.2	108.2 ± 1.2	106.4 ± 3.5[b]
MC + CA	93.0 ± 3.5[b]	123.8 ±3.6	107.3 ± 2.8	106.6 ± 4.2[b]
CR + CA	82.8 ± 2.5	131.5 ± 4.6	96.4 ± 4.1	112.5 ± 3.7
MCC	85.7 ± 1.9	120.4 ± 3.6	91.6 ± 2.9[a,b]	112.1 ± 3.5

[a]Significantly different from ND control; [b]significantly different from HFD control.

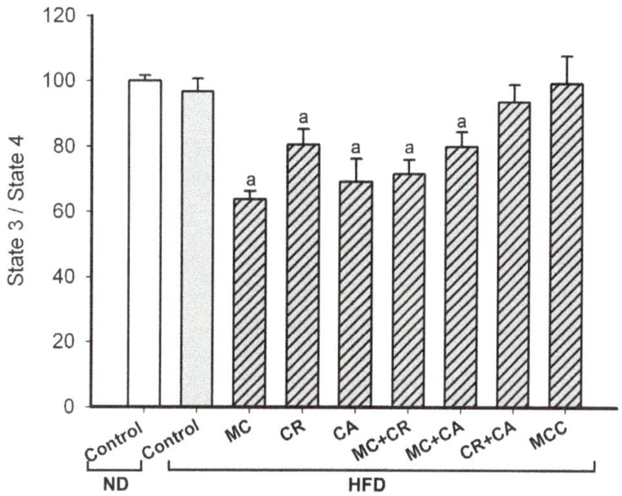

Figure 4. Effects of MCC and various combinations of its constituents on mitochondrial coupling efficiency of skeletal muscle in HFD-fed mice. Mice were sacrificed at 24 h after the last dosing of MCC as described in Materials and Methods. Mitochondrial respiratory of skeletal muscle was measured polarographically by a Clark-type oxygen electrode at 30˚C. The respiratory control ratio (RCR) was estimated by calculating the ratio of state 3 to state 4 respirations. Data were expressed as % control, by normalizing with ND control. Values given are means ± SEM, with n = 10 - 15. [a]Significantly different from ND control; [b]significantly different from HFD control.

that MCC (1.5 g/kg) did not produce detectable changes in various metabolic enzyme activities (PFK, *β*-HAD and CS) of skeletal muscle, MCC decreased the CPT activity (56%) as well as the mitochondrial coupling efficiency (28%) of skeletal muscle in HFD-fed mice.

4. Discussion

HFD-fed mice, as observed in the present and other studies [12], showed increases in body weight, the degree of

Table 4. Effect of MCC (1.5 g/kg) on various parameters in HFD-fed mice.

MCC (1.5 g/kg)	% stimulation (+) or % suppression (–) VS HFD control
Body weight	
BW change	–64[a]
Fat pad indices	
Total fat pad index	–22[a]
Subcutaneous fat pad index	–36[a]
Gonadal fat pad index	No significant difference
Mesenteric fat pad index	–66[a]
Plasma lipid and leptin levels	
Plasma TG	–65[a]
Plasma TC	–72[a]
LDL to HDL ratio	–127[a]
Glucose homeostasis	
24-h fasting	
Plasma glucose	–83[a]
Oral glucose tolerance test	
Glucose intolerance	–100[a]
Insulin sensitivity index	+29[a]
Metabolic enzyme activities in skeletal muscle	
PFK	No significant difference
β-HAD	No significant difference
CS	No significant difference
CPT	–56[a]
Mitochondrial coupling efficiency in skeletal muscle	
Coupling efficiency	–25[a]

[a]Significantly different from ND control; [b]significantly different from HFD control.

adiposity and plasma lipid contents, as well as impairments in glucose homeostasis and metabolic status of skeletal muscle. It has been shown that HFD caused an increase in free fatty acid uptake in skeletal muscle, with a resultant insulin resistance [13], which is a well-established risk factor of diabetes and metabolic syndromes. In the present study, MCC and various combinations of its constituents reduced the weight gain in HFD-fed mice, which was accompanied with an improvement on glucose homeostasis. Our earlier study has suggested that the weight loss effect produced by MCC is likely due to a modulation of fatty acid absorption and/or metabolism [8]. In the present study, emodin, which was found to ameliorate metabolic dysfunctions in HFD-induced obese mice [14], was used as a positive control. Consistent with the recent findings, emodin reduced the weight gain, adiposity and plasma lipid contents in HFD-fed mice (data not shown), suggesting the validity of the mouse model of HFD-induce obesity in the present study. Varied effects of MCC and its constituents or their combinations on total and differential adiposity, plasma lipid contents and metabolic status of skeletal muscle were observed. We therefore sought to define the role of each constituent of MCC in producing the weight loss effect and the associated metabolic changes in HFD-induced obese mice.

Despite the fact that all constituents of MCC (MC, CA and CR) independently suppressed the HFD-induced weight gain in mice, MC seems to be the most effective. The MC/CA/CR-induced weight reduction in HFD-fed mice may be attributed to the improvement in metabolic status of skeletal muscle, as indicated by as a reversal increase in PFK activity and an induction of mitochondrial uncoupling, with the degree of improvement produced by MC being larger than those of CA and CR. However, only CA and CR, but not MC, significantly reduced the total adiposity and visceral adiposity (as assessed by mesenteric fat pad index) as well as plasma LDL-C to HDL-C ratio. On the other hand, MC, when being combined with CR or CA, could reduce the degree of visceral adiposity or the LDL-C to HDL-C ratio respectively, in addition to decreasing body weight. Given that an increased visceral adiposity and an elevated plasma LDL-C to HDL-C ratio are predisposing factors of metabolic disorders [2], the combination of MC with CR or CA may be beneficial for lowering the risk of metabolic disorders in obese individuals. This postulation was strengthened by the observation that among the 2-component combinations, MC + CA and MC + CR treatments were more effective than that of CA + CR in weight reduction, possibly due to the induction of mitochondrial uncoupling in skeletal muscle of mice. While MC + CA reduced the extent of visceral adiposity and stimulated the PFK activity of skeletal muscle, MC + CR decreased the plasma LDL-C/HDL-C ratio. Conceivably, MCC treatment may produce a multiple effect on weight reduction, visceral adiposity suppression and plasma LDL-C/HDL-C regulation in HFD-induced obese mice. Unexpectedly, the weight reduction afforded by MCC (6.0 g/kg) was not accompanied with the suppression of visceral adiposity and induction of mitochondrial uncoupling in skeletal muscle in HFD-induced obese mice. Since an inducer of mitochondrial uncoupling has been shown to cause a dose-dependent and biphasic response in round spermatids [15], the failure of MCC to induce mitochondrial uncoupling in skeletal muscle may be related to the high dose of treatment. This postulation is supported by the finding that the weight reduction afforded by MCC treatment at a lower dose (1.5 g/kg) was associated with an induction of mitochondrial uncoupling in skeletal muscle as well as a suppression of visceral adiposity and a reduction of LDL-C/HDL-C ratio in HFD-induced obese mice. While the ability of MCC to modulate the metabolism of cholesterol remains unclear, the suppression of visceral adiposity is likely causally related to mitochondrial uncoupling in skeletal muscle, which oxidizes excessive fatty acids in HFD-fed mice. As visceral adipose tissue contains a large number of mitochondria [16], we cannot exclude the possibility that MCC may also induce mitochondrial uncoupling in visceral adipose tissue, with a resultant mobilization of lipid reservoir in adipose tissue. As an excessive accumulation of visceral adipose tissue is associated with metabolic abnormalities such as insulin resistance and high blood lipid contents [17], the reduction of fat mass of visceral adipose tissue is therefore beneficial for preventing metabolic diseases such as metabolic syndromes and type 2 diabetes [18]. In this regard, MCC treatment was found to improve glucose tolerance and insulin sensitivity in HFD-fed mice.

Contemporary anti-obesity approaches have been targeted at the reduction of intestinal absorption [19], the enhancement of fatty acid metabolic status in skeletal muscle [20] and the induction of mitochondrial uncoupling in skeletal muscle [21]. An earlier study on the weight loss effect of MCC revealed that MCC treatment (5.1 g/kg) decreased the weight gain in HFD-fed mice, presumably due to the reduction of intestinal lipid absorption in HFD-fed mice [8]. In the present study, we have further demonstrated that a lower dose of MCC (1.5 g/kg) induces mitochondrial uncoupling in skeletal muscle of HFD-fed mice and thus provides an extended view on the biochemical mechanism underlying weight loss effect of MCC. In this connection, an induction of mitochondrial uncoupling in skeletal muscle was found to augment the energy expenditure in uncoupling protein 1 up-regulated mice [22].

5. Conclusion

In conclusion, MCC treatment at a dose of 1.5 g/kg was found to reduce the HFD-induced weight gain and the associated metabolic abnormalities in HFD-fed mice. The finding suggests that MCC may offer a promising prospect for ameliorating the diet-induced obesity and the associated metabolic disorders in humans.

References

[1] Ahima, R.S. and Lazar, M.A. (2013) The Health Risk of Obesity-Better Metrics Imperative. *Science*, **341**, 856-858. http://dx.doi.org/10.1126/science.1241244

[2] Fontana, L.J., Eagon, C., Trujillo, M.E., Scherer, P.E. and Klein, S. (2007) Visceral Fat Adipokine Secretion Is Associated with Systemic Inflammation in Obese Humans. *Diabetes*, **56**, 1010-1013. http://dx.doi.org/10.2337/db06-1656

[3] Manninen, V., Tenkanen, L., Koskinen, P., Huttunen, J.K., Mänttäri, M., Heinonen, O.P. and Frick, M.H. (1992) Joint Effects of Serum Triglyceride and LDL Cholesterol and HDL Cholesterol Concentrations on Coronary Heartdisease Risk in the Helsinki Heart Study. Implications for Treatment. *Circulation*, **85**, 37-45. http://dx.doi.org/10.1161/01.CIR.85.1.37

[4] Wing, R.R. and Phelan, S. (2005) Long-Term Weight Loss Maintenance. *The American Journal of Clinical Nutrition*, **82**, 222S-225S.

[5] Caveney, E., Caveney, B.J., Somaratne, R., Turner, J.R. and Gourgiotis, L. (2011) Pharmaceutical Interventions for Obesity: A Public Health Perspective. *Diabetes*, *Obesity and Metabolism*, **13**, 490-497. http://dx.doi.org/10.1111/j.1463-1326.2010.01353.x

[6] Tseng, Y., Cypess, A.M. and Kahn, C.R. (2010) Cellular Bioenergetics as a Target for Obesity Therapy. *Nature Reviews Drug Discovery*, **9**, 465-482. http://dx.doi.org/10.1038/nrd3138

[7] Thrush, A.B., Dent, R., McPherson, R. and Harper, M.E. (2013) Implications of Mitochondrial Uncoupling in Skeletal Muscle in the Development and Treatment of Obesity. *FEBS Journal*, **280**, 5015-5029. http://dx.doi.org/10.1111/febs.12399

[8] Leong, P.K., Leung, H.Y., Wong, H.S., Chen, J., Ma, C.W., Yang, Y. and Ko, K.M. (2013) Long-Term Treatment with an Herbal Formula MCC Reduces the Weight Gain in High Fat Diet-Induced Obese Mice. *Chinese Medicine*, **4**, 63-71. http://dx.doi.org/10.4236/cm.2013.43010

[9] Siddiqua, M., Hamid, K., Rashid, M.H.A., Akther, M.S. and Choudhuri, M.S.K. (2010) Changes in Lipid Profile of Rat Plasma after Chronic Administration of Laghobanondo Rosh (LNR)—An Ayurvedic Formulation. *Biology and Medicine*, **2**, 58-63.

[10] Colberg, S.R., Simoneau, J.A., Thaete, F.L. and Kelley, D.E. (1995) Skeletal Muscle Utilization of Free Fatty Acids in Women with Visceral Obesity. *The Journal of Clinical Investigation*, **95**, 1846-1853. http://dx.doi.org/10.1172/JCI117864

[11] Crescenzo, R., Mainieri, D., Solinas, G., Montani, J.P., Seydoux, J., Liverini, G., Iossa, S. and Dulloo, A.G. (2003) Skeletal Muscle Mitochondrial Oxidative Capacity and Uncoupling Protein 3 Are Differently Influenced by Semistarvation and Refeeding. *FEBS Letters*, **544**, 138-142. http://dx.doi.org/10.1016/S0014-5793(03)00491-5

[12] Wang, C.Y. and Liao, J.K. (2012) A Mouse Model of Diet-Induced Obesity and Insulin Resistance. *Methods in Molecular Biology*, **821**, 421-433. http://dx.doi.org/10.1007/978-1-61779-430-8_27

[13] Martins, R., Nachbar, R.T., Gorjao, R., Vinolo, M.A., Festuccia, W.T., Lambertucci, R.H., Cury-Boaventura, M.F., Silveira, L.R., Curi, R. and Hirabara, S.M. (2012) Mechanisms Underlying Skeletal Muscle Insulin Resistance Induced by Fatty Acids: Importance of the Mitochondrial Function. *Lipids in Health and Disease*, **11**, 30. http://dx.doi.org/10.1186/1476-511X-11-30

[14] Feng, Y., Huang, S.L., Dou, W., Zhang, S., Chen, J.H., Shen, Y., Shen, J.H. and Leng, Y. (2010) Emodin, a Natural Product, Selectively Inhibits 11beta-Hydroxysteroid Dehydrogenase Type 1 and Ameliorates Metabolic Disorder in Diet-Induced Obese Mice. *British Journal of Pharmacology*, **161**, 113-126. http://dx.doi.org/10.1111/j.1476-5381.2010.00826.x

[15] Nakamura, M., Ikeda, M., Suzuki, A., Okinaga, S. and Arai, K. (1988) Metabolism of Round Spermatids: Gossypol Induces Uncoupling of Respiratory Chain and Oxidative Phosphorylation. *Biology of Reproduction*, **39**, 771-778. http://dx.doi.org/10.1095/biolreprod39.4.771

[16] Kraunsøe, R., Boushel, R., Hansen, C.N., Schjerling, P., Qvortrup, K., Støckel, P., Mikines, K.J. and Dela, F. (2010) Mitochondrial Respiration in Subcutaneous and Visceral Adipose Tissue from Patients with Morbid Obesity. *The Journal of Physiology*, **588**, 2023-2032. http://dx.doi.org/10.1113/jphysiol.2009.184754

[17] Girard, J. and Lafontan, M. (2008) Impact of Visceral Adipose Tissue on Liver Metabolism and Insulin Resistance. Part II: Visceral Adipose Tissue Production and Liver Metabolism. *Diabetes & Metabolism*, **34**, 439-445. http://dx.doi.org/10.1016/j.diabet.2008.04.002

[18] Knight, J.A. (2011) Diseases and Disorders Associated with Excess Body Weight. *Annals of Clinical & Laboratory Science*, **41**, 107-121.

[19] Caveney, E., Caveney, B.J., Somaratne, R., Turner, J.R. and Gourgiotis, L. (2011) Pharmaceutical Interventions for Obesity: A Public Health Perspective. *Diabetes*, *Obesity and Metabolism*, **13**, 490-497. http://dx.doi.org/10.1111/j.1463-1326.2010.01353.x

[20] Goto, T., Teraminami, A., Lee, J.Y., Ohyama, K., Fu-nakoshi, K., Kim, Y.I., Hirai, S., Uemura, T., Yu, R., Takahashi, N. and Kawada, T. (2012) Tiliroside, a Glycosidic Flavo-Noid, Ameliorates Obesity-Induced Metabolic Disorders via Activation of Adiponectin Signaling Followed by Enhancement of Fatty Acid Oxidation in Liver and Skeletal Muscle in Obese-Diabetic Mice. *The Journal of Nutritional Biochemistry*, **23**, 768-776. http://dx.doi.org/10.1016/j.jnutbio.2011.04.001

[21] Costford, S., Gowing, A. and Harper, M.E. (2007) Mitochondrial Uncoupling as a Target in the Treatment of Obesity. *Current Opinion in Clinical Nutrition & Metabolic Care*, **10**, 671-678. http://dx.doi.org/10.1097/MCO.0b013e3282f0dbe4

[22] Adjeitey, C.N., Mailloux, R.J., Dekemp, R.A. and Harpe, M.E. (2013) Mitochondrial Uncoupling in Skeletal Muscle by UCP1 Augments Energy Expenditure and Glutathione Content While Mitigating ROS Production. *American Journal of Physiology—Endocrinology and Metabolism*, **305**, E405-E415. http://dx.doi.org/10.1152/ajpendo.00057.2013

List of Abbreviations

Analysis of variance (ANOVA); area under the curve (AUC); body mass index (BMI); L-carnitine (CA); carnitine palmitoyl CoA transferase (CPT); citrate synthase (CS); pericarpium of *Citri reticulate* (CR); fasting plasma insulin (FPI); fasting plasma glucose (FPG); β-hydroxyacyl-Co A dehydrogenase (β-HAD); high-density lipoprotein cholesterol (HDL-C); high fat diet (HFD); insulin sensitivity index (ISI); low-density lipoprotein cholesterol (LDL-C); the fruit of *Momordica charantia* (MC); normal diet (ND); oral glucose tolerance test (OGTT); phosphofructokinase (PFK); triglyceride (TG)

12

Effect of *Qing'e Pill* plus *Salvia* on Non-Traumatic Osteonecrosis of the Femoral Head of Idiopathic Type in Earlier Stage: A Case Report of a Twelve-Month of Period

Bo Shuai, Yanping Yang*, Lin Shen#, Manxiang Wu

Department of Integrated Traditional Chinese and Western Medicine, Union Hospital, Tongji Medical College, Huazhong University of Science and Technology, Wuhan, China
Email: #bobo3137@126.com

Abstract

Background: Compromised circulatory and bone/lipid metabolic dysfunction are two major contributors to non-traumatic osteonecrosis of the femoral head (ONFH). *Qing'e pill* plus *Salvia* has significant anti-inflammatory and anti-atherosclerotic action, and it could also regulate bone formation and remodeling by suppressing osteoclasts. Case Report: We describe a case of a 62-year-old man with ONFH of idiopathic type in earlier stage that could not be adequately controlled with oral non-steroidal analgesics and restoring bone loss agents for past 3 years. After six months treatment with *Qing'e pill* plus *Salvia*, the plasma low-density lipoprotein (LDL), high-density lipoprotein (HDL), apolipoprotein A1 (apo A1), apolipoprotein B (apo B), total cholesterol (TC), triglycerides (TG), and blood viscosity were measured on an empty stomach. The Harris scores were maintained during a six months follow-up after discontinuation of *Qing'e pill* plus *Salvia*. Discussion: Our case has shown that plasma levels of inflammatory and atherosclerotic relaxed factors and the Harris scores may be controlled with herbal medication in ONFH of idiopathic type in earlier stage that could not be adequately controlled with oral non-steroidal analgesics and restoring bone loss agents.

Keywords

***Qing'e Pill*, Osteonecrosis, Femoral Head, Ischemic, Biomarker, Traditional Chinese Medicine**

*This author contributed equally to this work.
#Corresponding author.

1. Introduction

Abnormal lipid metabolism and bone marrow fat cells hypertrophy/proliferation play important roles in non-traumatic osteonecrosis of the femoral head (ONFH) [1]-[4]. Fat emboli and/or thrombi may further compromise circulation to the femoral head [5]-[7]. In addition, repair capacity and bone remodeling play important roles in the progression and severity of nontraumatic ONFH [8].

In ONFH treatment, non-steroidal analgesics, Hypolipidemics, Anticoagulants, Vasodilators, and restoring bone loss agents are of vital importance to prevent the above complications, as confirmed by the Ajmal M. [9]. The non-steroidal analgesics are generally achieved by administration of Coxibs. And the restoring bone loss agents are generally achieved by administration of oral Bisphosphonates and Alendronate agents or intramuscular calcitonin as well as by weight-bearing. However, there are patients who, for various reasons, are unable to meet dietary or weight-bearing requirements or who remain unresponsive to drug treatment.

We observed a positive effect of *Qing'e pill* plus *Salvia*, an herbal extract used in Traditional Chinese medicine, on lowering plasma levels of inflammatory and atherosclerotic relaxed factors and reducing symptom in ONFH patients of idiopathic type in earlier stage that were unresponsive to oral non-steroidal analgesics and restoring bone loss agents.

2. Case History

Patient characteristics and diagnosis: A 62-year-old man (weight, 81 kg; height, 176 cm; waist, 36 inches, left leg) with non-traumatic ONFH of idiopathic type in stage II according to Association Research Circulation Osseous (ARCO) stage conformed by MRI at Union hospital of Tongji Medical College of Huazhong University of Science and Technology (HUST).

Five kinds of herbal materials of *Qing'e pill* were purchased form the Pharmacy of Union hospital of Tongji Medical College of HUST. The ingredients of *Qing'e pill* include 160 g of fried *Psoralen* which steep in wine; 80 g of fried *Eucommia* which peeled and dipped in ginger; 60 g of peeled *Walnut*; 160 g of *Salvia*. The above specimens were crushed into fine powder, and pasted for the pills with 60 g of garlic (**Table 1**). All five herbs were identified and authenticated by Prof. Shen Lin (The Botany and Drug Department of Union Hospital of Tongji Medical College). The patients were given every two pills and twice a day for six months.

After six months of the medicine treatment, blood viscosity was regularized, but LDL/HDL ratio level was remained unchanged. The follow up was started for twelve's months continuously. At the end of follow up period, Apo B/apo A1 ratio and Harris Score was raised significantly, blood viscosity and total cholesterol were decreased significantly, and LDL/HDL ratio was still not difference significantly (**Table 2**).

The blood pressure (140 - 150/90 - 100 mmHg) was mild high with nosymptom which was monitored after follow up period and it become normal after 3 months with no treatment.

During Qing'e pill administration, there was normalization of abnormal laboratory parameters of hemorheology indexes including 1/s (mPa.S), 5/s, 50/s, 100/s and 200/s. Four months after the last dose of Qing'e pill, the indexes were decreased significantly (**Table 3**).

Finally it was concluded after four months follow up period, the patient Harris Score was increased (80) with 29.03%, and (90) 45.16 at 12 months. Symptoms such as hip pain, limited mobility, and daily activities have been improved significantly.

3. Discussion

Currently, non-surgical femoral head-salvage therapy in Western medicine treats patients with non-steroidal

Table 1. Components of modified Qing'e pill and total dose of each herb.

No. Herbal name	Processing	Contents (g)
1 Psoralen	steep in wine	160
2 Eucommia	fried, peeled and dipped in ginger	80
3 Walnut	peeled	60
4 Salvia miltiorrhiza	levigation	160
5 garlic	steaming	60

Table 2. Serial routine laboratory measurements and immunohematological results.

	Total cholesterol mg/dl	LDL/HDL ratio	Apo B/apo A1 ratio	CRP	Harris score
resentation					
0 mounth	235.70	1.80	0.90	9.86	62
1 mounth	238.12	1.85	0.87	8.97	72
2 mounth	210.63	1.93	0.82	8.53	78
3 mounth	-	-	-	-	78
4 mounth	203.45	1.74	0.77	8.03	80
5 mounth	-	-	-	-	84
6 mounth	193.72	1.83	0.71	6.03	86
7 mounth	-	-	-	-	86
8 mounth	-	-	-	-	86
9 mounth	-	-	-	-	86
10 mounth	-	-	-	-	88
11 mounth	-	-	-	-	90
12 mounth	190.55	1.73	0.69	6.89	90

During Qing'e pill administration, there was normalization of abnormal laboratory parameters including total cholesterol, Apo B/apo A1 ratio, CRP, and Harris Score. Four months after the last dose of Qing'e pill, Harris score rose to 80.

Table 3. Serial routine laboratory measurements of hemorheology indexes.

Shear rate of whole blood	1/s (mPa.S)	5/s (mPa.S)	50/s (mPa.S)	100/s (mPa.S)	200/s (mPa.S)
resentation					
0 mounth	44.38	38.83	27.48	24.33	20.35
1 mounth	38.57	32.13	24.13	20.57	17.64
2 mounth	32.72	29.78	19.08	22.46	18.83
3 mounth	-	-	-	-	-
4 mounth	28.27	26.17	16.25	19.07	15.78
5 mounth	-	-	-	-	-
6 mounth	29.87	25.83	16.46	18.72	15.98
7 mounth	-	-	-	-	-
8 mounth	-	-	-	-	-
9 mounth	-	-	-	-	-
10 mounth	-	-	-	-	-
11 mounth	-	-	-	-	-
12 mounth	30.08	26.12	17.72	19.11	16.07

analgesics, Hypolipidemics, Anticoagulants, Vasodilators and Bisphosphonates while emphasizing the restriction of weight-bearing on the affected hip joint. One kind of Hypolipidemics drugs, Simvastatin, will increase the differentiation from marrow stromal cells (MSCs) towards osteoblasts, promoting mineralization of bones while inhibiting the differentiation from MSCs towards adipocytes, which can suggest the prevention of osteonecrosis. However, long-term effective dose of these drugs may bring severe adverse reaction of livers and muscles [10]. Enoxaparin, which is of Anticoagulants, and Iloprost, which is of Vasodilators, can relieve the pain of early-staged primary ONFH patients with tendency of thrombosis and with low fibrinolytic activity, but cannot reverse the necrotic process [11] [12]. Alendronate, as an osteoclast inhibitor, can improve clinical symptoms; retard joint collapsing and replacement time. But it also brings esophageal and gastrointestinal adverse reactions after long-term usage. For the patients who are suffering from gingivitis, it may also result in osteonecrosis of mandibular [13]. Other non-surgical treatments include electromagnetic stimulation, extracorporeal shock wave therapy, hyperbaric oxygen therapy and other physical therapies. However, there is a lack of large-sample study for all these therapies.

In recent years, we have harvested significant progress in traditional Chinese medicine of non-surgical treatment for ONFH patients. It will bring good clinical effect with absence of destructions, invasions, pains, and side effects, and therefore is very safe and reliable for the patients. All these advantages made traditional Chinese medicine therapy an international trend for treatment of osteonecrosis of the femoral head, and highly accepted by the scholars and the patients. Hence, comprehensive pharmacodynamics research and evaluation on representative prescriptions and therapies based on traditional Chinese medicine theory and combined with understanding of modern medicine are needed to filter out valid prescriptions and the rules, which are urgent priority and future direction of further research for prevention and treatment of the ONFH of early stage.

In Chinese medicine, ONFH is one kind of bone erosion and rheumatism diseases. In "*Qing*'*e pill*" prescription, *Eucommia ulmoides oliv* is warm-natured, with the effect of making kidney and bones strong, so in the book "Ben Cao Ji Yan", there is such a description, "*Eucommia ulmoides oliv* is only herb to strengthen lower energizer, remove pains of foots and legs, and fix knees and loins." Also in another ancient book named "Ben Cao Jing Shu", it was said "*Psoralea corylifolia* can warm the kidney, raise 'Yang' from 'Yin', raise 'fire' from 'soil', can cure kidney weakness and difficulties in sitting up." In "Ju Fang Qing'e pill", it described that "Juglans regia can invigorating the kidney and promote blood circulation, garlic bulb can make the retention pass and dredging collaterals... The combination of these four kinds of herb is called '*Qing*'*e pill*', which can not only cure kidney weakness and difficulties in sitting up, but also strengthen bone and musculature, promote blood circulation, make hair dark, and bring a good look." With the use of *Salvia* miltiorrhiza which can activate blood circulation to dissipate blood stasis, we can harvest a very good effect in urinary system and circulatory system [14]. Compromised circulatory and bone/lipid metabolic dysfunctions were two major contributors to ONFH. *Qing*'*e pill*, which can significantly improve bone quality which has been recognized by most Chinese medical scholars, combined with Salvia which can activate blood circulation to dissipate blood stasis, can more effective for treating ONFH theoretically than one single. Our previous experimental studies have shown that this prescription can raise bone mineral density and biomechanical strength of an avascular necrosis of femoral head in rabbit model by inhibiting resorption activity of osteoclasts and promoting the proliferation of osteoblasts [15] [16], which results in production of more bony matrix and the balance of bone metabolism in rat model [17] [18]. Besides, this prescription brings an obvious effect in promoting of joint function, improving density of suffering hip and reversing the process of necrosis [19]-[22]. The MRI examination of this case was not different significantly before and after treatment, the patient was not deteriorating further on imaging. Our this case has also shown that plasma levels of inflammatory and atherosclerotic relaxed factors, blood viscosity, and the Harris scores may be controlled with herbal medication in ONFH patient of idiopathic type in earlier stage without any toxicity and side effects. Further studies are required to investigate the exact compound responsible for ONFH treatment.

Acknowledgements

The authors would like to thank L.V. Lin for his expertise and assistance in performing the blood collection, Wang Quanshen for his technical assistance.

Research Support

Innovation Fund of Huazhong University of Science and Technology (Item Number: 2013QN235); National Natural Science Foundation of China (Project Number: 81273907 and 81072493).

References

[1] Shuai, B., Shen, L., Yang, Y.P., Xie, J., Shou, Z.X. and Wei, B. (2010) Low Plasma Adiponectin as a Potential Biomarker for Osteonecrosis of the Femoral Head. *The Journal of Rheumatology*, **37**, 2151-2155. http://dx.doi.org/10.3899/jrheum.100342

[2] Hirata, T., Fujioka, M., Takahashi, K.A., Arai, Y., Asano, T., Ishida, M., Kuribayashi, M., Akioka, K., Okamoto, M., Yoshimura, N., Satomi, Y., Nishino, H., Fukushima, W., Hirota, Y., Nakajima, S., Kato, S. and Kubo, T. (2007) ApoB C7623T Polymorphism Predicts Risk for Steroid-Induced Osteonecrosis of the Femoral Head after Renal Transplantation. *Journal of Orthopaedic Science*, **12**, 199-206. http://dx.doi.org/10.1007/s00776-007-1110-9

[3] Motomura, G., Yamamoto, T., Miyanishi, K., Jingushi, S. and Iwamoto, Y. (2004) Combined Effects of an Anticoagulant and a Lipid-Lowering Agent on the Prevention of Steroid-Induced Osteonecrosis in Rabbits. *Arthritis & Rheuma-*

tology, **50**, 3387-3391. http://dx.doi.org/10.1002/art.20517

[4] Pengde, K., Fuxing, P., Bin, S., Jing, Y. and Jingqiu, C. (2008) Lovastatin Inhibits Adipogenesis and Prevents Osteonecrosis in Steroid-Treated Rabbits. *Joint Bone Spine*, **75**, 696-701. http://dx.doi.org/10.1016/j.jbspin.2007.12.008

[5] Miyanishi, K., Yamamoto, T., Irisa, T., Yamashita, A., Jingushi, S., Noguchi, Y. and Iwamoto, Y. (2002) Bone Marrow Fat Cell Enlargement and a Rise in Intraosseous Pressure in Steroid-Treated Rabbits with Osteonecrosis. *Bone*, **30**, 185-190. http://dx.doi.org/10.1016/S8756-3282(01)00663-9

[6] Kong, X.Y., Wang, R.T., Tian, N., Li, L., Lin, N. and Chen, W.H. (2012) Effect of Huogu II Formula with Medicinal Guide Radix Achyranthis Bidentatae on Bone Marrow Stem Cells Directional Homing to Necrosis Area after Osteonecrosis of the Femoral Head in Rabbit. *Chinese Journal of Integrative Medicine*, **18**, 761-768. http://dx.doi.org/10.1007/s11655-011-0940-7

[7] Zhang, W., Kanehara, M., Ishida, T., Guo, Y., Wang, X., Li, G., Zhang, B., Kondo, H. and Tachi, S. (2004) Preventive and Therapeutic Effects of Acupuncture on Bone Mass in Osteopenic Ovariectomized Rats. *The American Journal of Chinese Medicine*, **32**, 427-443. http://dx.doi.org/10.1142/S0192415X04002089

[8] Radke, S., Battmann, A., Jatzke, S., Eulert, J., Jakob, F. and Schutze, N. (2006) Expression of the Angiomatrix and Angiogenic Proteins CYR61, CTGF, and VEGF in Osteonecrosis of the Femoral Head. *Journal of Orthopaedic Research*, **24**, 945-952. http://dx.doi.org/10.1002/jor.20097

[9] Ajmal, M., Matas, A.J., Kuskowski, M. and Cheng, E.Y. (2009) Does Statin Usage Reduce the Risk of Corticosteroid-Related Osteonecrosis in Renal Transplant Population? *Orthopedic Clinics of North America*, **2**, 235-239. http://dx.doi.org/10.1016/j.ocl.2009.01.004

[10] Glueck, C.J., Freiberg, R.A., Sieve, L. and Wang, P. (2005) Enoxaparin Prevents Progression of Stages I and II Osteonecrosis of the Hip. *Clinical Orthopaedics and Related Research*, 164-170. http://dx.doi.org/10.1097/01.blo.0000157539.67567.03

[11] Jäger, M., Zilkens, C., Bittersohl, B., Matheney, T., Kozina, G., Blondin, D. and Krauspe, R. (2010) Efficiency of Iloprost Treatment for Osseous Malperfusion. *International Orthopaedics*, **35**, 761-765. http://dx.doi.org/10.1007/s00264-010-0998-4

[12] Lai, K.A., Shen, W.J., Yang, C.Y., Shao, C.J., Hsu, J.T. and Lin, R.M. (2005) The use of Alendronate to Prevent Early Collapse of the Femoral Head in Patients with Nontraumatic Osteonecrosis: A Randomized Clinical Study. *The Journal of Bone & Joint Surgery*, **87**, 2155-2159. http://dx.doi.org/10.2106/JBJS.D.02959

[13] Camporesi, E.M., Vezzani, G., Bosco, G., Mangar, D. and Bernasek, T.L. (2010) Hyperbaric Oxygen Therapy in Femoral head necrosis. *The Journal of Arthroplasty*, **25**, 118-123. http://dx.doi.org/10.1016/j.arth.2010.05.005

[14] Wu, W.Y. and Wang, Y.P. (2012) Pharmacological Actions and Therapeutic Applications of Salvia Miltiorrhiza Depside Salt and Its Active Components. *Acta Pharmacologica Sinica*, **33**, 1119-1130. http://dx.doi.org/10.1038/aps.2012.126

[15] Yang, Y.P., Shen, L., Zhou, P.Q. and Xie J. (2002) Effects of Blood Rheology on Patients with Necrosis of Femoral Head Caused by Alcohol with Bushen Huoxuefang. *Chinese Journal of Traditional Medical Traumatology & Orthopedics*, **10**, 28-30.

[16] Zhou, P.Q., Shen, L., Yang, Y.P. and Xie, J. (2004) Effects of Blood Rheology and Bone Mineral Density on Patients with Necrosis of Femoral Head Caused by Alcohol with Bushen Huoxuefang. *Chinese Journal of Traditional Medical Traumatology & Orthopedics*, **12**, 27-29.

[17] Yang, Y.P., Shen, L., Liu, S.R., Xie, J. and Zhou, P.Q. (2004) Effects of Bone Density on Experimental Rabbits with Avascular Necrosis of Femoral Head by Bushenhuoxuefang. *Chinese Journal of Traditional Medical Traumatology & Orthopedics*, **12**, 5-7.

[18] Zhou, P.Q., Shen, L., Yang, Y.P. and Xie, J. (2006) Effects of Bone Density and Biomechanics on Experimental Rabbits with Avascular Necrosis of Femoral Head by Bushenhuoxuefang. *Chinese Journal of Rehabilitation Medicine*, **21**, 1139-1143.

[19] Shen, L., Du, J.Y., Yang, J.Y., Yang, Y.P. and Gao, L. (1994) Effect of Qing'e Pill on Ovariectomy Osteoporosis Rats. *Traditional Chinese Medicinal Research*, **7**, 19-21.

[20] Xiong, Z.L., Guo, X.J., Xu, Y. and Li, F.M. (2002) Effect of Extracts from Qing'e Pill on the Proliferation and Differentiation of Osteoblast-Like Cells UMR106. *Pharmacology and Clinics of Chinese Materia Medica*, **18**, 3-5.

[21] Ling, J.Y., Shen, L., Liu, Q., Xue, S. and Zhu, R. (2013) Effect of Xiaoyu Zhixue Tablet on Expression of Platelet Membrane Glycoprotein I b α and Quality of Life in Patients with Menorrhagia. *Acta Medicinae Universitatis Scientiae et Technologiae Huazhong*, **42**, 601-604.

[22] Shuai, B., Shen, L., Yang, Y.P., Xie, J., Zhou, P.Q., Xu, X.J., Li, C.G. and Wu, M.X. (2012) Effect of Bushenhuoxue Decoction on the Osteogenic Differentiation of Bone Marrow Stromal Cells in the Steroid Induced Osteonecrosis of the Femoral Head. *Research of Integrated Traditional Chinese and Western Medicine*, **4**, 297-301.

13

Acute Kidney Injury: Treatment with Unani Medicine—Case Report

Muhammad Shakil Ahmad Siddiqui[1,2*], Khan Usmanghani[2]

[1]Rafah-e-Aam Dawakhana Ajmali (Clinics) and Rafah-e-Aam Herbal Laboratories, Karachi, Pakistan
[2]Faculty of Eastern Medicine, Hamdard University, Karachi, Pakistan
Email: [*]rafaheaam@gmail.com

Abstract

A male named Anwer Jamal, age 45 years, married, visited Clinic Rafaheaam Dawakhana Ajmali on March 29, 2013, with history of glomerulonephritis, inherited renal diseases, hypertension and previously hooked on voltaren 50 (Diclofenic Sodium, 50 mg) and was not on dialysis. Different diagnostic parameters showed the patient was suffering from acute renal failure according to the RIFLE criteria. AKI is life threatening when kidneys suddenly is unable to filter waste products from blood. The patient was treated and managed with herbal medicines according to Unani system of medicine. Reversal of the parameter such as serum creatinine from 7.90 mg/dl (6.58 fold high) to 0.81mg/dl within two weeks clearly shows the remarkable recovery in a short period of time. During this period the other related parameters e.g. blood urea nitrogen (BUN), serum albumin, albuminuria, blood pressure were also normalized whereas clinical sign and symptom exhibited improvement.

Keywords

Acute Kidney Injury, Diagnosis, Unani Treatment, Outcome

1. Introduction

Acute Kidney injury is characterized by the sudden impairment of function occurring over a period of hours and days. A diagnose of AKI is made on the basis of presence of elevated serum creatinine and/or blood urea nitrogen (BUN) levels and/or decreased urine out put, despite their well known limitation. Therefore, acute kidney injury is the abrupt loss of kidney function resulting in the retention of urea and other nitrogenous waste products and in the dysregulation of extra cellular volume and electrolytes. The acute kidney injury specifies the sudden reduction in kidney function and is associated with morbidity and mortality. The acute renal failure cases

*Corresponding author.

are quite increasing in those patients with critical illnesses and drug adverse reactions. The causes are attributed sepsis [1], chronic dialysis [2], and varied critical condition. The procedures in clinical care adopted are ventilation, vasoactive intravenous medications, nutritional support, and dialysis. The aim of this article is to exhibit the implication and usefulness of Unani (herbal) medicine synergistic effects to obtain optimal patient outcomes in the following case study of kidney injury. Unani medicine is comprehensive system of medicine prevalent in south Asia including Pakistan. In this system the naturally occurring substances, mostly herbal medicine are used for the treatment of different types of diseases including kidney. Single medicine (Muffradat) is preferred over compound (Murrakabat) formulations for balancing the homeostasis of the body [3].

2. Case Presentation

A 45-year-old man was visited to the Clinic at Rafaheaam Dawakhana Ajmali, Karachi, on March, 31, 2013, with the complain of recurrent right flank pain, generalized swelling, bilateral pedal edema, anorexia, constipation, insomnia epigastric pain, fatigue, nausea, vomiting and mild fever without shivering, head ache and history of dark brown urine 2 days before, no mass or tenderness in the renal pelvis. The patient had a history of extensive use of NSAID e.g. volteran 50 for lumber pain. The patient had a history of hypertension for the last 8 years; renal stone cleared 9 years back and no history of diabetes, tuberculosis and ischemic heard disease. Whereas pain in the right lumber since last many years. The patient had complained of hematuria and renal stone in 1997.

The patient had been evaluated at Hospital Sind Institute of Urology and Transplantation (SIUT), Karachi, on March 29, 2013, where he was evaluated for ultrasound of KUB, CBC, blood urea, serum creatinine, serum electrolytes and urine D/R. ultrasound study shows; right kidney mild echogenic, mild fullness at proximal ureter; no stone seen. left kidney is echogenic. CBC; Hb 12.5G/dl, Htc 35.9%, WBC 9.5 × $10E^9$/L, platelets 402 × $10E^9$/L, urea 139 mg/dl, serum creatinine 7.90 mg/dl, sodium 126 meq/L, potassium 4.2 meq/L, chloride 101 meq/L, bicarbonate 19 meq/L, in urine albumin^{3+} present. The blood pressure was 180/100 mm·Hg. No surgical history found. Patient has family history of kidney disease, hypertension, diabetes maternal and history of hypertension and cardiac disease in paternal. O/E_chest clear, cardiac S_1 $S_{2,}$ audible, no murmur, bilateral pedal edema present, P/A abdomen soft, no mass or hardness found. On examination at March 30, 2013, generalized swelling present, abdomen was soft no tenderness found and blood pressure was 180/110.

On March 31, 2013, the temperature was 99.0˚F, the blood pressure 140/80 mm·Hg, the pulse 68 bpm, the respiratory rate 14 breaths per minute. generalized and orbital edema moderate, skin dry, taste of mouth bitter, nausea mild, vomiting mild, no hiccup, right lumber pain moderate, urine output low, constipation moderate, abdomen was soft whereas rest of the examination was otherwise normal.

On 02 April, 2013, temperature was 99.0˚F, blood pressure 170/80 mm·Hg, pulse 70 b/min., lumber pain moderate, nausea mild, and no vomiting and mild headache present. Biochemistry was: BUN 72 mg/dl, Serum albumin 2.76 g/dl, serum calcium 7.97 mg/dl, serum electrolyte levels was sodium 130 mEq/l, potassium 4.4 mEq/l, chloride 96 mEq/l, bicarbonate 26 mEq/l. Urinalysis showed a pH of 6.0, specific gravity 1.015, protein 3.0 g/l$^{(+3)}$ Occult blood negative; there were 8 - 10 pus cells, red cells nil, no cast and moderate bacteria.

On 03 April, 2013, ultrasound report was both kidneys appear slightly echogenic. No lesion was seen in liver, gall bladder, common bile duct, pancreas, spleen and retroperitoneum. On 04 April, 2013, Serum creatinine level was 5.10 mg/dl.

On 5 April, 2013, temperature was 99.0˚F, BP. 160/90 mm·Hg., generalized and orbital edema moderate, lumber pain moderate, nausea mild, pulse 70 b/min., epigastric burning moderate, skin normal, nausea mild, no vomiting, urine output low, constipation mild.

On 08 April, 2013, temperature was 98.6, B.P. 140/80 mm·Hg., Pulse 70 b/min. generalized edema moderate, orbital edema moderate, sleep was normal, pedal edema mild, no nausea, no vomiting, right lumber pain mild and urine output increased.

On 12 April, 2013, temperature was 98.6˚F, B.P. 125/80 mm·Hg., pulse 72b/min., no generalized, orbital, pedal edema, right lumber pain mild, mild epigastric burning, no nausea, no vomiting, Mouth taste was normal, sleep normal.

On 15 April, 2013, laboratory reports was; BUN 5.6 mg/dl., S. creatinine 0.81 mg/dl., S. albumin 2.86 g/dl., HbA1c 5.4%; urine detail report was specific gravity 1020, pH 6.0, protein^{+3}, pus cells 8 - 10, RBC nil, cast granular 4 - 5/LPF, bacteria few.

20 April, 2013 temperature was 99.0˚F, B.P. 120/80 mm·Hg, no edema, lumber pain mild, no nausea, no vo-

miting, no epigastric burning, bowl movement normal, urine output normal but the medicine used continue for more days.

According to RIFLE criteria (**Table 1**) of kidney damages classification; the patient is frame on the elevation of serum creatinine basis. The patient's serum creatinine level was 7.90 mg/dl. This increase in the level of serum creatinine is 6.58 folds from the baseline 1.2 mg/dl. It is renal failure Stage 3.

The patient kidney functions and other tests are given in **Table 2**.

3. Unani (Herbal) Medicine [4]

Unani Prescription 1. ***Majun Mussafi Khas***: Chob Chini (*Smilax chinensi* Linn) 300 mg, Sana Makki (*Cassia senna* Linn) 200 mg, Turbud (*Ipomea turpenthum R.Br.*) 50 mg Nigand Babri (*Vitex negundo* Linn) 200 mg, and **Qurs Rasoot**: Rasoot (*Berberis aristata D.C.*) 160 mg, Haleela Zard (*Terminalia chebula* Retz half ripe fruit) 160 mg. at morning; **Qurs Podina**: Zinjabeel (*Zingiber officinale* Rosc) 100 mg, Kala Zeera (*Carum carvi* Linn) 100 mg, Podina (*Mentha piperita* Linn) 150 mg, Ajwain (*Trachyspermum ammi* (L.) Sprague) 150 mg, Filfil Daraz (*Piper longum* Linn) 0.2 mg. at noon after lunch; **Habb e Sibr** (*Aloe vera* L. Burm f.) 100mg for constipation, **Itrifal Kishnizi**: Haleela Zard (*Terminalia chebula Retz*) 0.43 mg, and Haleela Siyah (*Terminelia chebula* Retz. uripe fruit) 0.21 mg and Kashneez (*Coriandrum sativum* Linn) 0.21 mg, **Hab-e-Fishar** (*Rauwolfia serpentina* (L.) Benth ex Kurz) 1.20 mg (for blood pressure) at night after meal. This prescription was used for 4 days.

Unani Prescription 2. ***Majun Mussafi Khas***: Chob Chini (*Smilax chinensi* Linn) 300 mg, Sana Makki (*Cassia senna* Linn) 150 mg, Turbud (*Ipomea turpenthum R.Br.*) 50 mg Nigand Babri (*Vitex negundo* Linn) 150 mg, **Sherbet Bazoori**: Each dose 25 ml contains aqueous extract Kasni (*Cichorium intybus* Linn) 2.0 mg, Kharpazza (*Cucumis melo* Linn 2.0 mg), Badyan (*Foeniculum vulgare* Mill) 2.0 mg and Sodium bicarbonate Tablet after meal; **Itrifal Kishnizi**: Haleela Zard (*Terminalia chebula Retz*) 0.43 mg, and Haleela Siyah (*Terminelia chebula* Retz. uripe fruit) 0.21 mg and Kashneez (*Coriandrum sativum* Linn) 0.21 mg. at night administered for 16 days.

Unani Prescription 3. ***Jawarish Zarooni Saida***: Badiyan (*Foeniculum vulgare* Mill) 1.50 mg, Filfil Siyah (*Piper nigrum* Linn.) 1.50 mg, Ajwain (*Trachyspermum ammi* (L.) *Sprague*) 1.50 mg, Post Beikh Karafs (*Apium graveolence* Linn.) 1.50 mg, Qaranfal (*Caryophyllus aromatica* Linn.) 1.50 mg, Tukhme Gazer (*Daucus carota* Linn.) 1.50 mg, Tukhme Karafs (*Apium graveolence* Linn.) 1.50 mg, Tukhme Kharpaza *Cucumis melo* Linn.) 1.50 mg, Aqirqarha (*Anacylus pyrethrum DC.*) 0.6 mg, Bisbasa (*Myristica fragrans* Houtt) 0.6 mg, Dar Chini-

Table 1. Risk of renal failure, injury to kidney, failure of kidney function, loss of kidney function, and end-stage renal failure (RIFLE) and Acute Kidney Injury Network (AKIN) classification schemes for Acute Kidney Injury (AKI).

Rifle	Serum creatinine criteria	UO criteria	AKIN criteria	Serum creatinine criteria	UO criteria	Jamal case at base line HK SHAKIL	Jamal case at conclusion of therapy HK SHAKIL
Risk	Increase in serum creatinine ≥ 1.5 × baseline or decrease in GFR ≥ 25%	< 0.5 mL·kg^{-1}·h^{-1} for ≥ 6 h	Stage 1	Increasde in serum creatinine ≥ 0.3 mg dL^{-1} (≥ 26.4 mg·dL^{-1}) or increase ≥ 1.5 × base line	< 0.5 mL·kg^{-1}·h^{-1} for ≥ 6 h		
Injury	Injury increase in serum creatinine ≥ 2.0 × baseline or decrease in GFR ≥ 50%	< 0.5 mL·kg^{-1}·h^{-1} for ≥ 12 h	Stage 2	Increase in serum creatinine ≥ 2 × baseline	< 0.5 mL·kg^{-1}·h^{-1} for ≥12 h		
Failure	Failure increase in serum creatinine ≥ 3.0 × baseline or decrease in GFR ≥ 75%	< 0.3 mL·kg^{-1}·h^{-1} ≥ 24 h or anuria ≥ 12 h ≥ 12 h	Stage 3	Increase in serum creatinine ≥ 3 × baseline or serum creatinine ≥ 4.0 mg·dL^{-1} (354 μmol·L^{-1}) with an acute rise of at least 0.5 mg·dL^{-1} (44 μmol·L^{-1}) or initiation of RRT	< 0.3 mL·kg^{-1}·h^{-1} ≥ 24 h or anuria ≥ 12 h	On March 29, 2013 7.90 mg·dL^{-1}	On April 15, 2013 0.81 mg·dL^{-1}
Loss	Complete loss of kidney function 94 wk						
ESKD	Complete loss of kidney function 93 mo						

ESKD indicates end-stage kidney disease; GFR, glomerular filtration rate; RRT, renal replacement therapy.

Table 2. Pateint kidney function tests.

TEST	29-03-2013 Before treatment	02-04-2013	04-04-2013	15-04-2013 After treatment	06-04-2013 Follow up	08-05-2013 Follow up	12-05-2013 Follow up	Normal range
Hemoglobin	12.50							0.85 - 1.35 mg dL
Creatinine	7.90		5.10	0.81		0.87	0.76	0.85 - 1.35 mg dL
BUN	64.9	72.0		5.6				5.20 mg dL
Albumin, Serum		2.76		2.86				3.5 - 5.2 mg dL
Urine albumin	+3	+3		+3		0	0	NIL
Pus cells		10	10			2	6	1-2
RBC		0						NIL
Cast				5G				NIL
Bacteria		MOD		Few			Few	NIL
Calcium		7.79						8.6 - 10.2
Chloride		96						104 - 114 mEq/l
Sodium		130						136 - 146 mEq/l
Potassium		4.4						3.6 - 5.1 mEq/l
Bicarbonate		26						23 - 29 mEq/l
Blood Pressure	180/100	170/95	160/90	142/85	120/80			

(*Cinnamomum zeylanicum* Linn) 0.6 mg, bid for 15 days.

The patient was treated at Rafah-e-Aam Dawakhana Ajmali (Clinics), Karachi and was prescribed and administred the Unani (herbal) compound and simple medicine as mentioned earlier. The treatment was started on March 29, 2013, at first Unani preparation I for four days, thereafter, Unani preparation 2 was given for 16 days, and the patient recovered from creatinine and other biochemical and physiological parameters. In order to stabilize patient general health paradigm Unani preparation 3 was then continued for 15 days. During the treatment the following clinical and pathological features were observed.

4. Follow-Up

The follow up monitoring of the patient was carried out. On 08 May, 2013, test repeated report was serum creatinine 0.87 mg/dl. urine specific gravity 1020, pH 6.0, protein nil, blood nil, us cells nil, cast nil, crystals nil, bacteria nil. patient was evaluated clinically and blood pressure was 120/80 mm·Hg, no lumber pain, no edema, urine output was normal all other complains were also normal.

Whereas on June 12, 2013, the serum creatinine 0.76 mg/dl, and urinary creatinine 100.8 mg/dl. were reported, urine D/R specific gravity 1.030, pH 6.0, albumin negative, blood nil pus cell 4 - 6/HPF, RBC, casts, crystals were nil, bacteria reported few and 24 hrs. The creatinine clearance reported at 64.4 ml/min. (60 - 170 mg dL).

5. Discussion

Approximately (1% to 2%) free creatine in muscles irreversibly converts to creatinine which in turn released into blood and ultimately excreted by the kidney [5]. It has been cited in the literature that herbal treatment was initiated treatment by utilizing over the counter herbal dosage form design that resulted in the improvement of laboratory parameter for cases of chronic renal failure. Herbal Chinese Formula: *Rehmaniae* Rx, *Dioscoreae* Rz, *Corni* Fr, *Poria cocos* Rx, *Alismatis* Rz, *Cinnamomi* Cx, *Aconiti* Rx. Ayurvedic Herbal Formula: *Didymocarpus pedicellata, Saxifraga ligulata, Rubia cardifolia, Ocimum basilicum, Achyranthes aspera, Cyperus rotundus, Crataeva religiosa*, and *Uva ursi*. Nagasaka and associates [6] have reported four cases of chronic renal failure effectively treated with *Astragalis* radix. Where in it reduces serum creatinine level, but it did not improve BUN, proteinuria and anemia [7]. Zhong et all in a review article have cited that Traditional Chinese herbal medications are utilized for treatment of chronic kidney diseases in China and many other Asian countries. These are decoction of *Astragalus* with *Angelica sinensis, Rheum palmatum L* and its components: emodin and rhein, decoctions of *Radix bupleuri* and components of *R. bupleuri* (saikosaponin a and d), *Cordyceps sinensis* and its component H1-A, Extracts of *Tripterygium wilfordii* Hook and component Triptolide (PG490), have been used to treat glomerulonephritis, calcium influx inhibition, vasodilatation, antithrombosis, antioxidation, anti-inflammation, and immune regulation, decreases proteinuria and improves the plasma levels of total cholesterol and albumin in patients with nephrotic syndrome, treatment decreased proteinuria and glomerulosclerosis, decreased urinary protein excretion in a rat model of subtotal nephrectom [8].

Acute kidney injury has become increasingly prevalent in Pakistan and uncertainty about the incidence of acute kidney injury limits awareness of the problem and its treatment modes. The reason could be gastroenteritis, or infections, diarrhea, poisoning, malaria, or septic abortion. The treatment is costly in developing regions, so the herbal medicine therapy could be an alternate to eradicate causes of acute kidney injury, and here we report evidence-based management.

6. Conclusion

Unani herbal preparations have resolved acute kidney injury within 20 days, as analyzed by the BUN, serum creatinine and 24 hour serum creatinine clearance levels. Further follow up for another 15 days showed sustained improvement. Monitoring for another 15 days showed sustained improvement. Serum creatinine does not rise to abnormal levels until a large proportion of the renal mass is damaged, because the relationship between the glomerular filtration rate (GFR) and the serum creatinine level is not linear, especially early in disease. The data presented clearly represent where in creatinine level on March 29, 2013 at 7.90 mg dL and on April 15, 2013 it decrease to 0.81 mg dL. Similarly the urine output gave better results and also the patient kidney function tests consisting of such as hemoglobin, BUN, albumin serum, urine albumin, pus cells, RBC, Cast, bacteria, calcium chloride, potassium, sodium, bicarbonate, blood pressure, HbA_1C after herbal treatment came within the normal range and matched with controls. The early treatment can help to optimize management and avoid the preventable complications of acute kidney injury.

References

[1] Kosinski, M. (2009) What's Old Is New again: AKI and ARF. 2009 NTI and Critical Care Exposition. AACN. www.aacn.org
http://www.aacn.org/wd/nti/nti2009/docs/nti_program_schedule_booklet.pdf

[2] Uchino, J., Kellum, A., Bellomo, R., Gordon, S., Doig, Y., Morimatsu, H., Morgera, S., Schetz, M., Tan, I., Bouman, C., Macedo, E., Gibney, N., Tolwani, A. and Ronco, C. (2005) Acute Renal Failure in Critically Ill Patients A Multinational, Multicenter Study. *JAMA*, **294**, 813-818. http://dx.doi.org/10.1001/jama.294.7.813

[3] http://apps.who.int/medicinedocs/documents/s17558en/s17558en.pdf

[4] Kabir, H. (2003) Murakkabat (Unani Formulation). Shamsher Publication & Distributor, Aligarh, 63, 80.

[5] Newman and Price, F.C. (2001) Non Protein Nitrogen Metabolites. In: Burtis, C.A. and Ashwood, A.R., Eds., *Tietz Fundamental of Clinical Chemistry*, W.B. Saunders Company, Philadelphia, 414-422.

[6] Nagasaka, K., Fukuda, H., Watanabe, T. and Ngata, Y. (2012) Report on Four Cases of Chronic Renal Failure Effectively Treated with Astragali Radix. *Kampo Medicine*, **63**, 98-102. http://dx.doi.org/10.3937/kampomed.63.98

[7] Chang, C.H., Lin, C.Y., Tian, Y.C., Jenq, C.C., Chang, M.Y., Chen, Y.C., Fang, J.T. and Yang, C.W. (2010) Acute Kidney Injury Classification: Comparison of AKIN and RIFLE Criteria. *SHOCK*, **33**, 247-252.
http://dx.doi.org/10.1097/SHK.0b013e3181b2fe0c

[8] Zhong, Y., Deng, Y., Chen, Y., Chuang, P.Y. and He, J.C. (2013) Therapeutic Use of Traditional Chinese Herbal Medications for Chronic Kidney Diseases. *Kidney International*, **84**, 1108-1118.

14

Hepatoprotective and Antioxidant Effects of *Salvia officinalis* L. Hydroalcoholic Extract in Male Rats

Khakpour Shahrzad[1], Najari Mahya[2], Tokazabani Belasei Fatemeh[2], Khosravi Maryam[2], Farhadi Belasei Mohammadreza[3], Mahsa Hadipour Jahromy[1*]

[1]Tehran Medical Sciences Branch, Physiology and Pharmacology Research Laboratories of Medical Sciences Research Centre, Islamic Azad University, Tehran, Iran
[2]Tehran North Branch, Islamic Azad University, Tehran, Iran
[3]Ghazvin Medical Sciences University, Ghazvin, Iran
Email: [*]Jahromymh@yahoo.com

Abstract

The antioxidant effects of *Salvia officinalis* L. hydroalcoholic extract and also its hepatoprotective effects in male rats were evaluated. *Salvia officinalis* L. extract was administered intraperitoneally for 28 days. Serum levels of aspartate aminotransferase, alanine transferase and alkaline phosphates in rats coadministered with both isoniazid (INH) 50 mg/kg and *Salvia officinalis* L. extract at 250 mg/kg showed significant reduction when compared to INH group, but administration of *Salvia officinalis* L. extract 250 mg/kg alone and with INH has alleviated gamma-glutamyl transferase comparing to INH receiving rats. After treatment of rats with INH 50mg/kg, severe tissue necrosis, and inflammation of central vein in liver and lymphocyte proliferation were observed; in the experimental group receiving *Salvia officinalis* L. extract (250 mg/kg) mild dilution in central vein and sinusoids in liver were seen. In rats coadministered with *Salvia officinalis* L. extract 250 mg/kg and INH low sinusoids dilution was indicated. It seems that *Salvia officinalis* L. extract exhibited anti-oxidative and hepatoprotective effects.

Keywords

***Salvia officinalis* L., Antioxidant Effects, Rat**

1. Introduction

Oxygen free radicals or, more generally, reactive oxygen species (ROS) are believed to be involved in the etiol-

[*]Corresponding author.

ogy of certain diseases [1] [2]. The biological effects of ROS are controlled *in vivo* by enzymatic and non-enzymatic mechanisms. But, in some conditions, these effects cannot be controlled and lead cell damages. In such cases, exogenous antioxidants can be useful. Among the drugs, Isoniazid (INH) induces oxidative stress, which is one of the mechanisms responsible for cytotoxicity [3]. For these purposes, natural plant products have been used since ancient times. *Salvia officinalis* L. (Lamiaceae) is among the plants to which hypolipidaemic properties have been attributed by traditional medicine; it is a common aromatic plant, which is distributed widely in the Mediterranean and the Middle East countries. Studies on the leaves, roots and water soluble extractions of *Salvia officinalis* L. showed that they contain volatile fatty acids, diterpens, saponins, flavonoids, phenolic acids, resin and oestrogenic substances [4]-[7]. In the present study, we evaluate antioxidant effects of *Salvia officinalis* L. hydroalcoholic extract and its therapeutic effect to counteract liver damage in male rats.

2. Materials and Methods

Salvia officinalis L. plants were collected from Kordan area of Karaj in Iran. The aerial parts of plants were lyophilized and kept at −20˚C. Hydroalcoholic extract was prepared using food grade ethanol and deionised water (96 and 4%, respectively). Male Wistar rats (180 ± 20 g) were purchased from Tehran Pasteur Institute (Iran) and acclimated to our laboratory animal facilities for at least one week before the start of the experiments. During this period, the animals were maintained on a natural light/dark cycle at 20˚C ± 2˚C and given food and tap water *ad libitum*. The animals were kept and handled in accordance to our University regulations that follows the *Guidelines for the Human Use and Care of Laboratory Animals*. The rats were randomly divided into 8 groups (7 rats each) as follows: Group 1, healthy control rats received distilled water as sole drinking source; Group 2 received Isoniazid (INH), 50 mg/kg orally by gavage; Groups 3, 4 and 5 were treated intraperitoneally (IP) with *Salvia officinalis* L. hydroalcoholic extract with the doses 100, 250 and 400 mg/kg, respectively; Groups 6, 7 and 8 were coadministered with Isoniazid (50 mg/kg) and *Salvia officinalis* L. hydroalcoholic extract 100, 250 and 400 mg/kg, respectively. All the treatments were done for 28 days. Hepatotoxicity of Isoniazid, and *Salvia officinalis* L. hydroalcoholic extract effects were then evaluated. Also changes in aspartate aminotransferase (AST), alanine aminotransferase (ALT), alkaline phosphates (ALP), gamma-glutamyltransferase (GGT) levels were assessed. At the end of the experiment, animals were sacrificed by cervical dislocation and blood plasma was collected. A fresh piece of the liver from each rat with approximately 2 mm thickness, was rapidly immersed in Bouin's solution and kept for 24 h at 4˚C. Fixed tissues were then processed routinely for embedding in paraffin, sectioned (5 μm), deparaffinized and rehydrated using standard techniques. The extent of liver damage was evaluated based on morphological changes in liver sections stained with hematoxylin and eosin (H & E) using standard techniques.

Statistical Analysis

Data are expressed as means ± SEM. The comparison between the means of treatments and control group was performed using Student's *t*-test. *P* values ≤ 0.05 were considered statistically significant.

3. Results

3.1. Effects on Liver Enzymes

Serum level of AST in rats coadministered with both INH and plant extract at 250 and 400 mg/kg showed significant reduction when compared to INH group, that may indicate the antioxidant effects of the plant extract while no differences were seen with control (**Figure 1**). At all plant extract concentrations, specially at 250 mg/kg, serum ALT level significantly reduced when coadministered with INH compared to both INH and control group (**Figure 2**). Evaluation of GGT in all groups revealed that the plant extract at doses of 100 and 250 mg/kg alone and with INH 50 mg/kg, has alleviated the enzyme comparing to INH receiving rats (**Figure 3**). Coadministration of the plant extract at concentrations of 250 and 400 mg/kg with INH again showed significant reduction in ALP serum level statistically (**Figure 4**).

3.2. Liver Histopathology Study

Histopathology effects of the plant extract on rat liver have been also studied in all groups. All microscopic ob-

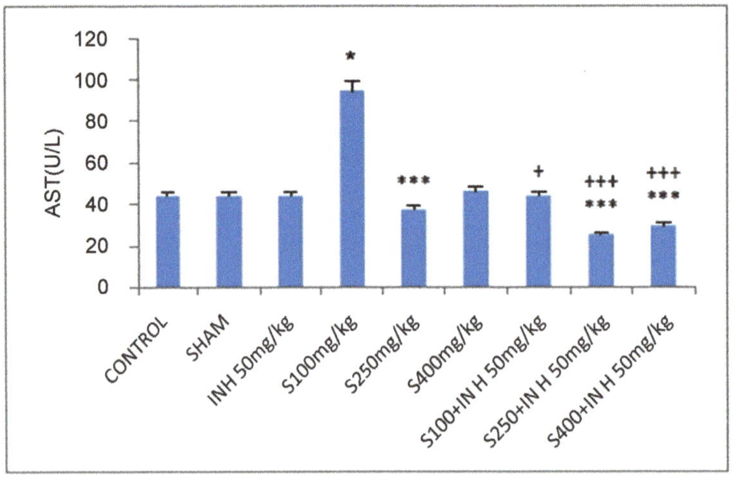

Figure 1. Serum level of AST in rats in different groups; s = plant extract, INH = Isoniazid. *: compared to control, +: compared to INH group. P < 0.001.

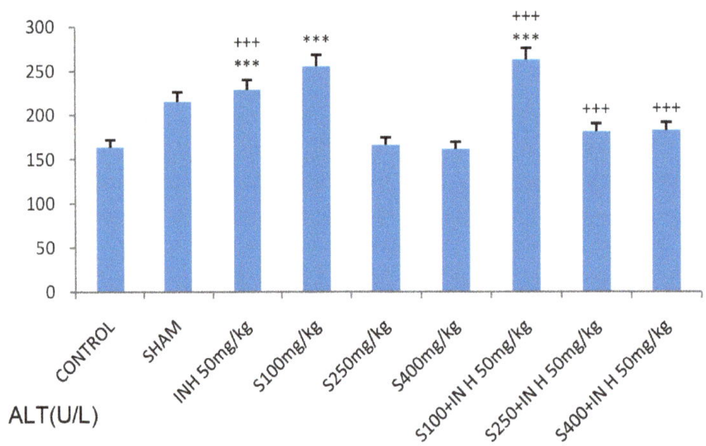

Figure 2. Serum level of ALT in rats in different groups; s = plant extract, INH = Isoniazid. *: compared to control, +: compared to INH group. P < 0.001.

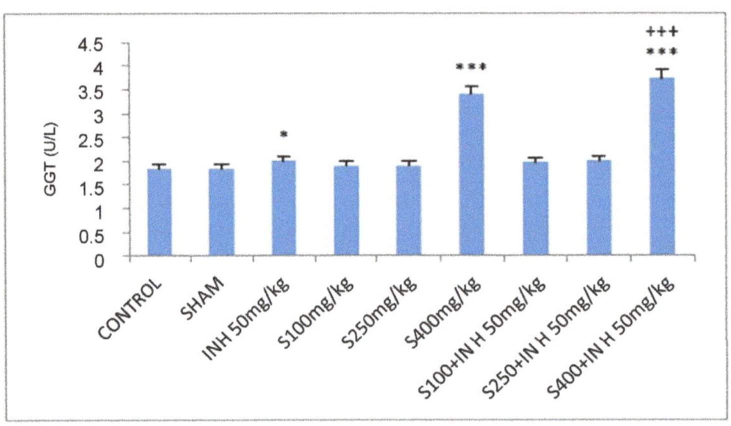

Figure 3. Serum level of GGT in rats in different groups; s = plant extract, INH = Isoniazid. *: compared to control, +: compared to INH group. P < 0.001.

servations have been performed and reported by a pathology expert. **Figure 5** shows the normal liver section stained with H & E. After treatment of rats with INH 50 mg/kg for 28 days, severe tissue necrosis, and inflammation of central vein in liver and lymphocyte proliferations were observed (**Figure 6**). **Figure 7** shows the mild dilution in central vein and sinusoids in rat liver received the plant extract 250 mg/kg. Finally the liver histopathology alterations in rats coadministered with the plant extract 250 mg/kg and INH is shown in **Figure 8** that indicating low sinusoids dilution.

4. Discussion

In the present study, the protective role of the plant extract on liver has been emphasized. Interestingly, at different plant concentrations, the biochemical parameter changes and histopathology studies revealed marked reduction in INH-induced hepatic damage. In this research, first hepatotoxicities in rats were produced by administering INH (50 mg/kg) orally for 28 days. A significant rise above the normal upper limits in the measured serum transaminases was considered a biochemical indication of liver injury. Increased oxidative stress play a role in the development of liver injury induced by INH [8] [9]. Previous reports in rats suggest that the hydra zine metabolite of INH which has subsequent effect on CYP2E1 induction is involved in the development of

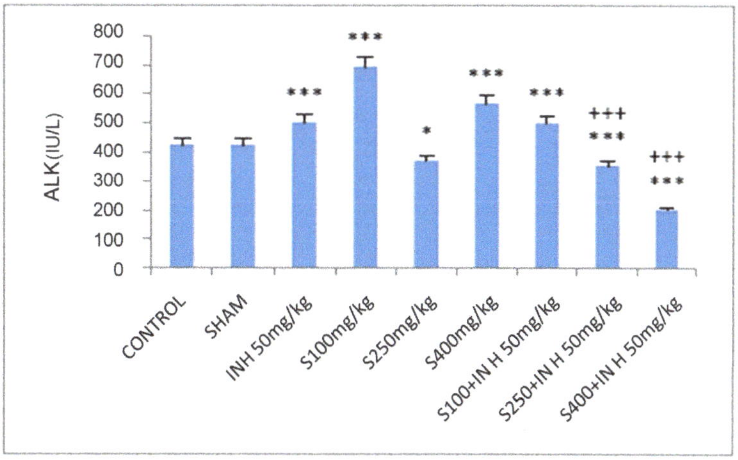

Figure 4. Serum level of ALK in rats in different groups; s = plant extract, INH = Isoniazid. *: compared to control, +: compared to INH group. $P < 0.001$.

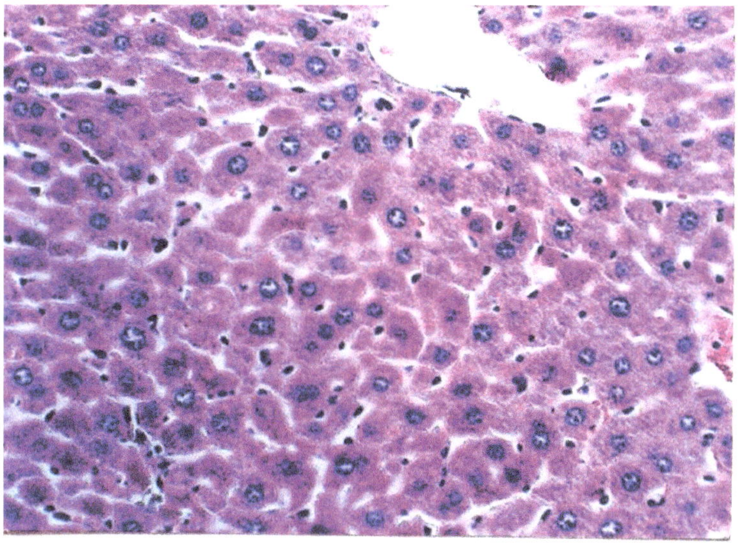

Figure 5. Microscopic photo of normal rat liver stained with H & E ×400.

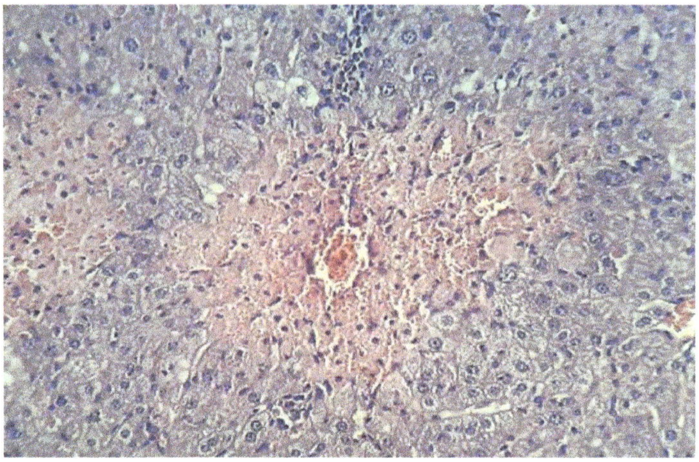

Figure 6. Microscopic photo of rat liver treated with INH 50 mg/kg stained with H & E ×200.

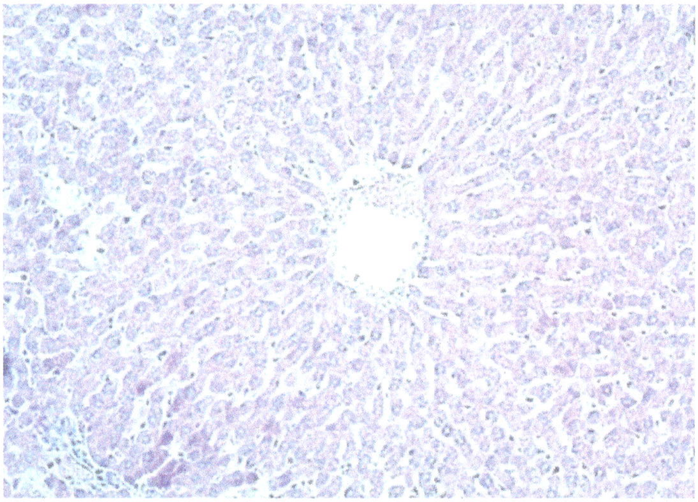

Figure 7. Microscopic photo of rat liver treated with plant extract 250 mg/kg stained with H & E ×200.

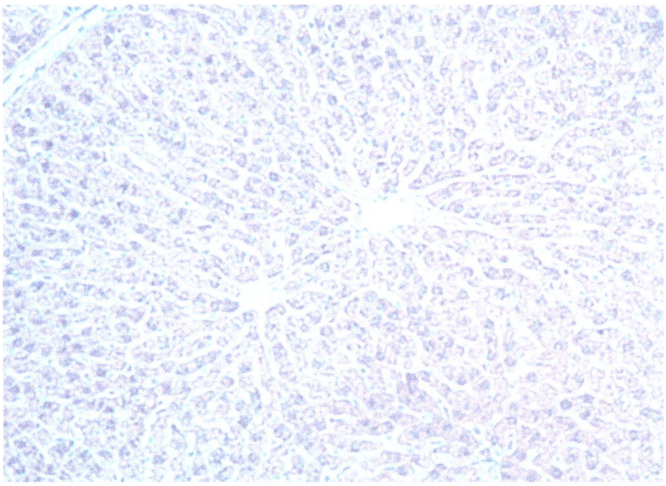

Figure 8. Microscopic photo of rat liver treated with both INH 50 mg/kg and plant extract 250 mg/kg stained with H & E ×200.

INH-induced hepatotoxicity, and also oxidative stress as one of the mechanism for INH induced hepatic injury [8]-[10].

Oxidative stress is involved in the pathogenesis of many complications in animals and humans. Excessive oxidative stress causes exceeding free radicals product especially reactive oxygen species (ROS). ROS has been known to produce cellular and tissue injury through covalent binding, DNA strand breaking, lipid peroxidation (LPO) and augment fibrosis [11] [12].

The liver is regarded as one of the central metabolic organs, regulating and maintaining homeostasis. The increase in the level of AST, ALT, ALP and GGT are important indices for hepatic damage. Amino transferases are present in high concentration in liver, an important class of enzymes linking carbohydrate and amino acid metabolism. In cases of liver damage with hepatocellular lesions and parenchymal cell necrosis, these marker enzymes are released from the damaged tissues into the blood stream [10] [12].

In the present study, the activities of these enzymes were found to increase in the hepatotoxic animals, and were significantly reduced in groups of the plant extract administered rats as compared to that of toxicant rats. This confirms the protective effect of the extract against INH induced hepatic damage. The effect was more pronounced with 250 mg/kg extract.

So far, hepatoprptective effects of many plant extract have been reported. Possible mechanism of all of the extracts including presenting herb as hepatoprotective may be due to their anti-oxidant effects or inhibition of cytochrome P450. This might be due to the high contents of polyphenoles present in the extract which could have reduced the production and/or accumulation of toxic derived metabolites [11] [13]-[19]. Histopathological examination of the liver section of the rats treated with INH showed intense centrilobular necrosis and vacuolization. The rats treated with the plant extract and extracts along with toxicant showed sign of protection against these toxicants to considerable extent as evident from formation of normal hepatic cards and absence of necrosis. The hepatoprotective effect of the extract may be explained depending on the fact that it contains polyphenolic compounds like toyon, cineole and camphor which may scavenge free radicals offering hepatic protection and its antioxidant potential mechanism suggesting that the extract of plant may be useful to prevent the oxidative stress induced damage. More research is required in this point of view to develop a suitable hepatoprotective drug from the plant extract. Purification of extracts and identification of the active ingredient may yield to introduce active hepatoprotective agents.

5. Conclusion

The results of this study indicate that *Salvia officinalis* L. extract has hepatoprotective action against INH induced hepatic damage in rats. This study suggests that possible mechanism of this activity may be due to free radical-scavenging and antioxidant activities which might be attributed to the presence of flavonoids in the extract.

References

[1] Temple, N.J. (2000) Antioxidants and Disease: More Questions than Answers. *Nutrition Research*, **20**, 449-459. http://dx.doi.org/10.1016/S0271-5317(00)00138-X

[2] Sa, C.M., Ramos., A.A., Azevedo, M.F., Lima., C.F., Fernandes-Ferreira, M. and Pereira-Wilson, C. (2009) Sage Tea Drinking Improves Lipid Profile and Antioxidant Defences in Humans. *International Journal of Molecular Sciences*, **10**, 3937-3950. http://dx.doi.org/10.3390/ijms10093937

[3] Yilmaz, H.R., Uz, E., Gokalp, O., Ozcelik, N., Cicek, E. and Ozer, M.K. (2008) Protective Role of Caffeic Acid Phenethyl Ester and Erdosteine on Activities of Purine-Catabolizing Enzymes and Level of Nitric Oxide in Red Blood Cells of Isoniazid-Administered Rats. T*oxicology and Industrial Health*, **24**, 519-524. http://dx.doi.org/10.1177/0748233708098128

[4] Miliauskas, G., Venskutonis, P.R. and Van Beek, T. (2004) Screening of Radical Scavenging Activity of Some Medicinal and Aromatic Plant Extract. *Food Chemistry*, **85**, 231-237.

[5] Slamenova, D., Masterova, I., Labaj, J., Horvathova, H., Kubala, P., Jakubikova, J. and Wsolova, I. (2004) Cytotoxic and DNA-Damaging Effects of Diterpenoid Quinines from the Roots of *Salvia officinalis* L. on Colonic and Hepatic Human Cells Cultured *in Vitro*. *Basic & Clinical Pharmacology & Toxicology*, **94**, 282-290. http://dx.doi.org/10.1111/j.1742-7843.2004.pto940605.x

[6] Lima, C.F., Andrade, P.B., Rosa, M.S., Fernandes, M.F. and Wilson, C.P. (2005) The Drinking of *Salvia officinalis*.

Infusion Liver Antioxidant Status in Mice and Rats. *Journal of Ethnopharmacology*, **97**, 383-389. http://dx.doi.org/10.1016/j.jep.2004.11.029

[7] Yurtseven. S., Cetin, M., Sengul, T. and Sogut, B. (2008) Effect of Sage Extract (*Salvia officinalis*) on Growth Performance, Blood Parameters, Oxidative Stress and DNA Damage in Partridges. *South African Journal of Animal Science*, **38**.

[8] Ravinder, P. Kim, V. Arbab, S. Kartar, S.and Satya, V.R. (2006) Effect of Garlic on Isoniazid and Rifampicin-Induced Hepatic Injury in Rats. *World Journal of Gastroenterology*, **12**, 636-639.

[9] Thattakudian Sheik Uduman, M.S., Sundarapandian, R., Muthumanikkam, A., *et al.* (2011) Protective Effects of Methanolic Extract of Annona Squamosa Linn in Isoniazid-Rifampicin Induced Hepatotoxicity in Rats. *Pakistan Journal of Pharmaceutical Sciences*, **24**, 129-134.

[10] Kaplowitz, N. (2001) Drug-Induced Liver Disorders: Implications for Drug Development and Regulation. *Drug Safety*, **24**, 483-490. http://dx.doi.org/10.2165/00002018-200124070-00001

[11] Srinivasan, R., Chandrasekar, M.J.N., Nanjan, M.J. and Suresh, B. (2007) Antioxidant Activity of Caesalpiniadigyna Root. *Journal of Ethnopharmacology*, **113**, 284-291. http://dx.doi.org/10.1016/j.jep.2007.06.006

[12] Gao, M., Li, Y. and Yang, J. (2011) Protective Effect of Pedicularisdecora Franch Root Extracts on Oxidative Stress and Hepatic Injury in Alloxan-Induced Diabetic Mice. *Journal of Medicinal Plants Research*, **5**, 5848-5856.

[13] Meral, I., Yener, Z., Kahraman, T. and Mert, N. (2001) Effect of Nigella Sativa on Glucose Concentration, Lipid Peroxidation, Antioxsidant Defense System and Liver Damage in Experimentally-Induced Diabetic Rabbits. *Journal of Veterinary Medicine. A, Physiology, Pathology, Clinical Medicine*, **48**, 593-599.

[14] Gupta, R.K., Kesari, A.N., Murthy, P.S., Chandra, R., Tandon, V. and Watal, G. (2005) Hypoglycemic and Antidiabetic Effect of Ethanolic Extract of Leaves of Annonasquamosa L. in Experimental Animals. *Journal of Ethnopharmacology*, **99**, 75-81. http://dx.doi.org/10.1016/j.jep.2007.06.006

[15] Kaleem, M., Asif, M., Ahmed, Q.U. and Bano, B. (2006) Antidiabetic and Antioxidant Activity of Annonasquamosa extract in Streptozotocin-Induced Diabetic Rats. *Singapore Medical Journal*, **47**, 670-675.

[16] Mujeep, M., Aeri, V., Bagri, P., *et al.* (2009) Hepatoprotective Activity of Methanolic Extract of Tylophoraindica Leaves. *International Journal of Green Pharmacy*, **3**, 125-127.

[17] Chaudhari, B.P, Chaware, V.J, Joshi, Y.R., *et al.* (2009) Hepatoprotective Activity of Hydroalcoholic Extract of *Momordicacharantia Linn.* Leaves against Carbon Tetrachloride Induced Hepatopathy in Rats. *International Journal of ChemTech Research*, **1**, 355-358.

[18] Gayatri, G., Ramesh Babu, J., Sumalatha, N., Venkateswarao, J. and Vidyadhara, S. (2011) Hepatoprotective Activity of Ethanolic Extract of Stachytarphetaindica on Wistar Rats. *International Journal of comprehensive Pharmacy* (*IJCP*), **1**.

[19] Saleem, T.S.M., Christina, A.J.M., Chidambaranathan, N., Ravi, V. and Gauthaman, K. (2008) Hepatoprotective Activity of Annonasquamosa Linn on Experimental Animal Model. *International Journal of Applied Research in Natural Products*, **1**, 1-7.

15

DALP Analysis on Genetic Diversity of *Panax notoginseng*

Xiuming Cui[1*], Hui Xiao[2], Jingjing Yang[1], Tina Dong[3], Karl Wah-Keung Tsim[3], Yuqin Sun[2], Yan Zhu[2]

[1]College of Life Science and Technology, Kunming University of Science and Technology, Kunming, China
[2]Wenshan Sanqi Research Institute, Wenshan College, Wenshan, China
[3]Department of Biology and Biotechnology Research Institute, The Hong Kong University of Science and Technology, Hong Kong, China
Email: [*]sanqi37@vip.sina.com

Abstract

***Panax notoginseng* (Burk) F.H. Chen is one of the most famous Chinese traditional medicinal plants, which belongs to *Panax genus* under *Araliaceae* family. At the present, *Panax notoginseng* cultivated is a mix colony. Using DALP makers, this article studied on genetic diversity of cultivated populations of *Panax notoginseng* in Wenshan County of Yunnan province and Napo country of Guangxi province. And the results showed that there were 260 polymorphic loci detected from the total of 292 in 13 populations, and there was great part of genetic diversity found between populations and the genetic differentiations were lower within populations. So there is broad prospect in good species breeding. And it can provide basic information for resource protection and sustainable use of *Panax notoginseng*.**

Keywords

***Panax notoginseng*, Genetic Diversity, DALP**

1. Introduction

Panax notoginseng (Burk) F. H. Chen is one of the most famous Chinese traditional medicinal plants, which belongs to *Panax notoginseng* under *Araliaceae* family. Wenshan prefecture is the major producing area, and it is about 400 years that *notoginseng* was cultivated [1]. In the process of cultivation and selection, some excellent genetic resource was lost. To protect that genetic resource and provide basic information for sustainable use of

[*]Corresponding author.

Panax notoginseng, we must strengthen the basic genetic research of *Panax notoginseng*. And it has to deeply understand the genetic differentiation of *Panax notoginseng*. Molecular maker is the most direct and accurate method for genetic diversity analysis, so we used DALP molecular maker in genetic diversity.

2. Materials and Methods

2.1. Materials

The three-year *panax notoginseng*' s leaves were collected from Yanshan base in Wenshan county of Yunnan province and Jingxi country of Guangxi province, except yellow *panax notoginseng* and purplish panax *notoginseng*' s leaves that were collected from Zhela base of Wenshan County, Yunnan province. The geographical location and the habitat overview of the population is showed in **Table 1**.

2.2. Methods

Using CTAB to extract Genomic DNA from leaves of *Panax notoginseng*. Detecting DNA concentration is diluted and preserving in −20°C. Getting 8 primers from 40 random primers that can get clear bands and react stably; they are PS01-PR02, PS02-PR01, PS04-PR01, PS04-PR02, PS05-PR02, PS08-PR01, PS09-PR01and PS10-PR01 (the primers' sequence is in **Table 2**).

Table 1. The habitats and localities of materials.

Code	Sampling position	Population	Altitude (m)	Longitude	Latitude
WM	Matang	PA	1470	104°5'	23°49'
WZ	Zhuilijie	PB	1430	204°24'	23°37'
WL	Laohuilong	PL	1450	104°36'	23°46'
WD	Dongshan	PI	1760	104°58'	23°54'
YC	Chongka	PD	1498	104°25'	23°32'
YZ	Zhela	PC	1580	104°35'	23°62'
YA	Aolongke	PE	1600	105°6'	23°6'
YP	Panlong	PJ	1510	104°31'	23°54'
MR	Renhe	PG	1600	106°7'	23°4'
MB	Bazhai	PH	1480	104°7'	23°0'
QB	Niejiao	PF	1992	103°87'	23°54'
GNP	Napo	PK	1100	105°57'	23°18'

"Code" is the abbreviation of "sampling position", for example, WM = Wenshan matang, YC = Yanshan chongka; PA—PL is the randomizing ID of the population.

Table 2. The number and sequence of primers.

Primer	No.	Sequence (5'-3')
Selective primers	PS01	5'-GTTTTCCCAGTCACGACAGC-3'
Selective primers	PS02	5'-GTTTTCCCAGTCACGACGAC-3'
Selective primers	PS03	5'-GTTTTCCCAGTCACGACACG-3'
Selective primers	PS04	5'-GTTTTCCCAGTCACGACCAG-3'
Selective primers	PS05	5'-GTTTTCCCAGTCACGACCAC-3'
Selective primers	PS06	5'-GTTTTCCCAGTCACGACTCAG-3'
Selective primers	PS07	5'-GTTTTCCCAGTCACGACCCAG-3'
Selective primers	PS08	5'-GTTTTCCCAGTCACGACGC-3' 5'-GTTTTCCCAGTCACGACCTAG-3'
Selective primers	PS09	5'-GTTTTCCCAGTCACGACCGC-3'
Selective primers	PS10	5'-AACAGCTATGACCATGA-3'
Reverse primers	PR01	5'-TTTCACACAGGAAACAGCTATGAC-3'
Reverse primers	PR02	

The PCR system for DALP analysis was as follows: dd H_2O 6.5 uL, 2.5 mmol/L dNTP 1 uL, 25 mmol/L Mg^{2+} 2 uL, 10 × PCR buffer 2.5 uL, 50 - 100 ng template DNA 2 uL, 5 pmol/L selective primer 1 uL, 5 pmol/L reverse primer 3 uL, 1U Taq polymerase in 20 uL reaction system. And the PCR program was as follow: pre-denaturation 5 min at 94˚C, denatured 30 s at 94˚C, annealed 30 s at 50˚C, 1 min at 72˚C, 12 cycles, and denatured 30 s at 94˚C, annealed 30 s at 50˚C, 30 s at 72˚C 28 cycles, then extend at 72˚C, 4˚C hold.

Using 0/1 matrix and POPGENE1.32 to calculate the Nei's genetic diversity index (H), Shannon information index (I), percentage of polymorphic bases (PPB), genetic differentiation (Gst), diversity index within population (Hs), total genetic diversity (Hs & Ht), the Nei's genetic distance (D) and genetic identity (I). Then the populations were calculated by the MEGA software.

3. Results

1% Agar gel electrophoresis showed that the bands of 192 samples' DNA extracted by CTAB method were the highest purity, best quality, clear and less fragments (As shown in **Figure 1**). The test results of DALP analysis as shown in **Figure 2** to **Figure 5**.

A total of 292 clear bands were amplified from 8 selected DALP primers, 260 (89.05%) of which were polymorphic. The PPB (79.08), Shannon index (0.2817) and the Nei's genetic diversity index (0.1172) of popula-

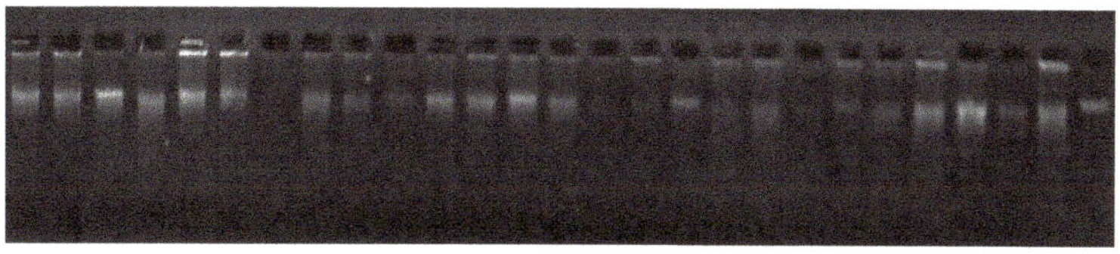

Figure 1. Total DNA extracted by CTAB method.

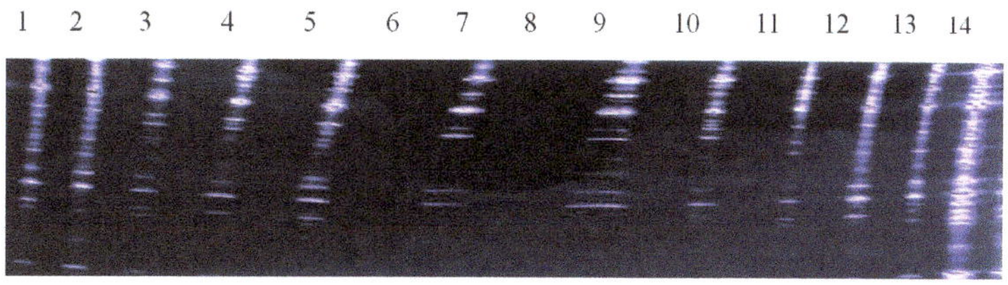

Figure 2. The PCR amplified results of *Panax notoginseng* cultivated in Wenshan prefecture by primer ps05-pr1.

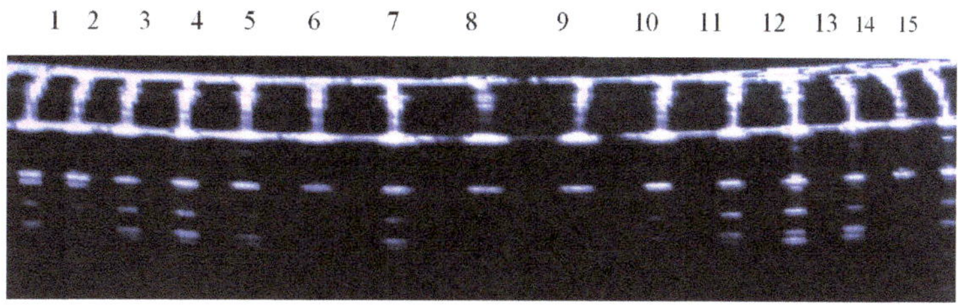

Figure 3. The PCR amplified results of *Panax notoginseng* cultivated in Guangxi province by primer ps05-pr1.

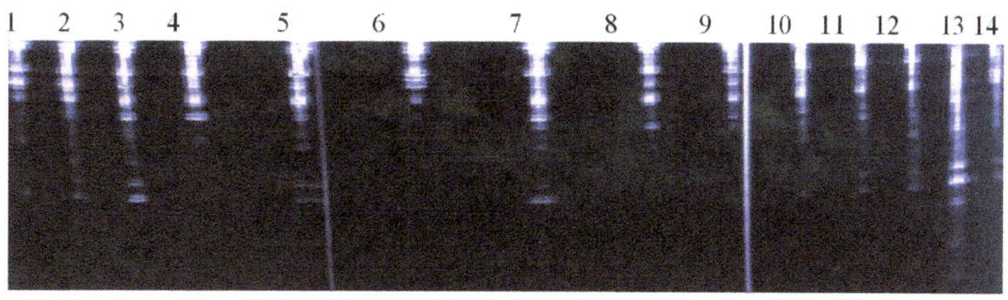

Figure 4. The PCR amplified results of yellow *Panax notoginseng* by primer ps05-pr1.

tions cultivated in Zhela (PC) were highest in Wenshan's populations. And The PPB (40.92), Shannon index (0.0868) and the Nei's genetic diversity index (0.0606) of populations cultivated in Bazhai (PH) were lowest in Wenshan's populations. And there were big difference between the highest one and the lowest one. Overall, the PPB, Shannon index and the Nei's genetic diversity index of Wenshan's populations were lower than Guangxi's populations' which had more genetic diversity. And the PPB, Shannon index and the Nei's genetic diversity index of *Panax stipuleanatus* which was contrast were next to Guangxi's populations (The results shown in **Table 3**).

Based on the proportion of genetic diversity level in Ht, Ht-Hs and Gst, we know that genetic differentiation between 10 populations cultivated in Wenshan was 0.7732. And it showed that there was 23.38% molecular variation only within populations and there was 77.32% molecular variation between populations, so there was more variation between populations. Genetic differentiation idex (0.1696) of the PK population cultivated in Napo Guangxi province was lowest. There was 83.04% molecular variation within population and only 16.96% molecular variation between populations. The degree of genetic diversity within population was lower than the total degree in 11 populations, and it showed that genetic diversity mainly existed between populations. Based on Wright (1931) [2], the migration number of every populations (Nm*) was over 1, which suggested that there existed sufficient genetic exchanges to prevent the genetic differentiation made by genetic drift among population. The sufficient genetic exchange number was inversely proportional to genetic differentiation level among populations in PD population of Longka and PK population of Napo, which's Nm* was over 1 and the genetic differentiation was low (The results shown in **Table 4**).

The analysis results of genetic distance showed that the genetic distance of every populations ranged from 0.0714 to 0.2408 (**Table 5**). The distance ranged from PB population to PC population was only 0.01. And genetic distance of Wenshan populations was close expecting PG. More distance excited between PK and other populations, especially PA which was over 0.1694. The cluster analysis showed that PB and PC classified one group, PD, PE and PF classified one group, PH classified with PI and PJ, and PG and PK were separate ones.

A total of 150 clear bands were amplified from 8 screened DALP primers, 120 (80%) of which were polymorphic in 96 samples from Wenshan, Guangxi, yellow *Panax notoginsseng*, purple *Panax notoginseng* and *Panax stipuleanatus*. From the **Table 6**, the genetic diversity analysis showed that PPB (81.82), Shannon index

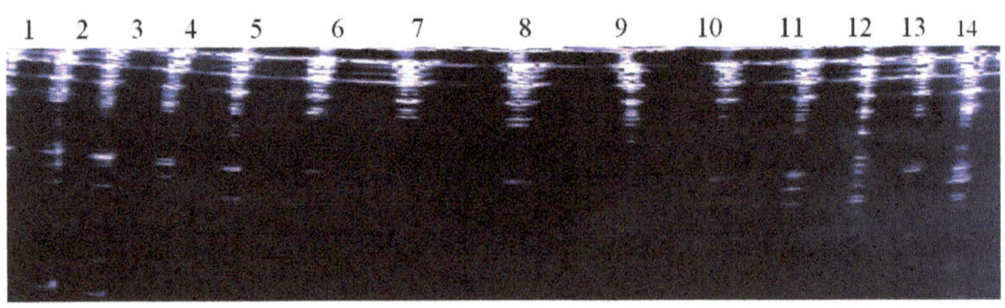

Figure 5. The PCR amplified results of purple *Panax notoginseng* by primer ps05-pr1.

Table 3. Genetic diversity of 11populations in *Panax notoginseng*.

Population	Total number of loci	No. of polymorphic loci	PPB	na*	ne*	The Nei's genetic diversity H*	Shannon index I*
PA	110	84	76.36%	1.3818	1.3055	0.1697	0.243
PB	148	105	70.92%	1.2364	1.1891	0.1051	0.1504
PC	120	94	79.08%	1.2636	1.2109	0.1172	0.2817
PD	135	73	54.54%	1.1818	1.1455	0.0808	0.2466
PE	128	80	62.5%	1.2091	1.1674	0.0928	0.264
PF	80	37	46.35%	1.1545	1.1255	0.0692	0.0989
PG	117	47	73.65%	1.2455	1.1964	0.1091	0.1562
PH	113	45	40.92%	1.1364	1.1091	0.0606	0.0868
PI	127	55	43.65%	1.1455	1.1164	0.0646	0.0926
PJ	138	82	60%	1.2	1.16	0.0889	0.1273
PK	110	90	81.82%	1.8182	1.396	0.2442	0.3782
stipuleanatus	140	112	80%	1.8	1.4168	0.2544	0.3896

Table 4. Analysis on genetic differentiation among populations.

Population	Ht	Hs	Dst	Gst	Nm*
PA	0.1534	0.0750	0.0784	0.5111	0.4783
SD	0.0395	0.0132	0.0263		
PB	0.0955	0.0455	0.05	0.5238	0.4545
SD	0.0304	0.0094	0.021		
PC	0.1091	0.0455	0.0636	0.5833	0.3571
SD	0.0344	0.0094	0.0248		
PD	0.0693	0.0477	0.0216	0.3115	1.1053
SD	0.0220	0.0109	0.0111		
PL	0.0773	0.0273	0.05	0.6471	0.2727
SD	0.0278	0.0061	0.0217		
PF	0.0659	0.0318	0.0341	0.5172	0.4667
SD	0.0229	0.007	0.0159		
PG	0.1102	0.0250	0.0852	0.7732	0.1467
SD	0.0386	0.0057	0.0329		
PH	0.0534	0.0295	0.0239	0.4468	0.6190
SD	0.0185	0.0066	0.0119		
PI	0.0614	0.0227	0.0387	0.6296	0.2941
SD	0.0229	0.0052	0.0177		
PJ	0.0864	0.0273	0.0591	0.6842	0.2308
SD	0.0309	0.0061	0.0248		
PK	0.2478	0.2058	0.042	0.1696	2.4476
SD	0.0312	0.022	0.0092		

*: *Ht* = Total gene diversity; *Hs* = Gene diversity within population; *Gst* = The coefficient of gene differentiaton; *SD* = Standard deviation; **Nm* = estimate of gene flow from Gst or Gcs. E.g., *Nm* = 0.5(1 - Gst)/Gst; See McDermott and McDonald, Ann. Rev. Phytopathol. 31:353-373 (1993).

Table 5. The Nei's genetic similarity (above the diagonal) and the genetic distance D (below the diagonal).

pop	PA	PB	PC	PD	PE	PF	PG	PH	PI	PJ	PK
PA	****	0.9311	0.9206	0.8779	0.8779	0.8555	0.8111	0.8593	0.882	0.8934	0.786
PB	0.0714	****	0.9499	0.9551	0.9551	0.9250	0.8472	0.8999	0.888	0.8837	0.809
PC	0.0827	0.0514	****	0.9345	0.9345	0.8941	0.8345	0.9222	0.904	0.8877	0.826
PD	0.1306	0.0459	0.0678	****	1.0179	0.9611	0.8494	0.8963	0.881	0.8536	0.825
PE	0.1303	0.0459	0.0678	−0.017	****	0.9611	0.8494	0.8963	0.881	0.8536	0.825
PF	0.1561	0.078	0.1119	0.0397	0.0396	****	0.8732	0.8673	0.871	0.8390	0.834
PG	0.2094	0.1658	0.1809	0.1632	0.1633	0.1355	****	0.8810	0.842	0.8254	0.824
PH	0.1517	0.1055	0.0810	0.1095	0.1097	0.1424	0.1267	****	0.943	0.9089	0.852
PI	0.1247	0.1179	0.1007	0.1267	0.1266	0.1372	0.1711	0.0580	****	0.9536	0.824
PJ	0.1127	0.1237	0.1192	0.1583	0.1583	0.1756	0.1919	0.0955	0.047	****	0.807
PK	0.2408	0.2114	0.1902	0.1921	0.1924	0.1811	0.1934	0.1594	0.193	0.2138	****

Table 6. The genetic variation among populations.

Population	Total number of loci	PPB	na*	ne*	H*	I*
Wenshan	110	70	1.7	1.3182	0.1965	0.3063
Guangxi	98	81.82	1.8182	1.396	0.2442	0.3782
YELLOW	133	50.91	1.5091	1.1774	0.1166	0.1893
PURPLE	102	37.27	1.3727	1.1585	0.1029	0.1633
stipuleanatus	118	79.6	1.8	1.4168	0.2544	0.3896

*: PPB = The percentage of polymorphic loci is; *na = Observed number of alleles; *ne = Effective number of alleles [Kimura and Crow (1964)]; *h = Nei's (1973) gene diversity; *I = Shannon's Information index [Lewontin (1972)].

(0.3782) and the Nei's genetic diversity index (0.2442) of Guangxi population were highest; the ones of Wenshan population were next to Guangxi population. And PPB (37.27), alleles number (1.3727), Shannon index (0.1633) and the Nei's genetic diversity index (0.1029) of purple *panax notoginseng* were minimum value in all populations, shows the amount of genetic variation is the lowest.

Based on the proportion of genetic diversity level in Ht, Ht-Hs and Gst, we know that species genetic differentiation was 0.5182. There was 48.12% molecular variation existed within populations, and more molecular (51.82%) variation existed between populations. In different population level, there was only 16.96% molecular variation existed among populations, and 83.04% one existed within populations in Guangxi's populations. There was 21.37% molecular variation existed among populations and 78.63% molecular variation existed in population in yellow fruit *notoginseng*. There was 14.76% molecular variation existed among populations, and 85.24% existed in population in *Panax stipuleanatus*. In the five populations, the genetic differentiation mainly existed among populations. Based on Wright (1931) [2], the migration number of every populations (Nm^*) was over 1, which suggested that there existed sufficient genetic exchanges to prevent the genetic differentiation made by genetic drift among population. The sufficient genetic exchange number was inversely proportional to genetic differentiation level among populations in all populations and the genetic differentiation was lowest, except Wenshan's population (**Table 7**).

The analysis results of genetic distance showed that the genetic distance of every populations ranged from 0.137 to 0.259 (**Table 8**). The distance ranged from *Panax notoginseng* to *Panax stipuleanatus* was farthest, which was over 0.5154. And genetic distance of *Panax notoginseng* cultivated in Wenshan was close to Guangxi one. The distance of yellow fruit *Panax notoginseng* was close to purple fruit *Panax notoginseng* which was 0.5001.

And The cluster analysis using UPGMA method showed that Wenshan's *Panax notoginseng* and Guangxi's classified one group, yellow fruit *Panax notoginseng* and purple fruit *Panax notoginseng* classified one group, *Panax notoginseng* was Separate clustering (**Figure 6**).

4. Discussion

Intraspecific genetic variation decides the evolution trend of species [3]. The more genetic diversity, the more extensive evolution [4]. So it is the basic for sustainable use of genetic resources that maintain the intraspecific

Table 7. The genetic diversity analysis of populations.

Population	Ht	Hs	Gst	Nm^*
Wenshan	0.1963	0.0946	0.5182	0.4649
SD	0.0325	0.0099		
Guangxi	0.2478	0.2058	0.1696	2.4476
SD	0.0312	0.022		
Yellow fruit	0.1181	0.0929	0.2137	1.8393
SD	0.0235	0.0137		
Purple fruit	0.0899	0.071	0.2197	1.8712
SD	0.0224	0.0145		
stipuleanatus SD	0.2549	0.2173	0.1476	2.887
	0.0301	0.0227		

*: *Ht* = Total gene diversity; *Hs* = Gene diversity within population; *Gst* = The coefficient of gene differentiaton; *SD* = Standard deviation; $^*Nm$ = estimate of gene flow from Gst or Gcs. E.g., Nm = 0.5(1 - Gst)/Gst; See McDermott and McDonald, Ann. Rev. Phytopathol. 31:353-373 (1993).

Table 8. The Nei's genetic similarity (above the diagonal) and the genetic distance D (below the diagonal).

pop	Wenshan	Guangxi	Pingbian	Purple fruit	Yellow fruit
Wenshan	****	0.8720	0.7718	0.8598	0.8710
Guangxi	0.1370	****	0.8327	0.8320	0.8491
Pingbian	0.2590	0.1831	****	0.7667	0.7729
Purple fruit	0.1511	0.1839	0.2656	****	0.9674
Yellow fruit	0.1381	0.1636	0.2576	0.0331	****

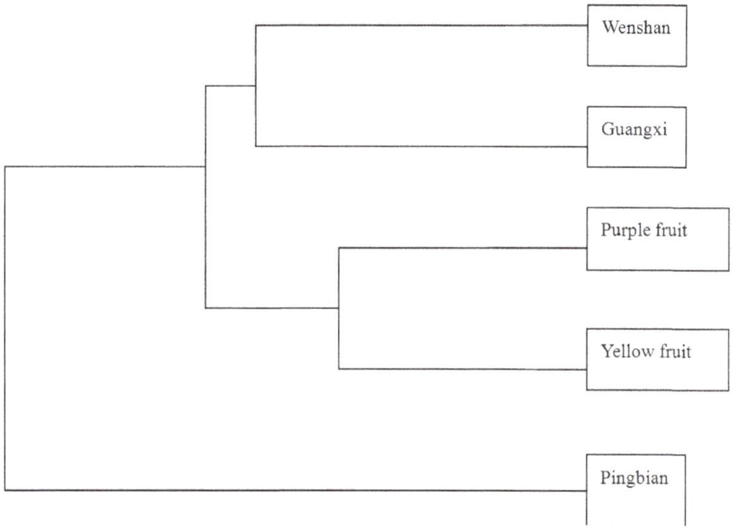

Figure 6. The UPGMA clustering dendrogram of populations.

genetic variation. The results of DALP analysis showed that *Panax notoginseng* and its allied species were abundant in genetic diversity which had strong evolution potential. Based on Ruozhu QU [5], the stable group had high Gst value, but the unstable one had low Gst value. The genetic differentiation index of Wenshan's populations and Guangxi's ones were over 0.3439, which showed that more genetic variation existed among populations, so they had great genetic differentiation and stable population. Many researches showed that the genetic diversity of endangered species was lowed, and the lack of diversity was the important reason to endanger [6]-[11]. So for *Panax notoginseng*, we must protect its genetic diversity at first, to build the resource garden and breed good varieties. The study provides basic information for resource pretection and sustainable use of *Panax notoginseng*.

Acknowledgments

We wish to thank Mr. X. M. Cui who is my tutor for thesis guide. This work is supported by Wenshan Sanqi Research Institute in Yunnan province.

References

[1] Zheng, G.Z. and Yang, C.R. (1999) The Biology and Application in *P. notoginseng.* Scientific Press (Ch).

[2] Sewall, W. (1931) Evolution in Mendelian Populations. *Genetics*, **2**, 97.

[3] Li, T.W. and Li, C.H. (2003) RAPD Analysis on Genetic Diversity of 5 Nihan Populations. *Biodiversity Species*, **2**, 118 (Ch).

[4] Ge, S. (1994) Isoenzyme in Plant Evolutionary Biology. In: Chen, J.K. and Yang, J., Eds., *Plant Evolutionary Biology*, Wuhan University Press, Wuhan, 153 (Ch).

[5] Qu, R.Z., Hou, L., Lve, H.L. and Yan, L.H. (2004) The Gene Flow of Population Genetic Structure. *Heredity*, **3**, 377 (Ch).

[6] O'Brien, S.J., Wildt, D.E., Goldman, D., Merril, C.R. and Bush, M. (1983) The Cheetah Is Depauperate in Genetic Variation. *Science*, **221**, 459. http://dx.doi.org/10.1126/science.221.4609.459

[7] O'Brien, S.J., Nash, W.G., Wildt, D.E., Bush, M.E. and Benveniste, R.E. (1985) A Molecular Solution to the Riddle of the Giant Panda's Phylogeny. *Nature*, **317**, 140. http://dx.doi.org/10.1038/317140a0

[8] Su, B. (1994) Protein Electrophoresis Study on Genetic Diversity of Giant Panda. *Sciences Bulletin*, **39**, 742 (Ch).

[9] Su, B. (1995) The Genetic Diversity of *Ailurus fulgens*. Genetic Research in China.

[10] Wayne, R.K., Bruford, M.W., Girman, D., Rebholz, W.E.R., Sunnucks, P. and Taylor, A.C. (1994) Molecular Genetics of Endangered Species. *Creative Conservation*, 92 (Ch).

[11] Zhang, Y.P., Wang, W., Su, B., Fan, Z.Y., Zhang, H.M. and He, T.M. (1995) The Screening and Application on Microsatelite DNA of Giant Panda. *Animal Research*, **16**, 301 (Ch).

16

Pi Wei Xiang Biao Li and the Trajectory of Zuyangming

Electra Peluffo

Faculty of Medicine, Universidad de Valencia, Valencia, Spain
Email: acupuntura@electrapeluffo.com

Abstract

In this paper, it is studied the reason why Zuyangming (stomach meridian) travels the body through yin territory in contrast with the other eleven main meridians governed by the quantitative-qualitative yinyang synchronicity of meridians and territories to discover. Zuyangming meets this principle only partially (in face and leg) and that's why the reasons for this exception in the thoraco-abdominal trajectory are attempted to be deciphered here. Ancient traditional medical texts describe the internal and external routes of meridians and the relations between the *spleen stomach* pair, which *Su Wen* 8 transforms into *spleenstomach*, mentioning the membranous binding (connective tissue today) which unifies both viscera. In addition, the embryological studies of the human fetus provided information on yuan—source of life—and the development of tissues (fascia and membranes) during fetal organic evolution, allowing us to understand many of the classical ideas about life, health and disease. Reflections in this paper conclude that zuyangming internalizes its resplendent yang energy, and thus compensates for the predominant presence of yin energy (yin organs in yin territory), keeping the inter organic harmony of energy blows.

Keywords

Zuyangming; Zutaiyin; Stomach and Spleen Meridians; Membranes; Connective Tissue; *Su Wen*; *Ling Shu*; *Shang Han Lun*; *Nan Jing*

1. Introduction

The author started studying Chinese Medicine under Professor Ye Chenggu at Guan An Men Hospital in Beijing between 1965 and 1967, time during which the subject concerning this study already caught her attention. Subsequently, in 1982 she attended classes individually, at that same Hospital, under the direction of Professor Gao Lishan with whom she consulted the difference shown by the stomach meridian along its path. Dr Gao pointed out that the question itself revealed a clear understanding of the energetic physiology of the Chinese Medicine. However, it was only after long years of practice and studies on Classic Medicine text that the author was able to develop a hypothesis about why the stomach meridian does not follow the **yinyang** rule of territorial distribution.

Working Hipothesis

Ancient Chinese Medical texts provide detailed information, both theoretical and practical, on meridians and their trajectories; these data when elaborated, allow us to develop a hypothesis that explains the reasons why the stomach meridian path differs from the **yinyang** rule governing the energetic channels trajectories.

The Medicine Classics revealed the interorganic physical relationship through membranes (currently known as connective tissue) between the members of the pair linking spleen and stomach as shown in the internal path of the respective meridians and their functions, concepts accepted until now.

This work emphasizes the Chinese classic conception of energy and cosmic resonance, as well as the relationship between the **yangming** (the innermost of the **yang** energy levels) and **taiyin (**the outermost of **yin** levels) which shows the bond not only material, anatomical but also functional; being the principle of complementary opposition, so dear to Chinese thought, fully respected.

The thoraco abdominal cavity (anterior face of the body and therefore **yin**) is home to almost all the **zang fu** (organs and viscera) that give the area a greater **yin** energy charge, which according to our hypothesis, is sought to get counteracted by the presence of hollow and peristaltic **yang** bowels whose main representative is the stomach **yangming**, resplendent energy, energy that is internalized when getting in contact with **taiyin**.

2. Material and Method

Analytical reading of chapters deals with the subject in both ancient and modern translations-interpretations of Classics: Su Wen, Ling Shu, Nan Jing, Huai Nan Zi and Shang Han Lun, listed in References.

3. Zuyangming Trayectory

Stomach meridian, **zuyangming**, starts in the nose through which it goes up and down, covers the upper gums and teeth, comes in front of the ears and rises up to the scalp; this journey through the face allows it to include all the organs of the senses. It goes down to the neck (St.9) and shoulder along the horizontal branch of the jawbone and turns towards the spine to meet the **yang** meridians in GV.14. After that it reaches the clavicle, and from there one branch penetrates the anterior trunk and moves forward crossing the diaphragm so as to, in CV13, enter the stomach and keep descending until the groin among **yin** meridians (all of them with an ascending direction) and returning to **yang** areas, travelling along thigh, leg and foot (2nd and 3rd toe) (**Figures 1-3**).

The twelve main meridians get together or pair up to form the six levels of energy that exchange their breaths. Out of this confluence six energetical dynamics are born, among them **yangming-taiyin** [1] *spleenstomach* which is the one before us today.

Zuyangming—stomach—is shining **yang**, radiant and being the innermost of all **yang** meridians in the six energetic levels concept, gets to contact coupled **zutaiyin** (spleen) to interchange their opposite and complementary energies.

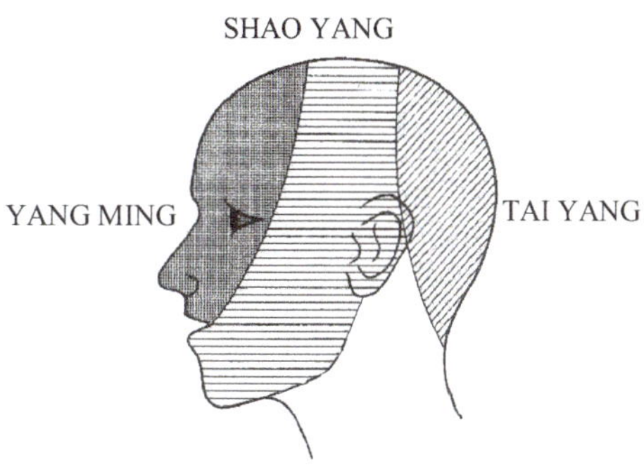

Figure 1. Head. Yang areas.

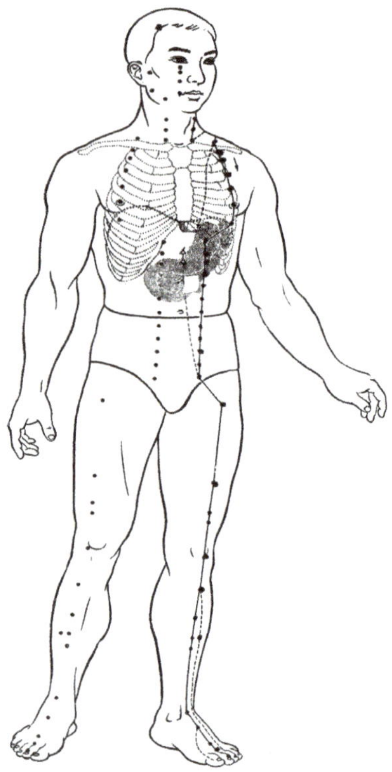

Figure 2. Zuyangming.

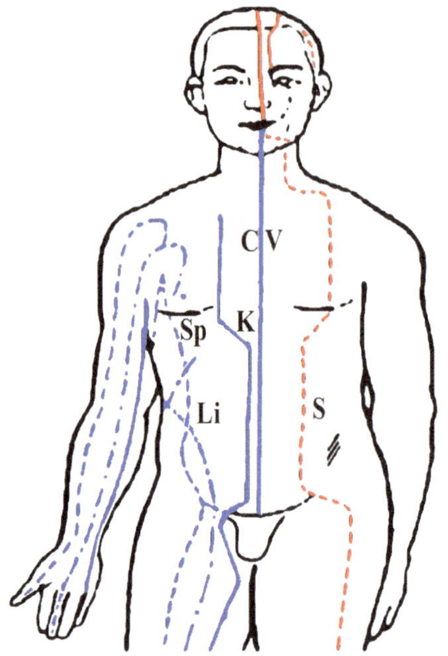

Figure 3. Left, **zuyangming**. Right, **yin** meridians.

Internal Routes of Zuyangming and Zutaiyin

The inner route of **Zuyangming** is told to us by *Ling Shu* 10: "... in **Quepen** (St.12), one branch descends along the thorax and spirally envelops the spleen. Another branch begins at the stomach exit and descends through the stomach lining until St.30 **Qichong** (also **Qijie**) [2]. When mentioning the lining of the stomach, is it referring to mesentery, hypodermic fascia?

Almost all texts accept *Ling Shu* version except *Lei Jing Tu Yi* (*Classics of Categories*) which details that the branch going down through the abdomen cover, descends slightly laterally to the kidney meridian, and begins at the same level as **Huangshu** Kid.16, right by the navel [3]. Both references correspond to **yin** transits.

There is a difference in language regarding the energetical relationship between an organ and its meridian and with coupled organ and meridian. If it is said that the meridian belongs or penetrates (**shu**) certain organ that means the meridian is completely rooted in it, in a reciprocal relation of mutual belonging. For instance, the liver and the liver meridian constitute a whole like a basin between a river and its lakes, inseparable.

The relationship between the inner trajectory of a meridian and the paired organ which it spirally envelopes (**luo**) is different. The connection is not so intimate any more, the river contours, envelopes a rock, it does not penetrate it: stomach spirally [4] envelopes around the spleen. And also spleen spirally envelopes (**luo**) stomach (**Figures 4** and **5**).

Wang Bing (710-804) in his *Su Wen* compilation says "**zuyangming** [5], stomach vessel, descends through the diaphragm, touches the stomach and envelopes the spleen…" This spiral connection as it is told in the Classics is established by membranes, sheaths. *Su Wen* 29 in its final lines describes the connection between spleen and stomach through tissues and membranes that keep the two organs attached so that body fluids **jin ye**, can circulate through both of them.

And thus, the density of the *spleenstomach* relationship is highlighted thanks to the membranes that gather them together with the same density of relationships on earth, so intimate they reach physical contact, and that enables the control of that which flows between those two membranes.

When the Emperor asks *Su Wen* 29 [6]-whether the **jin ye** actually go through this kind of tissue or membrane to reach the entire body and specially until the viscera, **Qi Bo** answers that **zutaiyin** (spleen) runs through the stomach and establishes a **shu** dependency relationship with the spleen (penetrates it) and a **luo** relationship with the throat (envelopes it). Thus, **taiyin** makes the **qi** circulate in the three **yin** levels: **tai**, **shao** and **jueyin**.

Zuyangming is the obverse movement **biao**, that is towards the outside, is the sea of the 5 **zang** and the 6 **fu**, responsible for the circulation of **qi** through the three **yang** levels: **tai, shao and yangming**.

Clear is the responsibility of *spleenstomach* in front of the six great meridians, three **yin**, and three **yang** and also in front of the twelve main meridians.

Spleen and stomach interact so as to share the circulatory function of the **yin yang** meridians because although it is assured in *Su Wen* 29 that both **zang** and **fu** get **qi** through the **yangming** (stomach makes **jinye**-body fluids-circulate) this would not happen without the intervention of the spleen, that makes this simultaneous **yangyin** movement irrigate the whole body.

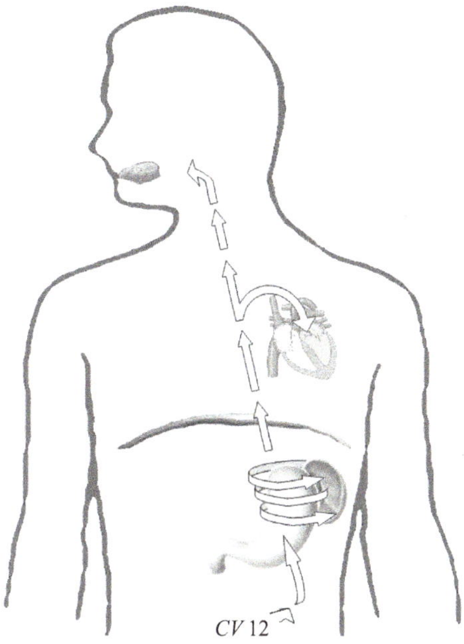

Figure 4. Internal route **zutaiyin**.

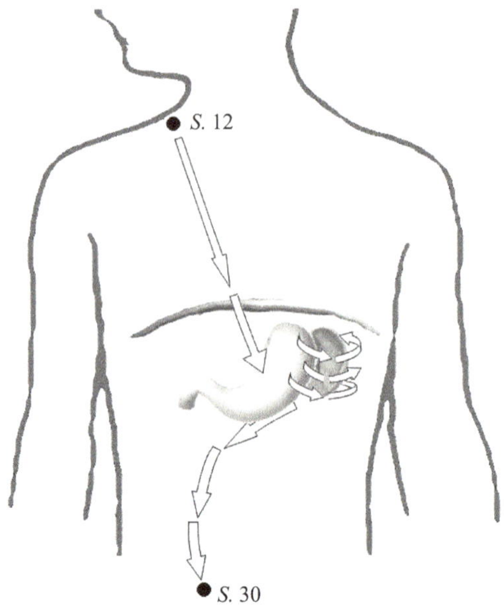

Figure 5. Internal route **zuyangming.**

4. Membranes. Yuan: Source, Origin

Chinese people paid attention to human embryology because they were interested in concepts such as "beginning, root, origin" …many Chinese ideographs imply the notion of origin or root or basic part: **yuan** source, basic idea in the source theory in *Ling Shu* 1 and in *Nan Jing* 66. They wanted to know where things came from, the source or origin of life, and embryology gave them an essential information, because fetal organic development and its connective tissues, fascias, membranes allowed them to understand many of the classic ideas upon life, health and illness [7]. This evolution of the embryo was already announced in *Huai Nan Zi* 7 [8] which describes the human being development based on a previous text, *Guan Zi* [9] from IV century BC where membranes and mesenteric fascias were not discussed as shown in *Huai Nan Zi.*

These mentions of the Classics show that, from ancient times, the anatomical presence of the interorganic membranes linking spleen and stomach together with their internal trajectories were well known.

The connective tissue is a versatile organic system, quite widespread and omnipresent which, being both well known and well analyzed by modern medicine, interconnects all parts of human body in each level, from the macro to microscopic one and can be found even in the simplest of the organelles, in each cell and in each texture or body framework.

Of greater importance for Eastern medicine—both theoretical and practical—are the now known properties these tissues show: to generate energy and to conduct it.

The Chinese conceived and sensed the energy of the **qi** watching the winds and their movements both in time and space.

Ganying, the cosmic resonance, the stimulus and the response to stimulus, is an essential ingredient in the Chinese thought. Resonances were not, are not abstract, there is always a material subtract so that they can occur. Joseph Needham [10] highlights the Chinese predilection for "action from a distance."

It is registered that in China in the year 132 an apparatus to detect earthquakes was designed, that device used the concept of action from a distance, the resonance already mentioned in *Huai Nan Zi* chapter 6 as a purely vibrational phenomenon of the **qi** [11]. Knowing these data, it is not noteworthy that Chinese attributed field effects—to generate and to drive energy—to the connective tissue and its numerous variants in the body.

5. Western Conception, Eastern Conception

Let us start from the acceptance that Chinese medicine is a complete and independent medical system.

We the Western medicine doctors, are instructed (taught and learned) through topics of learning in which Anatomy, organs, materiality have an undoubted predominance. And by this, please do not understand that I am suggesting that Physiology should not be studied; on the contrary a lot of it, all of it should be studied! But we have to accept that the Western comprehension of the Eastern way of presenting the body and its functioning is always interfered by our outstanding organic references which, for instance, lead to translate the names of the meridians using organ denominations whereas the original Chinese medicine defines them using their topography (hand or foot), quality (**yin yang**) and quantity (**tai**, **shao**, **jue**). Confusion prevails, even admitting that Eastern concepts are difficult to translate and to explain especially if homologation with our way of thinking is sought [12].

6. Classical Texts

Classical texts provide data which explain this territorial "anomaly" of **zuyangming** transiting through **yin** areas.

Su Wen 8 narrates the dialog between **Huang Di** and **Qi Bo** describing how is this set arranged; it is an interdependent set form by the six **fu** (viscera) and the five **zang** (organs) totaling *eleven* elements although *twelve* are mentioned: heart, lung, liver, gall bladder, **tanzhong**, *spleen*, *stomach*, large intestine, small intestine, kidneys, **sanjiao**, bladder. When we join *spleenstomach* together they are reduced to *eleven.*

The bond between the *spleenstomach* pair is unique because they share dynamism: rise and fall, reception and distribution, dryness and humidity whereas all the other **zangfu** perform only one function for each viscus. *Spleenstomach* being in the sixth place of the organic list of eleven, ranks in the central position (the earth) that is to say the center framed by five function-organs from above and other five from below leaving the spleen quite close to the **yang** function of the six **fu**. It is interesting to note that *spleenstomach* is needed for **zangfu**, **yinyang**, meridians, blood, essences and **qi** renewals, that is why earth in central place means that it does not take a special place but it is in all places which can be hinge or pivot between two qualities of **qi** [13].

The same Chapter 8 of *Suwen* [14] states that *spleenstomach* constitutes the silo and the barn from where the five flavors will emerge. *Spleenstomach* collects and distributes as well, without losing sight that between these two movements the transformations—digestion and assimilation—are developed.

Let us remember that in this enumerative list, the fifth place is for **tan zhong**, the sea of energy, where **xuli**, great stomach **luo**, pours. **Tan zhong** constitutes a knot of life in the center of the chest, a concentration of **qi** energy that gets distributed along all the meridians; this task explains why **tanzhong** (nurtured by **xuli,** great stomach **luo**) is in the fifth position, the center place, unity-meeting of life. It makes sense that **piwei** is in the sixth place because six corresponds with the maintenance of life. The sixth place, in this case the one in the middle, is to nurture the six **fu** from an already established space. Number six is what shares, it is the organized flow.

The dynamism of *spleenstomach* is similar to that of **cang lin** storage places and barns, as can be read in *Su Wen* as we mentioned above. It is interesting to decipher the meaning of these two sinograms, understanding them will bring us closer to the *spleenstomach* unitary function we are talking about here: **cang** is the place where a large amount of grain is placed, the silo, as in a gathering, a meeting, a being together, the grain is arranged for its shared cooking and in taking [15].

Lin is the place where the grain is taken (barn) to be kept and then distributed, a double process: collect from distribute to. And this double process (rise and fall) also represents the double aspects of the **piwei** pair. Surely, *spleenstomach*, a pair that balances in the central area (middle triple warmer) constitutes the best example of the earth-heaven interrelation of organs, of the earth-heaven dialectic within a visceral set.

And from this singularity we know that stomach **wei** is basically [16] **yang**, a **fu** which transforms and transports towards others **fu** and that spleen **bi** is a **zang** that storages and produces essences to be distributed, and it is added to the **fu** group because of its capacity to transform, promote, distribute and transport like the five **fu** but in a **zang** manner: storing and elevating the clear and pure thus called "root of storages and barns". For Chinese medicine, a **zang** rather than being a visceral mass or an organ is a movement, a dynamic, a quality of energies, one of the ways of running one of the five polarities needed for the establishment and the maintenance of existence, one of the five **wu xing** phases.

Cang lin expresses the double task of collecting and distributing to the desired place whenever it is needed. The spleen distributes the afflux of body liquids, essences and nurturing elements toward flesh and towards the 4 limbs which host the twelve meridians trajectories, that is to say to the whole body. This double aspect function is unique and helps us to understand that spleen works as a **zang** storing and elaborating the essences which then distributes to the whole body and that stomach has a **fu** task transforming and transporting to other **fu**. Thus *spleenstomach* is a center between the exterior and the interior with the help of other viscera, because there is no dynamism that can work by its own.

According to *Nei Jing* theory, **yang** rises and forms the heaven and **yin** descends to form the earth. This definition can help us to clarify the "biology" of the meridians whose external route, generally more or less vertical, show us a route, let us say only material, because what is important is the direction in which the energy circulates inside them, the content and the sense of circulation in the paths rather than the "pipelining", that is to say the dynamics of it, the function.

We mentioned above that **wei** is mainly **yang** in its function and thus its energy descends. The Chinese thought develops the concept of complementary opposite which, in essence, is telling us that a **yang** element carries in itself (and seeks to carry) a portion of **yin**, being the reverse also true. So, **yang** stomach has a **yin** component, the spleen, its pair, which it interchanges and shares functions with. The stomach meridian **zuyangming** starts in the head and descends until the feet, **yang** route that, in part, runs through **yin** territory. The spleen meridian z**utaiyin** starts in the feet and ascends along the inner face of the leg until the thorax, **yin** route and territory. Along the road they relate and interchange energy through their functions. Should this be possible if **zuyangming** circulated in the body in an "orthodox" way through the back or flank, both **yang** territories?

In *Suwen* 9 it is assured that the spleen together with the stomach and intestines (large and small) plus the triple heater and the bladder constitute the roots of silos and barns, the residence of the reconstruction [17]. At its base, all depends on **taiyin**, freely communicated with the earthy energies. Spleen is **zang**, but this description places it in the **fu** group and so *spleenstomach* represents a unit which does not appear in other organic pairs. This unit which differentiates *spleenstomach* is also expressed in its meridians that run very close in thorax and abdomen, despite of the different **zang fu** categorization of the organs they represent and the different circulatory direction. Spleen ascends and stomach descends.

The stomach is a **yang** store and barn: it receives food, breaks it into nutritious essences which still in the process of differentiating the five flavors, get sent to the spleen, it also commands the *descent* of waste to be eliminated through the intestines, **sanjiao** and bladder. It is **fu** but it also works as a **zang** because it absorbs, stores and processes. Stomach **fu** and spleen **zang**, **yinyang** pair of complementary opposites, show-in my opinion-more complementarity than opposition.

Su Wen 29 mentions the **biao li** obverse-reverse relation of **zutaiyin-zuyangming** because the *spleenstomach* is not an outside-inside bond (**nei-wai**) but the *dynamism which facilitates the connections* between the inner and the outer. The inner is the heaven in each of us which we do not have access to, and the outer is appearance and everything around it, the world [18]. It is important to understand the difference between *nei-wai* and *biao-li*, complex perhaps but very enriching. The physical has a external **wai** space to its disposal and everything not related to space is inner or interior, **nei**. They are **yin-*yang*** forms, spleen and stomach beat together, and because of that *Suwen* 8 presents them as *spleenstomach.* They are very close together despite being different, or maybe just because of that, one is **yin** and commands the lower part and the other one, **yang**, commands the upper part, this could seem opposite to the ascent-descent movement of each one which actually refers to the movement of empting and filling, filling and emptying, one after the other as is the case with the annual seasons: in spring-summer **yang** ascends and **yin** descends and in fall-winter **yin** ascends and **yang** descends. This dynamism is specifically represented in the body by the complementary alternation of the *spleenstomach* function, prototype of the **yinyang** link, *heavenearth*. The only way to put heaven and earth in contact is that heaven descends energies and earth ascends them. In this topic at hand, the earth is represented by the stomach that rules the centrifugal dynamism of descent and by the spleen which commands the centripetal movement of ascent.

This was already announced by **Lao Zi** in *Dao De Jing* [19] II

...high and low determine one another, but always through **wuwei**, that is without a manifested "action," because if it were product of a voluntary acting it would mean that something descended because the opposite ascended.

In the trunk, the diaphragm determines the boundary between upper **yang** and lower **yin** (**yang** above and **yin** below) and also the lumbar spine in some cases, the sacrum can have a **yin** quality in spite of belonging to a **yang** space. The interior or inner side of the body corresponds to **yin** and the exterior one to **yang**.

In the trunk, **zuyangming** (St. earth phase) runs through **yin** territory along a path parallel to the one of **zushaoyin** (K. water phase) and not far from **zujueyin** (Liv wood phase). Registered is the anecdote of doctor **Liu**

Zi who, when treating a patient, missed the stomach meridian and mistakenly jabbed the needle into the liver one, quite close in thorax and abdomen [20].

In the face, stomach meridian is clearly located in the less **yang** area where it controls all the sensory organs. Also in the leg it gets close to **yin**, considering the tibia edge as a border line between the **yin** and **yang** areas.

In the energy levels distribution, **yangming** is the innermost of the external and carries its strength and brightness to the **yin**. Its connection with GV.14 reinforces its **yang** which decreases from top down, and is needed by St. in its exchange with **yin** spleen and it is also needed to supply Large Intestine, **xuli** (its great **luo** vessel) and **tangzhong**, to nourish the lung and also to make energy available for its long route.

Stomach, sea of liquids and cereals, is one of the four seas: brain is sea of marrows, **tanzhong** is sea of energy and **chong mai**, sea of the twelve meridians and the blood but…attention, please! in the series of seas stomach is the only **fu**, all the rest are **zang**, that is **yin**.

All these connections demonstrate how difficult is to talk of one meridian alone for it is never isolated: its *raison d'être* is to belong to an energy network.

Knowing the energy network the meridians weave to establish deep interorganic relationship, allows us to understand the inseparable links between organs, viscera, meridians and their functions, so constituting an indivisible whole. This body framework is a characteristic approach of Chinese Medicine which addresses the body as a unit where each part represents the whole and vice versa, not giving the anatomical either/or functional division that Western medicine describes isolating ones from others and hence, their functions.

The net or mesh meridians (and the whole organism is a meridian) weave allows to maintain the organic functional union, there are no individualities, everything is one, unity prevails.

Yangming is **yang**, powerful and bright like the sun. Its function is not exteriorized but, on the contrary, it closes towards the interior to penetrate the **yin** to which it brings its richness and splendor. This movement explains why, in texts, **yangming** is frequently described as the "interior of the exterior" of the body: the digestive body tract is exterior because it receives food and expels the rest outside after digesting it; **yangming** (stomach-large intestine) is the level in which the ingested solids and liquids are taken to the **yin** organs to be transformed. The intermediate step to do that is regulated by the hinge level **shaoyang** (GB-TW) which joins the digestive process *in toto* where **yangming** represents movement and homeostatic balance in the *internal* digestion paths.

7. Complementary Opposition.

Shan Hang Lun classic text says that **yangming** interiorizes towards the **yin** as much energy as blood because it corresponds to the deepest level of the **yang** meridians and offers its strength and dynamism: moving, processing, moving the chyle forward, absorbing essences. For all of these, it needs **taiyin** (Sp) which, in association with humidity balances out **yangming** affinity for dryness. **Taiying** and **yangming** deal with the delicate and labile stability that characterizes the digestive process and, generally, the whole organism. **Yangming**, with plenty of blood and energy contributes to dry the organs up and prevent humidity which is not only the impregnation of fluids but also a temperature parameter: humidity is cold, dryness is hot therefore these two **yangming-taiyin** energies balance out each other.

Yangming is one of a dry-hot nature and does not want dryness. **Taiyin** (cold and humid) does not want humidity and is afraid of humidity because it is rooted in earth and in humidity itself, and so it is understandable that desires some dryness, the one its pair, the stomach, can give. Humidity affects circulation, blocks it, this explains why the spleen cannot carry on with its task of transport and distribution. At flesh level, humidity produces edema and flabbiness.

At the same time, stomach escapes from dryness because its own dry nature needs humidity and liquids to perform its fermentation, maceration and transformation tasks. *Suwen* 4 summarizes saying that *spleenstomach* are not very cold, not very hot, not very dry and not very humid.

In this dynamism, we must not forget the participation of **chongmai** meridian which ascends from St.30 joined to the kidney meridian making use of the solid and liquid substances which gastric physiology provides.

8. Conclusions

There is a territorial categorization that governs the network of the meridians paths.

Thorax, abdomen, and pelvis (thoracoabdominal region) host almost the totality of **yin** organs and **yang** viscera and all the **yin** foot and hand meridians run the area, and this circumstance gives a **yin** energetic predominance to the area.

I understand that **zuyangming** in its shinning condition takes its breath to areas with **yin** predominance so as to maintain dynamic balances. Stomach is the sea of liquids and cereals, **yin** material. That is to say, that **zuyangming** with its route of shinning **yang** re-harmonizes the **yin** excess in the mentioned territory.

According to the description of the meridian internal routes made by classic medicine doctors, membranes joining stomach and spleen keep the unity of those which thus fulfill their mission, described since ancient times. They are well defined functions executed by *spleenstomach* that share **yinyang** activities: receive, process, store, dry, and moisten.

Nowadays, a decisive role among the action ways of acupuncture is attributed to the connective tissue in its wide variety (membranes included). This does nothing else but confirms the capacity of observation and syncretism of ancient Chinese scholars.

These certainties and reviews transmitted by the Chinese classics, portray, explain what is perceived in the interior of the body (anatomy) and what is acknowledged in organic systemic functions (physiology) in accordance with the role of each organ and each organic pair, always according to the Chinese concept of organism.

Anyway, the *spleenstomach* exception confirms the **yinyang** territorial categorization rule for the meridians trajectories according to the functions of the **zang fu** whose energies they drive.

References

[1] Peluffo, E. (2013) Medicina China. Claves Teóricas. Miraguano Ediciones, Madrid, 105.

[2] Milsky, C. and Andrès, G. (2009) Traduction & Commentaires *Ling Shu*. Edition La Tisserande, Paris.

[3] Matsumoto, K. and Birch, S.G. (1988) Hara Diagnosis: Reflections on the Sea. Paradigm Publications Brookline Massachussetts, 53.

[4] Matsumoto, K. and Birch, S.G. (1988) Hara Diagnosis: Reflections on the Sea. Paradigm Publications Brookline Massachussetts, 49.

[5] Unchuld, P. and Tessenow, H. (2011) Huang Di Nei Jing Su Wen. Annotated Translation. University of California Press, Berkeley Los Angeles, 490.

[6] Veith, I. (1966) The Yellow Emperor's Classic of Internal Medicine. University of California Press. Berkeley, London, 235.

[7] Matsumoto, K. and Birch, S.G. (1988) Hara Diagnosis: Reflections on the Sea. Paradigm Publications, Brookline, 153.

[8] Major, J.S., Queen, S.A., Meyer, A.S. and Roth, H. (2010) The Huainanzi. Columbia University Press, Columbia.

[9] Rickett, W.A. (2001) *Guanzi* Study and Translation. Cheng & Tsui Company, Boston, Worcester.

[10] Needham, J. (1969) La science Chinoise et l'occident (Le grand Titrage) Éditions du Seuil.

[11] Cheng, A. (2002) Historia del Pensamiento Chino edicions bellatera Barcelona.

[12] Lu, H.H., Wang, Y.N., Song, Y.Y. and Lu, J. (2013) The Easter Cultural Signature of Traditional Chinese Medicine: Empirical Evidence and Theoretical Perspectives. *Chinese Medicine*, **4**, 79-86. http://scirp.org/journal/cm http://dx.doi.org/10.4236/cm.2013.43012

[13] Larre, C. and de la Vallée, E.R. (2004) Spleen and Stomach. Monkey Press, 117.

[14] de la Vallée, E.R. et Larre, C. (1993) Suwen Les Once Premiers Traités. Maisonneuve Moulins-lès-Metz (France).

[15] Larre, C. and de la Vallée, E.R. (2004) Spleen and Stomach. Monkey Press.

[16] Porkert, M. (1974) The Theoretical Foundations of Chinese Medicine. Systems of Correspondence. The MIT Press, Cambridge, Massachusetts and London England.

[17] de la Vallée, E.R. et Larre, C. (1993) Suwen. Les Once Premiers Traités. Maisonneuve-Moulins-lès-Metz (France).

[18] Larre, C. and Rochat de la Vallée, E. (2004) Spleen and Stomach. Monkey Press.

[19] Waley, A. (1958) The Way and Its Power. A Study of the Tao Tê Ching and Its Place in Chinese Thought. Grove Weidenfeld, New York.

[20] Lu, G.-D. and Needham, J. (2002) Celestial Lancets. A History of Rationale of Acupuncture and Moxa. Routledge Curzon, London.

17

Different Acupuncture for Neurodynia and Skin Lesions with Acute Herpes Zoster

Guohua Lin[1], Yunkuan Yang[2], Hongxing Zhang[3], Lixia Li[4*], Chuyun Chen[4], Yue Liu[5], Xushan Cha[1], Qian Li[1]

[1]The First Affiliated Hospital of Guangzhou University of Traditional Chinese Medicine, Guangzhou, China
[2]Chengdu University of Traditional Chinese Medicine, Chengdu, China
[3]Wuhan NO.1 Hospital, Wuhan, China
[4]Guangzhou Hospital of Traditional Chinese Medicine, Guangzhou, China
[5]The Second Hospital of Traditional Chinese Medicine of Guangdong Province, Guangzhou, China
Email: *llixia@126.com

Abstract

Objective: To analyze the effectiveness of different acupuncture-moxibustion therapies for neurodynia and skin lesions of acute herpes zoster. Patients and Methods: From April 2007 to October 2009, 500 patients with clinical acute herpes zoster were included in the study. They were randomly divided into five groups as follow: electroacupuncture (E); electroacupuncture + cotton-pave moxibustion (EC); electroacupuncture + fire acupuncture (EF); electroacupuncture + tapping combined with cupping (ET); control group of western medicine (WM). Results: The time of staunch bleb, scab and scab-off had no obvious statistical difference in the five groups; however, five methods could obviously reduce symptoms of herpes zoster and improved general symptoms. Within five days of treatment, compared to control group, the other four methods could more quickly ameliorate the general symptom of herpes zoster, and EF was superior to EC. In addition to electroacupuncture group, the treatment groups could relieve neuralgia and shortened duration of pain, which was superior to control group treatment. In addition, within first 3 days of treatment, the efficacy of treatment with E, EF or ET was superior to that of EC, and EF was better to E. After five days or end-of-treatment, the efficiency of odynolysis by treatment with EF, ETor EC was no more than E. The incidence of neurodynia was reduced after treatment with EC, EF or ET at 30th, 60th and 90th day, and pain of postherpetic neuralgia was relived. Conclusion: It is a certain advantages for organism reparation, abatement of neurodynia, and reduction of postherpetic neuralgia by acupuncture treatment.

Keywords

Herpes Zoster, Acute, Neurodynia, Acupuncture Treatment

*Corresponding author.

1. Introduction

Acute herpes zoster is caused by reactivation of latent varicella zoster virus (VZV or human herpesvirus 3). The virus can persist for years in the dorsal root ganglia of cranial or spinal nerves after resolution of original infection. As cellular immunity wanes with age or immunocompromise, the virus can be transported along peripheral nerves, producing an acute neuritis [1] [2]. Herpes zoster is characterized by a painful, unilateral vesicular eruption usually in a restricted dermatomal distribution [3].

Pain associated with herpes zoster infection can be classified as acute herpetic neuralgia, subacute herpetic neuralgia, and postherpetic neuralgia [4]. Pain is the most common symptom of acute herpes zoster and may precede skin changes by days or weeks [5] [6]. Moreover, pain is typically described as a sharp or stabbing sensation, burning sensation, or even "allodynia" (pain evoked by normally non-painful stimuli such as light touch) [6].

Pain associated with herpes zoster infection can cause significant suffering, particularly in elderly persons. Symptoms may be severe enough to interfere with sleep, appetite, or sexual function. In addition, symptoms may persist from months to years and cause profound psychosocial dysfunction, disability, and despair. The difficulty in treating herpes zoster means increased costs for individuals and health services [7] [8].

The treatment of herpes zoster is aimed primarily at earlier healing of lesions and prevention of complications. Randomized controlled trials and systematic reviews have found that oral antiviral agents (acyclovir, famciclovir and valaciclovir) are effective to relive pain at 1 - 3 months and to reduce the prevalence of postherpetic neuralgia at 6 months, although the effect is moderate. These drugs must be administered within 3 days from the onset of symptoms and have a good safety profile. Netivudine has a similar effect [9]-[12]. Other drugs such as levodopa, amantadine, amitriptyline, and idoxuridine are of unknown effectiveness in preventing herpes zoster complications. Moreover, corticosteroids drug are considered to be ineffective or even harmful [12]. Drugs considered to have a moderate effect in treating established postherpetic neuralgia are gabapentin and tricyclic antidepressants [11] [13] [14].

Despite these treatment options, many patients experience refractory pain and frequent adverse effects, especially elderly patients with cardiovascular disease. Therefore, pain associated with herpes zoster infection remains a challenge for effective management. Acupuncture and other methods from Traditional Chinese Medicine such as bloodletting and moxibustion have not been evaluated for this disorder. However, some Chinese case series report good treatment results but lack rigorous design [15]-[17]. We began a pain program at our primary care institution and collected cases with herpes zoster-associated pain to determine if these techniques could be helpful. This subject has been reviewed by the ethics committee of Chengdu University of Traditional Chinese Medicine.

2. Methods

2.1. Clinical Data

Diagnostic criteria: Traditional Chinese medicine diagnostic criteria has referred to diagnostic criteria of snake strand sore in "Diagnosis curative standard of tradition Chinese medicine disease"; Western medicine diagnosis standard has referred to diagnostic criteria of herpes zoster in *Cecil Textbook of Medicine*.

Inclusion criteria: Age range was from 18 to 70 years; the patients had herpes 1 to 7 days, and were not treated with antiviral or relieve pain drugs; all patients signed the information consent form, and agreed to accept the all therapeutic methods and obey arrangement.

Exclusion criteria: Special types of herpes zoster, including herpes zoster ophthalmicus (HZO), herpes zoster oticus (HZO), herpes zoster viscera, herpes zoster meninx, generalized herpes zoster, or no rash type herpes zoster; pregnant or lactating women; patients of anaphylaxis or drug allergy; scar diathesis; primary disease or systemic failure including cardiovascular, blood vessel of brain, liver, kidney and hematopoietic system, diabetes patients, cancer or mental patients, connective tissue disease and hemophilia, patients with bleeding tendency; patients with critical illness who were difficult to evaluate effectiveness and safety of treatment; patients who were treated with the corticosteroids or immunity inhibitor within one month.

2.2. General Information

All cases were come from the first affiliated hospital of Guangzhou university of Chinese traditional medicine,

Guangzhou hospital of traditional Chinese medicine, two Chinese medicine hospital in Guangdong Province, Chengdu Second People's Hospital, The affiliated hospital of Chengdu University of Traditional Chinese Medicine, traditional Chinese medicine research institute in Sichuan province and combining Chinese and Western Medicine Hospital of Wuhan at the time range from April 2007 to October 2009. A multicentric random trial(allocation concealment and central random are did in GCP center of Chengdu University of Traditional Chinese Medicine) was adopted, the 500 conforming cases who equally divided into five groups as follow: electroacupuncture (E); electroacupuncture + cotton-pave moxibustion (EC); electroacupuncture + fire acupuncture (EF); electroacupuncture + tapping combined with cupping (ET); control group (WM) with conventional western medicine therapy.

In E group, there were 45 male and 53 female cases included 4 cases with scab falling off, other 2 cases were eliminated; in EC group, there were 44 male and 56 female cases included 6 cases with scab falling off ; in EF group, there were 39 male and 58 female cases including 6 cases with scab falling off, and other 3 cases were eliminated; in ET group, there were 40 male and 56 female cases including only 1 case with scab falling off, and other 4 cases were rejected; in control group with conventional western medicine therapy group, there were 36 male and 62 female cases, including 3 dropping cases, and other 2 cases were eliminated. In five groups, the mean age was 43.76 ± 15.34, 46.98 ± 13.61, 45.20 ± 15.06, 44.33 ± 15.07 and 46.51 ± 15.30 years, respectively. Besides these, the time between feeling uncomfortable and medical consultation were 6.15 ± 4.11, 5.56 ± 3.14, 5.63 ± 2.70, 5.77 ± 3.05 and 5.24 ± 2.52 days, respectively. Meanwhile, the VAS scores of five groups were respectively 59.23 ± 25.71, 53.84 ± 25.95, 52.45 ± 28.11, 56.63 ± 25.44 and 57.20 ± 27.17 before treatment.

All indicators between the two as described above had no significant differences ($P > 0.05$), so, there was comparable between any two groups.

2.3. Treatment

All included patients kept the clean skin on parts of herpes zoster and protected skin lesions.

E: The main points included Ashi, Jiaji (on one side of sick), Zhigou and Houxi acupoints. The clients were adopted left and side-lying position, after routine disinfection, the Ashi acupoint was treated with acupuncture round pain; Jiaji point were treated with oblique insertion toward the spinal column; Zhigou and Houxi acupoints were dealt with coup droit. All points were inserted with needles at depths range from 0.8 to 1.0 cm, after result that patients suffered needling sensation response, the all cases were stimulated with Hans acupoint nerve stimulator (HANS; LH202H, China) which was operated in a standard method that adopted alternating current with frequency of 2/100 HZ and current of 2 ~ 5 mA, and a strength that all patients could bear.

EC: The cases were treated with cotton-pave moxibustion based on the E as described above. The clients were adopted lying position, then Ashi point was completely exposed to medical workers, after sterilization with iodine, the cotton wool that was tore into thin slices as cicada's wings (without a hole, 3×3 cm^2), was covered on the part of Ashi point, lit and burnt out rapidly. The acupuncture treatment was applied every 3 times.

EF: The patients were treated with fire acupuncture based on the E as described above. The clients were adopted lying position, then Ashi point was sterilized with iodine. Herpes central was penetrated with needle of moderate thickness that was heated until red and white, at depths range from 0.2 to 0.3 cm. Based on the number of herpes, early onset of herpes which selected numbers range from 3 to 5 were first pierced, and each was done 2 times. Postoperation, liquid of herpes zoster was drained then, the location was pressed for 30 s and coated with a flower oils.

ET: The cases were treated by combination tapping with cupping and E as described above. The clients were adopted sitting and side-lying position, after routine disinfection, the Ashi point was treated with plum blossom-needle tapping with slightly blooding. Cupping was pressed on the both ends of parts of collateral puncture and impairment. After bleeding by 3 to 5 ml and leaving the cupping for 5 to 10 min, the cupping was taken away and routinely sterilized.

Control: Valaciclovir and vitamin B1 were used through taken orally by 300 mg each with 2 times per day and 10 mg each with 2 times per day, respectively. The course of treatment consulted the E as described above.

2.4. Outcomes

Pain intensity (PI, VAS marking; mm): the tender spot was observed and noted in the 24 hours before the treatment. The interval range from 0 to 100 mm presented a level of pain intensity from indolence (0 mm) to maximum pain (100 mm) that patients could feel. We noted the pain intensity at first 10 days before treatment and at 11th day, respectively.

Duration of pain: we noted the time from pain presented to pain completely went away.

Incidence of postherpetic neuralgia PHN: we noted the postherpetic neuralgia PHN at 30th day.

2.5. Statistics

Values were shown mean ± SEM. The significance of differences between all groups was evaluated using one-way ANOVA with a post-hoc Student-Newman-Keuls multiple comparisons test. Chi-square test was used in enumeration data. Duration of pain analyses was adopted Log Rank test. Statistical analyses were performed using SPSS Software (V18.0, SPSS, USA), and a P-value < 0.05 was considered to be statistically significant.

3. Results

3.1. The Time of Staunch Bleb, Scab and Scab-Off

As shown in **Table 1**, the time of staunch bleb, scab and scab falling off had no statistical significance between any two groups ($P > 0.05$). So, five treatment methods showed a similar efficacy in time of staunch bleb, scab and scab falling off.

3.2. Aggregate Score of Herpes Zoster before and after Treatment

Before treatment, there were no statistical significance between five groups ($P > 0.05$), so it was comparability between the groups. However, at 5th days, the result ($P < 0.01$) was opposite compared to the pre-treatment, as described above. Compared to control group, the other four groups had statistical significance ($P < 0.01$), moreover, cotton-pave moxibustion group was superior to fire acupuncture group ($P < 0.05$). End-of-treatment, compared to control group, the other four groups had statistical significance ($P < 0.01$), the result as like as it as described above ($P < 0.01$ or $P > 0.05$), and there were statistical significance between pre-treatment and after 5 days treatment ($P < 0.01$). However, there was a difference between before and after treatment ($P > 0.05$). In summary, the five methods could reduce obviously the symptom of acute herpes zoster, and ameliorated the general symptoms. Within the first five days of treatment, compared to control, the other four methods could ameliorated more quickly the general symptom of herpes zoster, and fire acupuncture was superior to cotton-pave moxibustion (**Table 2**).

Table 1. The time of staunch bleb, scab and scab-off.

Group	Cases	Staunch vesicle (days)	Scab (days)	Scab-off (days)
E	94	5.02 ± 2.48	9.13 ± 3.90	21.49 ± 8.98
EC	94	4.54 ± 1.95	8.49 ± 3.47	20.87 ± 8.14
EF	91	4.87 ± 2.03	9.04 ± 4.57	20.13 ± 8.86
ET	95	5.05 ± 2.32	9.45 ± 4.90	21.06 ± 9.45
WM	95	4.83 ± 2.30	9.91 ± 3.63	24.27 ± 12.67

Table 2. Aggregate score of herpes zoster before and after treatment.

Group	Case (n)	pre-treatment	Treatment (within 5 days)	After treatment	Difference between treatment (5 days) and pre-treatment	Difference between before and after treatment
E	94	13.97 ± 3.31	8.27 ± 3.55	3.50 ± 2.79	5.70 ± 4.02	10.47 ± 3.79
EC	94	13.62 ± 3.50	8.77 ± 3.27	3.76 ± 2.56	4.85 ± 3.61	9.86 ± 3.82
EF	91	13.86 ± 3.69	7.44 ± 3.83	3.41 ± 2.80	6.42 ± 4.48	10.45 ± 4.44
ET	95	13.52 ± 3.94	8.11 ± 4.34	3.59 ± 3.03	5.41 ± 5.10	9.93 ± 4.51
WM	95	14.77 ± 3.30	10.23 ± 3.88	4.59 ± 3.02	4.54 ± 3.45	10.18 ± 3.36

3.3. Duration of Pain

As shown in **Table 3**, the pain lasting time had statistical significance between control and other four groups ($P < 0.01$). In addition, there was statistical significance between other three groups and ET group ($P < 0.01$ or $P < 0.05$). However, the pain lasting time had no statistical significance between any two groups for E, EC and EF groups as described above ($P > 0.05$). Therefore, the former four groups could obviously reduce the pain lasting time compared to western medicine group. However, the effects in three groups, including the E group, EC and EF group, were better compared to ET group.

3.4. VAS of Treatment

As shown in **Table 4**, there was no statistical significance between any two groups ($P > 0.05$). In addition, there was statistical significance between prior to the treatment and end-of-treatment between any two groups ($P < 0.01$). Meanwhile, at day 3, 5, 7 of their hospitalisation and end-of-treatment, there were significant difference between any two groups ($P < 0.01$). Besides that, there were statistical significance between former four groups and control group ($P < 0.01$). However, there were no statistical significance between any two groups of four groups included E, EC, EF and ET ($P > 0.05$). In summary, the five methods could reduce gradually the pain of nerve, the effects of former four methods was better compare to western medicine method. Moreover, at first 3 days of treatment, both the E, ET and EF had better therapeutical efficiency compared to EC, and the EF was superior to alone electroacupuncture.

3.5. Different VAS of Pre-treatment and Post-Treatment

After treatment for 5 days, there were statistical significance between the four groups and control group ($P < 0.01$). In addition, E, ET and EF were superior to EC ($P < 0.01$). Besides, E was better to ET and EF ($P < 0.01$). However, there was no statistical significance between pre-treatment and post-treatment. In short, the five methods could reduce gradually the pain of nerve, and former four methods had a better efficiency than control group. Furthermore, the three groups, including the E, ET and EF, which had better analgesic effect compared to EC, and E was superior to the EF and ET (**Table 5**).

3.6. VAS of during Follow-Up Period

As shown in **Table 6**, follow-up tests were applied at 22th, 30th, 60th and 90th day after treatments, respectively.

Table 3. Duration of pain.

Group	Case (n)	Duration of pain (days)
E	94	15.87 ± 11.86
EC	94	16.66 ± 8.80
EF	91	15.89 ± 12.00
ET	95	17.65 ± 13.53
WM	95	28.26 ± 19.69

Table 4. VAS of treatment.

Group	Case (n)	Pre-treatment	Treatment (3 days)	Treatment (5 days)	Treatment (7 days)	After treatment
E	94	58.88 ± 25.89	36.60 ± 24.18	22.88 ± 19.68	13.30 ± 17.52	4.03 ± 9.27
EC	94	54.09 ± 26.35	41.19 ± 24.61	27.30 ± 22.21	14.46 ± 16.76	6.05 ± 12.46
EF	91	52.67 ± 27.82	34.95 ± 23.98	23.63 ± 21.79	14.60 ± 16.65	5.01 ± 10.12
ET	95	56.17 ± 25.17	36.13 ± 23.17	25.96 ± 22.51	17.26 ± 19.49	5.16 ± 10.98
WM	95	58.01 ± 26.97	47.59 ± 23.96	34.73 ± 21.54	25.89 ± 19.43	14.30 ± 16.15

Table 5. Different VAS of pre-treatment and post-treatment.

Group	Case (n)	Difference between treatment (5 days) and pre-treatment	Difference between before and after treatment
E	94	36.00 ± 28.63	54.86 ± 25.84
EC	94	26.79 ± 23.26	48.03 ± 28.72
EF	91	29.04 ± 29.93	47.66 ± 27.73
ET	95	30.21 ± 25.18	51.01 ± 25.41
WM	95	23.28 ± 23.24	43.71 ± 27.55

Table 6. VAS of during follow-up period.

Group	Case (n)	22th day	39th day	60th day	90th day
E	94	1.44 ± 5.32	0.60 ± 3.52	0.27 ± 1.85	0.11 ± 1.03
EC	94	2.05 ± 7.03	1.04 ± 5.03	0.59 ± 4.01	0.53 ± 3.70
EF	91	2.33 ± 9.32	1.36 ± 7.40	0.22 ± 2.10	0 ± 0
ET	95	1.80 ± 8.22	1.13 ± 6.11	0.32 ± 2.28	0 ± 0
WM	95	8.18 ± 12.97	5.47 ± 10.72	2.21 ± 7.80	1.16 ± 6.03

There were statistical significance between the other four groups and control group ($P < 0.01$ or $P < 0.05$). Meanwhile, the E was superior to EF at 22th and 30th day ($P < 0.01$ or $P < 0.05$). In brief, levels of pain in E, ET, EF and EC groups were lighter compared to that in control group, and E was superior to EF group.

3.7. Incidence of Postherpetic Neuralgia

As shown in **Table 7**, Follow-up test were performed at 30th, 60th and 90th day after treatment, respectively ($P < 0.01$ or $P < 0.05$), in addition, postherpetic incidences in neuralgia E, ET, EF and EC groups were less compared to that in control ($P < 0.01$ or $P < 0.05$).

4. Discussion

Traditional Chinese medicine techniques such as acupuncture and moxibustion could be integrated with orthodox Western medicine therapies to fill the effectiveness gap in some pain problems included herpes zoster-associated pain to prevent or reduce pain with minimal adverse effects of treatment. The acute herpes zoster research is the first clinical study to investigate the effectiveness of an acupuncture treatment for acute herpes zoster pain in direct comparison to a standard analgesic treatment with gabapentine and to a sham laser acupuncture treatment in a three-armed, randomized controlled clinical trial. Compared to previous studies of acupuncture in the treatment of herpes zoster, this study has a more rigorous methodology and will include more patients.

In our study, for the time of staunch bleb, scab and scab falling off, there were no obvious statistical difference in E, EC, EF, ET and control groups, however, five methods could obviously reduce symptoms of herpes zoster and improved the general symptoms. At first five days of treatment, compared to control method, the other four methods could more quickly ameliorate the general symptoms of herpes zoster, and EF was superior to EC.

Acute herpes zoster is relieved during treatment; moreover, EC, EF and ET methods could reduce the neuralgia and shortened the duration of pain, which were superior to that treating with western medicine. In addition, at first 3 days of treatment, the efficacy of treatment with E, EF or ET was superior to that of EC, and EF method was better than E After the fifth day of treatment or end-of-treatment, the efficiency of relieve pain by treatment with EF, ET or EC was no more than alone E. The incidence of neurodynia was reduced after EC, EF or ET treatment at 30th, 60th and 90th day, and pain of postherpetic neuralgia was relived.

In my paper, base line of all cases in electro-acupuncture group was basically in compliance with the control

Table 7. Incidence of postherpetic neuralgia.

group	Case (n)	Follow-up (30th day)		Follow-up (60th day)		Follow-up (90th day)	
		No	Yes	No	Yes	No	Yes
E	94	90 (95.74)	4 (4.26)	92 (97.87)	2 (2.13)	93 (98.94)	1 (1.06)
EC	94	89 (94.68)	5 (5.32)	92 (97.87)	2 (2.13)	92 (97.87)	2 (2.13)
EF	91	87 (95.60)	4 (4.40)	90 (98.90)	1 (1.10)	91 (100.00)	0 (0.00)
ET	95	90 (94.74)	5 (5.26)	93 (97.89)	2 (2.11)	95 (100.00)	0 (0.00)
WM	95	63 (66.32)	32 (33.68)	86 (90.53)	9 (9.47)	90 (94.74)	5 (5.26)

group. Valaciclovir [18] was used in here, which had a bioavailability with 54.5%. So, it had a gender certainly as control.

In fact, the efficiency that local Ashi point was treated with stimulation of acupuncture which worked through a conducting system of cortex-meridians and collaterals-viscera. Varicella zoster viruses are almost lurked in spinal nerve root, namely locate in Du meridian and Jiaji points. In here, the partial skin lesions, painful place and relevant Jiaji points of ganglion are where pathogenic factors exist in, which could be thought as an Ashi point storing herpes zoster [19]. Jiaji point locates in between Du meridian and Sun meridians of foot, we can regulate the Yang-Heavy of Du meridian, Sun meridians of foot and the whole body, which makes it to reach the objective of regulation of meridians and collaterals and viscera.

5. Conclusion

In conclusion, it is a certain advantage for repairation of organism, abatement of neurodynia, and reduction of postherpetic neuralgia by acupuncture treatment, and the efficiency of combination electroacupuncture and fire acupuncture is better to that of the only electroacupuncture in the early days. However, at the end of the treatment period, the efficiency of electroacupuncture + cotton-pave moxibustion, electroacupuncture + fire acupuncture or electroacupuncture + tapping is no more than that of the only electroacupuncture. Further studies are required to determine the pre-clinical utility of this method.

References

[1] Burke, B.L., Steele, R.W., Beard, O.W., Wood, J.S., Cain, T.D. and Marmer, D.J. (1982) Immune Responses to Varicella-Zoster in the Aged. *Archives of Internal Medicine*, **142**, 291-293. http://dx.doi.org/10.1001/archinte.1982.00340150091017

[2] Meier, J.L. and Straus, S.E. (1992) Comparative Biology of Latent Varicella-Zoster Virus and Herpes Simplex Virus Infections. *The Journal of Infectious Diseases*, **166**, S13-S23. http://dx.doi.org/10.1093/infdis/166.Supplement_1.S13

[3] Gnann Jr., J.W. and Whitley, R.J. (2002) Herpes Zoster. *The New England Journal of Medicine*, **347**, 340-346. http://dx.doi.org/10.1056/NEJMcp013211

[4] Dworkin, R.H. and Portenoy, R.K. (1996) Pain and Its Persistence in Herpes Zoster. *Pain*, **67**, 241-251. http://dx.doi.org/10.1016/0304-3959(96)03122-3

[5] Gilden, D.H., Dueland, A.N., Cohrs, R., Martin, J.R., Kleinschmidt-DeMasters, B.K. and Mahalingam, R. (1991) Preherpetic Neuralgia. *Neurology*, **41**, 1215-1218. http://dx.doi.org/10.1212/WNL.41.8.1215

[6] Bowsher, D. (1995) Pathophysiology of Postherpetic Neuralgia: Towards a Rational Treatment. *Neurology*, **45**, S56-S57. http://dx.doi.org/10.1212/WNL.45.12_Suppl_8.S56

[7] Lydick, E., Epstein, R.S., Himmelberger, D. and White, C.J. (1995) Herpes Zoster and Quality of Life: A Self-Limited Disease with Severe Impact. *Neurology*, **45**, S52-S53. http://dx.doi.org/10.1212/WNL.45.12_Suppl_8.S52

[8] Graff-Radford, S.B., Kames, L.D. and Naliboff, B.D. (1986) Measure of Psychological Adjustment and Perception of Pain in Postherpetic Neuralgia and Trigeminal Neuralgia. *Clinical Journal of Pain*, **2**, 55. http://dx.doi.org/10.1097/00002508-198602010-00009

[9] Lancaster, T., Silagy, C. and Gray, S. (1995) Primary Care Management of Acute Herpes Zoster: Systematic Review of Evidence from Randomized Controlled Trials. *The British Journal of General Practice*, **45**, 39-45.

[10] Volmink, J., Lancaster, T., Gray, S. and Silagy, C. (1996) Treatments for Postherpetic Neuralgia—A Systematic Re-

view of Randomized Controlled Trials. *Family Practice*, **13**, 84-91. http://dx.doi.org/10.1093/fampra/13.1.84

[11] Alper, B.S. and Lewis, P.R. (2002) Treatment of Postherpetic Neuralgia: A Systematic Review of the Literature. *The Journal of Family Practice*, **51**, 121-128.

[12] Alper, B.S. and Lewis, P.R. (2000) Does Treatment of Acute Herpes Zoster Prevent or Shorten Postherpetic Neuralgia? *The Journal of Family Practice*, **49**, 255-264.

[13] Backonja, M. and Glanzman, R.L. (2003) Gabapentin Dosing for Neuropathic Pain: Evidence from Randomized, Placebo-Controlled Clinical Trials. *Clinical Therapeutics*, **25**, 81-104. http://dx.doi.org/10.1016/S0149-2918(03)90011-7

[14] Rice, A.S. and Maton, S. (2001) Gabapentin in Postherpetic Neuralgia: A Randomised, Double Blind, Placebo Controlled Study. *Pain*, **94**, 215-224. http://dx.doi.org/10.1016/S0304-3959(01)00407-9

[15] Owen, W. and Deadman, P. (1994) Treatment by Acupuncture for Herpes Zoster. *Journal of Chinese Medicine*, **45**, 1-2.

[16] Wu, J. and Guo, Z. (2000) Twenty-Three Cases of Postherpetic Neuralgia Treated by Acupuncture. *Journal of Traditional Chinese Medicine*, **20**, 36-37.

[17] Xuan, L. (2000) Treatment by Moxibustion for Herpes Zoster. *Journal of Chinese Medicine*, **64**, 17-18.

[18] Page, C.P., Curtis, M.J., Walker, M.J. and Hoffman, B.B. (2006) Integrated pharmacology. 3rd Edition, Elsevier (Mosby), Philadelphia, 87-160.

[19] Arora, A., Mendoza, N., Brantley, J., Yates, B., Dix, L. and Tyring, S. (2008) Double-Blind Study Comparing 2 Dosages of Valacyclovir Hydrochloride for the Treatment of Uncomplicated Herpes Zoster in Immunocompromised Patients 18 Years of Age and Older. *The Journal of Infectious Diseases*, **197**, 1289-1295. http://dx.doi.org/10.1086/586903

18

Acute and Long-Term Treatments with an Herbal Formula V-Vital Capsule Increase Exercise Endurance Capacity in Weight-Loaded Swimming Mice

Pou Kuan Leong[1], Hoi Yan Leung[1], Wing Man Chan[1], Ji Hang Chen[1], Hoi Shan Wong[1], Chung Wah Ma[2], Shi Yu Zou[2], Kam Ming Ko[1*]

[1]Division of Life Science, The Hong Kong University of Science & Technology, Hong Kong SAR, China
[2]Infinitus (China) Company Ltd., Guangzhou, China
Email: [*]bcrko@ust.hk

Abstract

Fatigue is a self-limiting response arising from physical and/or mental weariness, with a consequent personal and economic morbidity on work performance and social relationships. Anti-fatigue intervention is therefore urgently sought. "Qi-invigorating" Chinese tonic herbs, which can improve the energy status in the body according to the theory of traditional Chinese medicine, may produce beneficial effects in fatigue individuals. The herbal formula V-Vital capsule (VVC), which comprises 3 "Qi-invigorating" herbs, namely the root of *Rhodiola rosea*, *Eleutherococcus senticosus* and *Panax quinquefolium*, may produce anti-fatigue effect. In the present study, we investigated the effect of acute/long-term VVC treatment (acute: 0.75, 0.2 and 3.75 kg/day × 1 dose; long-term: 0.075 and 0.25 g/kg/day × 14 doses) on weight-loaded swimming female ICR mice. The weight-loaded swimming time until exhaustion, indicative of exercise endurance capacity, was recorded. Plasma levels of glucose, non-esterified fatty acid (NEFA), lactate and reactive oxygen metabolites (ROM) were measured in the exhausted mice. Glycogen levels in skeletal muscle and liver tissues were also measured. Mitochondrial function status [such as adenine nucleotide translocase (ANT) activity and coupling efficiency] was assayed. Results showed that acute VVC treatment increased the exercise endurance capacity in weight-loaded swimming mice. The ability of acute VVC treatment to enhance the exercise endurance was associated with increases in plasma glucose levels as well as glycogen levels in skeletal muscles and liver tissues, presumably due to the utilization of plasma lactate for gluconeogenesis and/or glycogen synthesis in the liver. While acute VVC treatment reduced the plasma ROM level in weight-loaded swimming mice, it increased the ANT activity. In this regard, the enhancement in exercise endurance afforded by acute

[*]Corresponding author.

VVC treatment might be due to an increase in the glucose supply to the skeletal muscle, the amelioration of systemic oxidative stress and the improvement in mitochondrial function of skeletal muscle. Consistent with the results obtained in acute VVC treatment experiment, the long-term VVC treatment enhances the exercise endurance in weight-loaded swimming mice. The ensemble of results suggests that VVC may offer a promising prospect for enhancing the exercise endurance and alleviating fatigue in humans.

Keywords

Fatigue, Exercise Endurance, *Rhodiola rosea*, *Eleutherococcus senticosus*, *Panax quinquefolium*

1. Introduction

Fatigue, which is a self-limiting response arising from physical and/or mental weariness, can be classified into three categories, namely secondary fatigue, physiologic fatigue and chronic fatigue [1]. Secondary fatigue refers to the weariness secondary to medical condition. While physiologic fatigue refers to an unbalance status of work and rest that can be recovered by taking rest, chronic fatigue is a pathological condition characterized by a persistent (or relapsing) debilitating and clinically unexplained fatigue that leads to a substantial impairment in functional status [2]. Chronic fatigue is a heterogeneous syndrome, characterized by a variety of pathophysiological features including neuroendocrine abnormalities, increased susceptibility to infections, obesity and chronic stress [2]. Despite the diversity of these pathophysiological anomalies, the disruption of structural and functional integrity of mitochondria has been shown to be crucially involved in the development of chronic fatigue, presumably due to an inadequate/inefficient energy supply to skeletal muscle [3] [4]. In order to sustain the energy demands in cytosol of muscle cells, the ATP synthesized in the mitochondria is exchanged with cytosolic ADP by adenine nucleotide translocase (ANT). In addition, the ANT-mediated ATP/ADP exchange was found to be critical for the maintenance of ATP synthase activity [5]. In view of the consequent personal and economic morbidity arising from the negative impacts of fatigue on work performance and social relationships [1], anti-fatigue intervention is urgently sought.

In an effort to develop safe interventions for fatigue, traditional Chinese medicine, which has a long history of use in safeguarding health, has attracted a lot of interest. In the realm of tradition Chinese medicine theories, Qi is a manifestation of energy status of the body [6]. In this connection, "Qi-invigorating" Chinese tonic herbs may produce beneficial effects in fatigue individuals. In support of this, recent studies have demonstrated that an extract of "Yang-invigorating" herb or a compound isolated from "Qi-invigorating" herb can enhance the mitochondrial ATP generation capacity in cultured cardiomyocytes as well as in mitochondria isolated from hearts of drug/herbal extract-treated rats [7] [8]. V-vital capsule (VVC) is an herbal formula comprising three "Qi-invigorating" herbs, namely, the root of *Rhodiola rosea*, the root of *Eleutherococcus senticosus* and the root of *Panax quinquefolium*. With respect to the increased capacity of mitochondrial ATP generation afforded by "Yang/Qi-invigorating" herbs [7] [8], VVC may offer a prospect for ameliorating physical and/or mental fatigue.

To evaluate the effectiveness of anti-fatigue intervention, force swimming test is a commonly adopted model for assessing the exercise endurance of mice [9] [10]. During the exercise, the supply of metabolic fuel molecules [such as glucose and non-esterified fatty acids (NEFA)] to skeletal muscle [11], the mobilization of energy reserves (such as glycogen in skeletal muscle and liver) [11] as well as the efficiency of mitochondrial respiration in skeletal muscle [12] determine the exercise endurance capacity. In the present study, we endeavored to examine the effect of acute and long treatment with VVC on exercise endurance and the associated changes in various biochemical parameters in mice using a weight-loaded forced swimming test. To assess the availability of fuel molecules, plasma levels of glucose and NEFA were measured. To examine the energy reserve, glycogen levels in skeletal muscle and liver tissues were also measured. In addition, various metabolites such as lactate (arising from the anaerobic glycolysis) and reactive oxygen metabolites (ROM, which is indicative of systemic oxidative stress) in plasma were measured. To assess the energy metabolic status of skeletal muscle, mitochondrial adenine nucleotide translocase (ANT) activity as well as state 3 and state 4 respiration rates of isolated mitochondria of skeletal muscle were assayed. The mitochondrial coupling efficiency was then estimated by computing the ratio of state 3 to state 4 mitochondrial respiratory rates.

2. Materials and Methods

2.1. Chemicals and Reagents

Lactate oxidase, horseradish peroxidase, bovine serum albumin (BSA) and 2,2'-azino-bis(3-ethylbenzothiazoline-6-sulfonic acid) diammonium salt (ABST) were purchased from Sigma Chemical Co. (St. Louis, MO, USA). NEFA assay kits were purchased from Wako Pure Chemical Industries, Ltd. (Okasa, Japan). Glucose assay reagent was obtained from Sigma Chemical Co. The VVC were manufactured and supplied by Infinitus (China) Company Ltd. (Guangzhou, China). All other chemicals were of analytical grade.

2.2. Animal Care

Male ICR mice (8 - 10 weeks old, 30 - 25 g) were maintained under a 12-hour dark/light cycle at about 22°C, and allowed food and water *ad libitum* in the Animal and Plant Care Facility at the Hong Kong University of Science and Technology (HKUST). All experimental protocols were approved by the University Committee on Research Practice at HKUST.

2.3. Animal Treatment

In the acute VVC treatment, male ICR mice were randomly assigned to 4 groups, with 10 - 15 mice in each group: (1) control; (2) VVC (0.75 g/kg); (3) VVC (2.5 g/kg); (4) VVC (3.75 g/kg). Control mice received water (vehicle) only. Thirty min post-dosing, the mice were subjected to weight-loaded swimming test. Mice were sacrificed under phenobarbital anesthesia after the swimming test.

In the long-term VVC treatment, male ICR mice were randomly assigned to 6 groups, with 10 - 15 mice in each group: (1) non-swimming control; (2) non-swimming VVC (0.075 g/kg); (3) non-swimming VVC (0.25 g/kg); (4) swimming control; (5) swimming VVC (0.075 g/kg); (6) swimming VVC (0.25 g/kg). Immediately after the 1st weight-loaded swimming test (*i.e.* week 0), mice were intragastrically administered with VVC (0.075 and 0.25 g/kg/day) 5 days per week for 2 weeks (*i.e.* 10 doses) while control mice received water (vehicle) only. Mice were then subjected to weight-loaded swimming test once a week for 2 weeks (*i.e.* at week 1 and week 2), at 30 min post-dosing with VVC. Mice were sacrificed under phenobarbital anesthesia after the last swimming test.

2.4. Weight-Loaded Swimming Test

The exercise endurance capacity was assessed by weight-loaded swimming test. Swimming exercise was conducted with mice carrying a load of 6% of their body weight. The exhaustion time was defined as the inability of weight-loaded mice to rise to the water surface for 7 seconds. Swimming exercise was carried out in a tank (20 × 25 × 33 cm), which was filled with water to a depth of ~28 cm and maintained at 25°C ± 1°C. The tank was shaken at a speed of 40 rpm. To avoid the influence of circadian rhythm on physical activity, swimming exercise was done during 11:00 to 17:00, a period in which a minimal variation of endurance capacity has been reported in mice. Hairs of mice were wet with detergent water (1% w/v) to reduce surface tension. The swimming time (second) until exhaustion was recorded.

2.5. Preparation of Blood/Tissue Samples

Blood samples were drawn from phenobarbital-anesthetized mice by cardiac excision using syringes rinsed with 0.5% heparin in saline (w/v). Plasma samples were obtained by centrifuging whole blood samples at 1500 ×*g* for 10 min at 4°C. Plasma samples were then subjected to biochemical analysis.

Minced gastrocnemius muscle tissues were digested by collagenase solution [0.075% (w/v) in buffer] at 4°C for 20 min. After removing the collagenase solution by centrifugation, the digested muscle tissues were mixed with 20 mL of ice-cold homogenizing buffer (100 mM KCl, 50 mM MOPS, 10 mM EGTA, pH 7.2) and subjected to homogenization with a Teflon-glass homogenizer at 4,000 rpm for 25 - 30 complete strokes. Then the homogenates were centrifuged at 600 ×*g* for 10 min at 4°C. The resultant supernatant was nucleus-free fraction [13].

Mitochondrial pellets were prepared from nucleus-free fractions of muscle homogenates by centrifugation at 9200 ×*g* at 4°C for 30 min. The mitochondrial pellets were then resuspended in a buffer containing 250 mM sucrose, 50 mM Tris, pH 7.5 [13].

2.6. Biochemical Analysis

Plasma fuel molecules. Plasma glucose levels were measured using an assay kit utilizing the coupled hexokinase-catalyzed and glucose-6-phosphate dehydrogenase-catalyzed reactions, with a resultant NAD reduction. Absorbance changes at 340 nm of the assay mixture were monitored spectrophotometrically by Victor^3 Multi-label Counter (Perkin Elmer, Turku, Finland). Plasma NEFA level was measured using assay kit.

Glycogen levels in the liver and skeletal muscle. Liver and skeletal muscle tissues were weighed and then subjected to acidic hydrolysis with 2 M HCl at 100˚C for 2 hours. The acidic hydrolyzed tissue samples were neutralized with 2 M NaOH and then centrifuged at 2150 ×*g* at 4˚C for 10 min. The glucose level of the supernatant, which contained glucose releasing from glycogen hydrolysis, was measured using assay kit.

Plasma lactate level. Plasma lactate level was measured using a reaction cocktail made up of lactate oxidase, horseradish peroxidase and ABST in a buffer [0.1 M citric acid, 1 mg/mL BSA, 0.1% $CaCl_2$ (w/v), 0.02% sodium azide (w/v), pH 6.0]. Absorbances at 405 nm of the assay mixtures were measured spectrophotometrically by Victor^3 Multi-label Counter.

Plasma reactive oxygen metabolites (ROM) level. The extent of exercise-induced changes in systemic oxidative stress was assessed by the measurement of plasma ROM level. Aliquots (40 μL) of plasma samples were mixed with 20 μL of 100 mM N, N-dimethyl-p-phenylenediamine (DMPD) and 1.97 mL of incubation buffer (0.1 M sodium acetate, pH 4.8). The reaction mixtures were incubated at 37˚C for 60 min in dark. Absorbances at 505 nm of the reaction mixtures were measured using Victor^3 Multi-Label Counter. The standard calibration curve was obtained by mixing 5 μL of *tert*-butylhydroperoxide (t-BHP) (up to 100 μM) with 20 μL phosphate-buffered saline, 5 μL of 2.52 mM $FeCl_2$ and 2 mL of DMPD. The amounts of hydroperoxyl compounds in plasma were estimated from the standard calibration curve and expressed in t-BHP equivalents [14].

Measurement of mitochondrial respiration. Mitochondrial respiratory rate was measured polarographically by a Clark-type oxygen electrode (Hansatech Instruments Ltd., Norfolk, UK) at 30˚C. Mitochondrial fraction (~0.5 mg protein/mL) was incubated in a buffer containing 30 mM KCl, 6 mM $MgCl_2$, 75 mM sucrose, 1 mM EDTA, 20 mM KH_2PO_4 and 0.1% (w/v) fatty acid-free BSA, pH 7.0. Substrate solution containing 10 mM glutamate and 2.5 mM malate was added, and after a stable state 2 respiration had been established, state 3 respiration (coupling) was initiated by the addition of ADP (final concentration 0.6 mM). When all of the added ADP was used up for ATP generation, oligomycin (ATP synthase inhibitor) was added to induce the state 4 respiration (uncoupling). The mitochondrial coupling efficiency was estimated by calculating the ratio of state 3 to state 4 respirations [13].

Adenine nucleotide translocase (ANT) function. ANT function was assessed by noting the transportation of ATP (out) and ADP (in) through mitochondrial inner membrane [4]. The mitochondrial ATP level (**a**) was first measured. Secondly, the same mitochondrial fraction was mixed with a buffer (pH = 5.5 ± 0.2; serving as an artificial cytosol) containing ADP, which activates the ANT to transport ADP to the mitochondrial matrix. After 10 min of incubation, the mitochondrial ATP level (**b**) was measured again. The value of ANT_{in} was estimated by measuring the fractional increase in mitochondrial ATP as follow: $ANT_{in} = [(b - a)/a]$. Thirdly, the same mitochondrial fraction was mixed with a buffer (pH = 8.9 ± 0.2) containing no ADP, which activates the ANT to transport ATP from the mitochondrial matrix to the artificial cytosol. After 10 min of incubation, the mitochondrial ATP level was measured again (**c**). The value of ANT_{out} was estimated by measuring the fractional decrease in ATP as follows: $ANT_{out} = [(c - a)/a]$

2.7. Statistical Analysis

Data were analyzed by one-way Analysis of Variance (ANOVA), except the data of the swimming time in long-term VVC treatment, were analyzed by mixed ANOVA. Post-hoc multiple comparisons were performed using Least Significant Difference. P values < 0.05 were regarded as statistically significant.

3. Results

3.1. Effects of Acute VVC Treatment on Weight-Loaded Swimming Time in Mice

Acute VVC treatment (2.5 and 3.75 g/kg) 30 min prior to weight-loaded swimming increased the weight-loaded swimming time by ~1-fold (104% and 104%, respectively) until exhaustion in mice (**Figure 1**).

3.2. Effects of Acute VVC Treatment on Plasma Levels of Fuel Molecules in Non-Swimming and Weight-Loaded Swimming Mice

Acute VVC treatment (0.75, 2.5 and 3.75 g/kg) dose-dependently increased plasma glucose level (22%, 40% and 54%, respectively) in non-swimming mice (**Figure 2**). However, acute VVC treatment decreased the plasma NEFA level (29%, 33% and 47%, respectively) in a dose-dependent manner. Weight-loaded swimming until exhaustion decreased plasma levels of glucose (25%) and NEFA (32%) when compared with the non-swimming control. Acute VVC treatment increased plasma glucose level (44%, 46% and 31%, respectively) and decreased plasma NEFA level (21% and 25% at 2.5 and 3.75 g/kg, respectively) in weight-loaded swimming mice.

3.3. Effects of Acute VVC Treatment on Skeletal/Hepatic Glycogen Levels in Non-Swimming and Weight-Loaded Swimming Mice

Acute VVC treatment did not produce any detectable changes in hepatic/skeletal muscle glycogen in

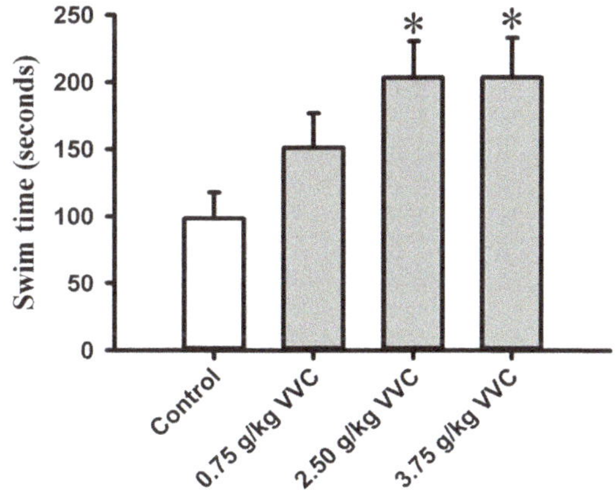

Figure 1. Effects of acute VVC treatment on weight-loaded swimming time in mice. Mice were intragastrically administered with VVC (0.75, 2.5 and 3.75 g/kg). At 30 minutes post-dosing, the mice were subjected to weight-loaded swimming test, as described in Materials and Methods. The swimming times of mice until exhaustion were recorded. Data were expressed as swimming time (second). Value given are means ± SEM, with n = 10 - 15. * Significantly different from drug-untreated control.

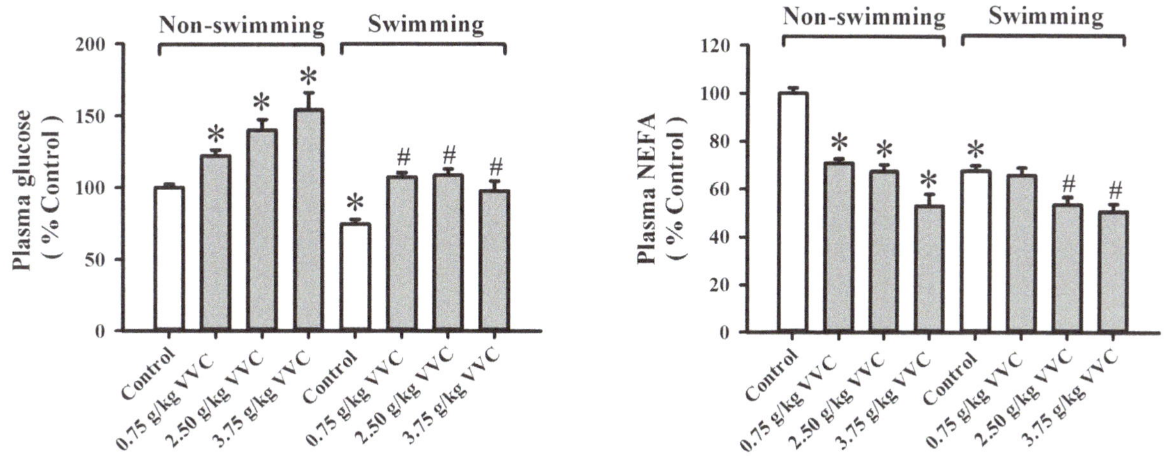

Figure 2. Effects of acute VVC treatment on plasma levels of fuel molecules in non-swimming and weight-loaded swimming mice. Mice were sacrificed after weight-loaded swimming until exhaustion. Plasma glucose level (Non-swimming control = 71.62 ± 2.61 mg/mL) and plasma non-esterified fatty acid (NEFA) level (Non-swimming control = 1.44 ± 0.05 mEq/L) were measured, as described in Materials and Methods. Data were expressed as % control, by normalizing with the value of non-swimming control. Value given are means ± SEM, with n = 10 - 15. * Significantly different from non-swimming control; # Significantly different from swimming control.

non-swimming mice. Weight-loaded swimming until exhaustion depleted skeletal muscle (49%) but not hepatic glycogen level in mice (**Figure 3**). Acute VVC treatment caused increases in skeletal muscle and hepatic glycogen levels in weight-loaded swimming mice, with maximal stimulation being 60% and 87% at the doses of 2.5 and 3.75 g/kg, respectively.

3.4. Effects of Acute VVC Treatment on Plasma Levels of Metabolites in Non-Swimming and Weight-Loaded Swimming Mice

Acute VVC treatment did not change plasma lactate levels in non-swimming mice. Weight-loaded swimming until exhaustion increased plasma lactate level (45%) (**Figure 4**), which was associated with the decrease in

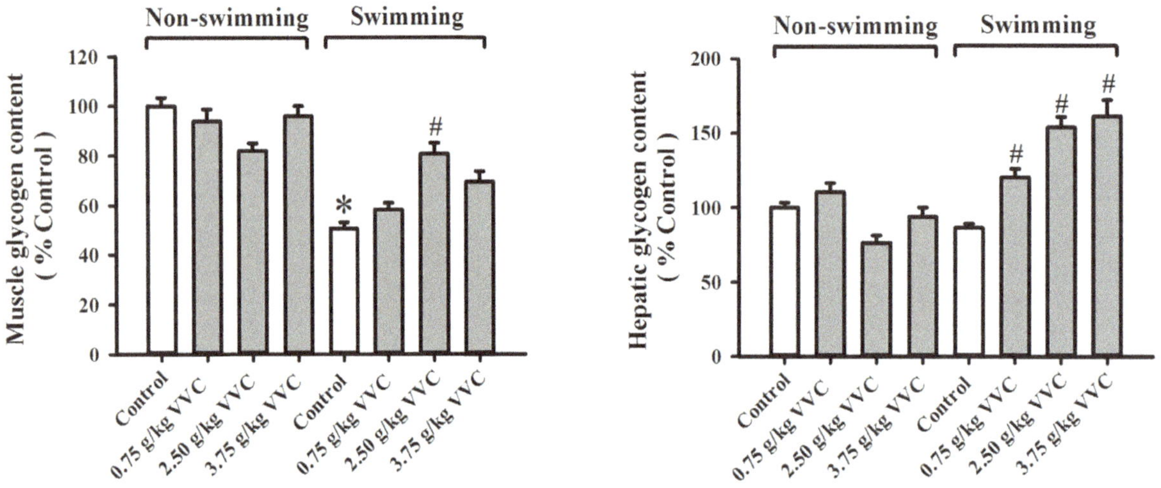

Figure 3. Effects of acute VVC treatment on skeletal/hepatic glycogen levels in non-swimming and weight-loaded swimming mice. Mice were sacrificed after weight-loaded swimming until exhaustion. Skeletal glycogen level (Non-swimming control = 0.52 ± 0.03 μmol glucosyl unit/unit g tissue) and hepatic glycogen level (Non-swimming control = 5.95 ± 0.41 μmol glucosyl unit/unit g tissue) were measured, as described in Materials and Methods. Data were expressed as % control, by normalizing with the value of non-swimming control. Value given are means ± SEM, with n = 10 - 15. * Significantly different from non-swimming control; # Significantly different from swimming control.

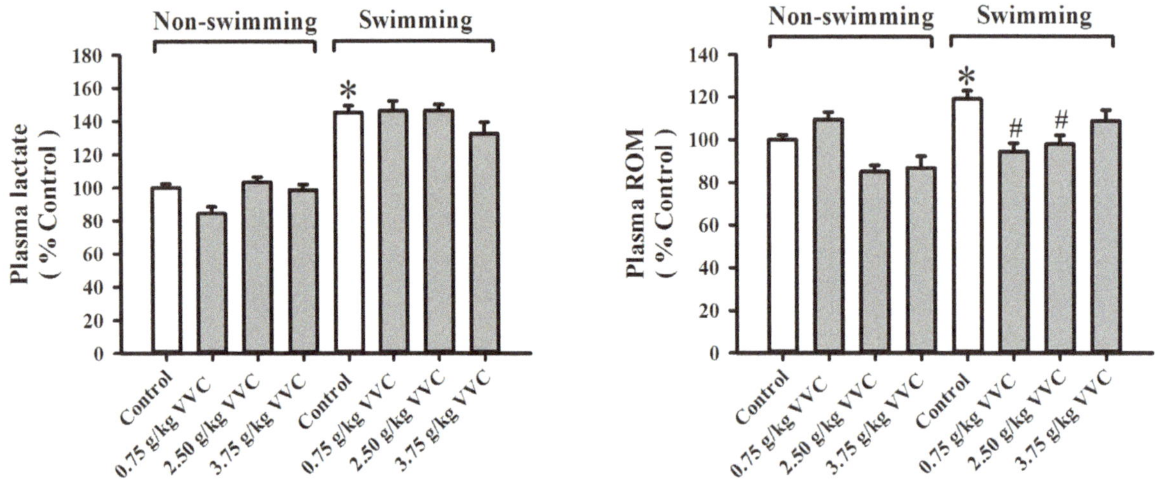

Figure 4. Effects of acute VVC treatment on plasma levels of metabolites in non-swimming and weight-loaded swimming mice. Mice were sacrificed after weight-loaded swimming until exhaustion. Plasma lactate level (Non-swimming control = 4.33 ± 0.24 mM) and plasma reactive oxygen metabolites (ROM) level (Non-swimming control = 105 ± 4.39 μmol tBHP equivalent) were measured, as described in Materials and Methods. Data were expressed as % control, by normalizing with the value of non-swimming control. Value given are means ± SEM, with n = 10 - 15. * Significantly different from non-swimming control; # Significantly different from swimming control.

plasma glucose level in weight-loaded swimming. Despite the fact that acute VVC treatment increased in plasma glucose level in weight-loaded swimming mice, plasma lactate levels were not affected. Acute VVC treatment also did not alter plasma ROM level in non-swimming mice. Weight-loaded swimming until exhaustion increased plasma ROM level (19%) in mice which was found to be reduced by acute VVC treatment (21% and 18% at 0.75 and 2.5 g/kg, respectively).

3.5. Effects of Acute VVC Treatment on Mitochondrial Functional Status of Skeletal Muscle in Non-Swimming and Weight-Loaded Swimming Mice

Acute VVC treatment did not produce any detectable change in the mitochondrial coupling efficiency of skeletal muscle in non-swimming mice (**Figure 5**). Weight-loaded swimming until exhaustion decreased mitochondrial coupling efficiency (24%) in mouse skeletal muscle. Acute VVC treatment at 0.75 g/kg significantly increased mitochondrial coupling efficiency (37%) in weight-loaded swimming mice. Acute VVC treatment (0.75, 2.5 and

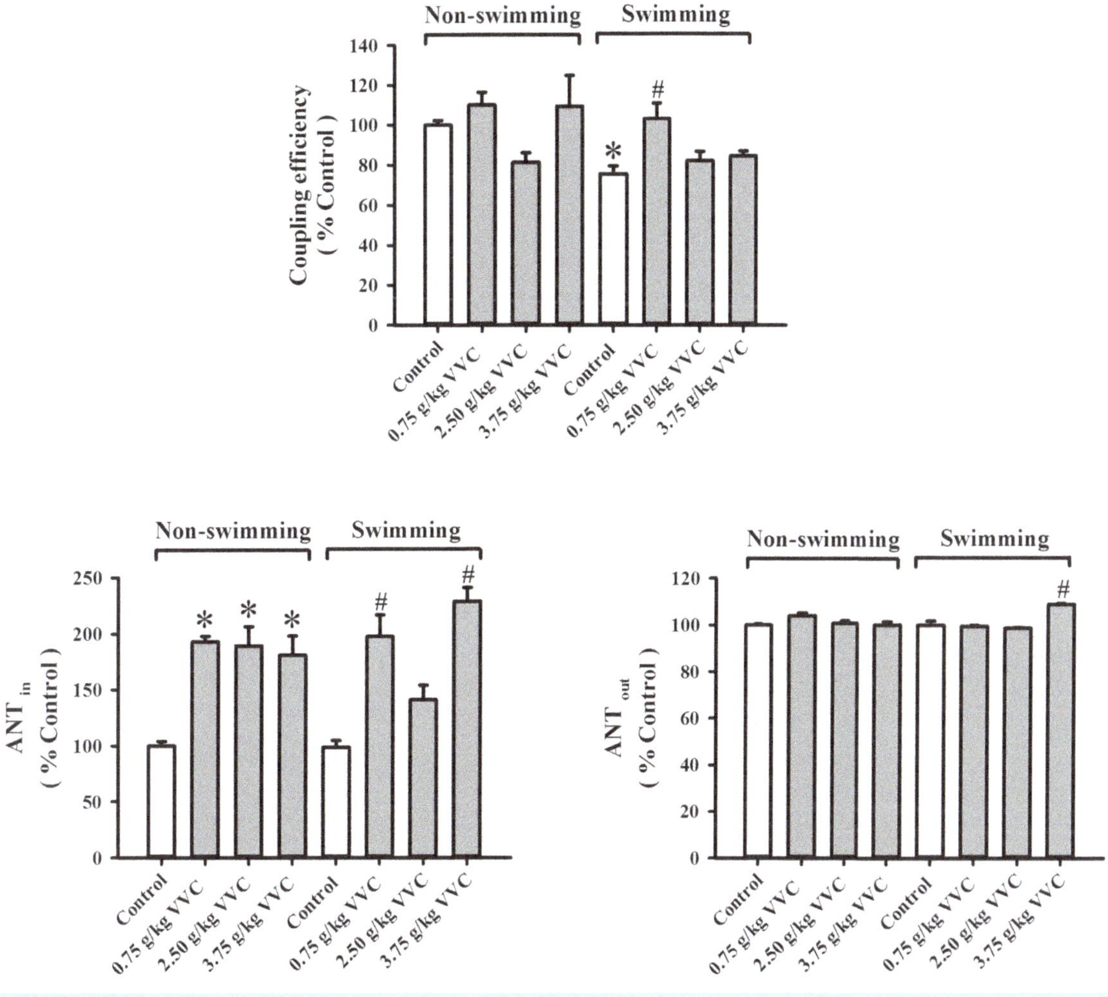

Figure 5. Effects of acute VVC treatment on mitochondrial functional status of skeletal muscle in non-swimming and weight-loaded swimming mice. Mice were sacrificed after weight-loaded swimming until exhaustion. Mitochondrial respiratory rates of skeletal muscle was measured polarographically by a Clark-type oxygen electrode at 30°C. The coupling efficiency was estimated by calculating the ratio of state 3 to state 4 respirations (Non-swimming control = 2.51 ± 0.07). The effectiveness of adenosine nucleotide translocase (ANT) of skeletal muscle was also assessed, as described in Materials and Methods. ANT_{in} (which indicates the effectiveness of ADP influx in mitochondria; Non-swimming control = 9.02 ± 1.00) and ANT_{out} (which indicates the effectiveness of ATP outflux from mitochondria; Non-swimming control = 0.94 ± 0.01) were measured. Data were expressed as % control, by normalizing with the value of non-swimming control. Values given are means ± SEM, with n = 5 - 10. *Significantly different from non- swimming control; # Significantly different from swimming control.

3.75 g/kg) significantly increased mitochondrial ANT_{in} activity (93%, 89% and 81%, respectively) in skeletal muscle of non-swimming mice, but it did not affect the ANT_{out} activity. While weight-loaded swimming until exhaustion did not alter mitochondrial $ANT_{in/out}$ activities, acute VVC treatment increased the ANT_{in} activity (101% and 92% at 0.75 and 3.75 g/kg, respectively) in weight-loaded swimming mice. The ANT_{out} activity seemed to be slightly but significantly increased (9%) in acute VVC-treated (3.75 g/kg) and weight-loaded swimming mice.

3.6. Effects of Long-Term VVC Treatment on the Weight-Loaded Swimming Time of Mice

Long-term treatment (0.075 and 0.25 g/kg) for 2 weeks progressively increased the weight-loaded swimming time of mice, with the effect produced by the low dose of VVC being more prominent at 1 week post-treatment and the extent of prolongation in weight-loaded swimming time being 35.6% for both doses at 2 weeks post-treatment (**Figure 6**).

3.7. Effects of Long-Term VVC Treatment on Various Biochemical Parameters in Non-Swimming and Weight-Loaded Swimming Mice

Long-term VVC treatment did not produce any significant changes in the levels of plasma glucose, muscle glycogen, plasma metabolites as well as mitochondrial coupling efficiency in skeletal muscle of non-swimming mice, except a decrease in plasma NEFA (15% at 0.25 g/kg), increases in hepatic glycogen (29% and 25% at 0.075 and 0.25 g/kg, respectively) as well as a dose-dependent increase in mitochondrial ANT_{in} activity in skeletal muscle (95% and 115% at 0.075 and 0.25 g/kg, respectively) (**Table 1**). Consistent with the results obtained from acute VVC treatment, weight-loaded swimming until exhaustion significantly decreased the plasma glucose as well as NEFA levels (25% and 32%, respectively), skeletal muscle glycogen level (46%) and hepatic glycogen level (37%). The weight-loaded swimming-induced depletions in plasma fuel molecules and energy reserves were associated with increases in plasma levels of metabolites, such as lactate (30%) and ROM (39%). While the long-term VVC treatment at low dose increased the mitochondrial ANT_{in} activity (79% vs. swimming control) in skeletal muscle of weight-loaded swimming mice, the long-term VVC treatment at high dose further increased the glycogen level (44% vs. swimming control) as well as mitochondrial coupling efficiency (83% vs swimming control) in skeletal muscle. The plasma ROM level was reduced (19% vs. swimming control) in VVC-treated (0.25 g/kg) weight-loaded swimming mice.

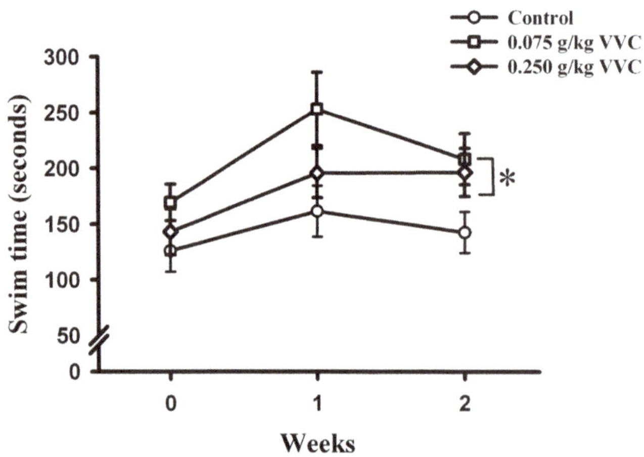

Figure 6. Effects of long-term VVC treatment on the weight-loaded swimming time of mice. Mice were subjected to weight-loaded swimming test every week (including the week 0) during the 2-week period of experiment, as described in Materials and Methods. The swimming times of mice until exhaustion were recorded. Immediately after the 1st weight-loaded swimming test (*i.e.* week 0), mice were intragastrically administered with VVC (0.075 and 0.25 g/kg/day) 5 days per week for 2 weeks (*i.e.* 10 doses), while control mice received water (vehicle) only. Data were expressed as swim time (second). Value given are means ± SEM, with n = 10 - 15. * Significantly different from drug-untreated control.

Table 1. Effects of long-term VVC treatment on various biochemical parameters in non-swimming and weight-loaded swimming mice.

	Non-Swim			Swim		
	Control	VVC		Control	VVC	
		0.075 g/kg	0.25 g/kg		0.075 g/kg	0.25 g/kg
Fuel molecules						
Plasma glucose	100 ± 2.4	108 ± 4.9	107 ± 3.2	74.5 ± 3.3[a]	61.0 ± 2.1	68.0 ± 3.5
Plasma NEFAs	100 ± 2.4	98.1 ± 3.0	84.8 ± 2.2[a]	68.2 ± 3.3[a]	65.8 ± 209	74.3 ± 3.2
Energy reserves						
Muscle glycogen	100 ± 2.2	93.3 ± 2.5	99.5 ± 2.7	53.8 ± 2.1[a]	65.5 ± 4.1	77.6 ± 4.4[b]
Hepatic glycogen	100 ± 2.3	129 ± 5.7 [a]	125 ± 3.9[a]	62.6 ± 2.4[a]	74.7 ± 3.8	84.1 ± 4.5
Metabolites						
Plasma lactate	100 ± 1.7	91.0 ± 4.0	90.9 ± 3.7	130 ± 4.1[a]	123 ± 3.4	115 ± 2.8
ROM	100 ± 2.8	95.9 ± 2.9	90.1 ± 3.3	139 ± 5.2[a]	126 ± 2.9	113 ± 2.9[b]
Mitochondrial functional status in skeletal muscle						
Coupling efficiency	100 ± 2.7	88.1 ± 14.7	87.7 ± 5.4	67.1 ± 10.2	90.9 ± 5.1	123 ± 17.8[b]
ANT_{in}	100 ± 4.5	195 ± 15.6[a]	215 ± 22.0[a]	144 ± 14.2	258 ± 32.8[b]	110 ± 7.7
ANT_{out}	100 ± 0.4	101 ± 0.2	102 ± 0.8	99.8 ± 0.2	100 ± 0.1	101 ± 0.3

a. significantly different from non-swimming control; b. significantly different from swimming control.

4. Discussion

Acute VVC treatment increased the exercise endurance capacity in mice, as indicated by the increase in the swimming time of weight-loaded swimming mice. The ability of VVC to enhance exercise endurance is consistent with the experimental observations that all component herbs of VVC (*i.e.*, the root of *Rhodiola rosea*, *Eleutherococcus senticosus* and *Panax quinquefolium*) independently increased the exercise endurance capacity in rodents. In this regard, the treatment with *Rhodiola rosea* extract was found to increase the swimming performance in both weight-unloaded and loaded rats [15] [16]. While the *Eleutherococcus senticosus* extract could increase the swimming time in forced swimming mice [17], the treatment with a protein fraction (containing proteins ranging from 8 - 66 kDa) isolated from *Panax quinquefolium* was able to increase the exercise endurance in weight-loaded swimming mice [18].

Force swimming-induced exhaustion, as observed in the present and other studies [9] [10], was found to be accompanied by depletions in plasma fuel molecules, suggestive of their involvement in muscle fatigue. In the present study, acute VVC treatment was found to increase the plasma level of glucose, with a concomitant decrease in plasma NEFA level, in both non-swimming and swimming mice. While the adipose tissue-derived NEFA is the major oxidative fuel molecule in skeletal muscle during low intensity exercise (such as weight-unloaded swimming) [19], plasma glucose is the major fuel molecule in skeletal muscle during high intensity exercise (such as weight-loaded swimming) [20]. As such, the enhancement in exercise endurance, as assessed by weight-loaded swimming, afforded by VVC may be due to the increase in plasma glucose supply to skeletal muscle for the anaerobic glycolysis. The lactate arising from anaerobic glycolysis then can undergo Cori cycle in the liver, with a resultant synthesis of glucose or glycogen. Given that high intensity exercise was found to time-dependently increase the plasma lactate level in rodents [21], VVC-treated mice, of which the swimming time is longer than those of VVC-untreated mice, should be expected to exhibit a higher plasma lactate level. However, VVC treatment did not increase the plasma lactate level in swimming mice, suggesting that plasma lactate may be utilized for gluconeogenesis and/or glycogen synthesis in the liver. This postulation is further strengthened by the observation that the glycogen levels in skeletal muscle and liver were elevated in VVC-treated weight-loaded swimming mice.

The increased production of metabolites [e.g. H^+ ion, lactate and reactive oxygen species (ROS)] during high intensity exercise was also found to be associated with muscle fatigue [22]. High plasma levels of H^+/lactate were conventionally considered as the major cause of muscle fatigue [23]. As mentioned earlier, VVC may facilitate the metabolism of lactate in the liver, leading to a postponed increase in plasma lactate level, which in turn enhances the exercise endurance. Recent studies have shown that low pH [24] [25] and high lactate level [26] [27] may have less inhibitory effect on the muscle contraction than that of previously assumed. The muscle fatigue may be mainly caused by the reduction of sarcoplasmic reticulum (SR) Ca^{2+} release [28]. With this notion in mind, ROS, which could reduce the maximum Ca^{2+}-activated force in skeletal muscle, the SR Ca^{2+} release and the Ca^{2+} sensitivity of contractile proteins [28], are hypothesized to play a critical role in muscle fatigue. In this connection, the acute VVC treatment-induced amelioration of systemic oxidative stress in swimming mice, as evidenced by a reduction of plasma ROM, may also contribute to the enhancement on exercise endurance. In support of this, a constituent of VVC, *Rhodiola rosea*, was also found to reduce swimming-enhanced oxidative stress in rat, possibly via its ROS scavenging capability and induction of the antioxidant defense system [15].

Acute VVC treatment improved the mitochondrial function in swimming mice, as indicated by increases in mitochondrial coupling efficiency and $ANT_{in/out}$ activities. An earlier study suggested that the mitochondrial function in skeletal muscle was positively correlated with the physical exercise performance in humans [29]. In this regard, the VVC-induced enhancement in exercise endurance may also be attributed to the improvement of mitochondrial function in skeletal muscle of swimming mice. In addition, a recent study showed that the PGC-1α-mediated activation of ANT reduced the production of mitochondrial ROS in cultured endothelial cells, with a resultant protection against oxidant-induced apoptosis [30]. Therefore, the activation of ANT by VVC may also be involved in the attenuation of systemic oxidative stress.

Consistent with the results obtained in acute VVC treatment, we further demonstrated that a long-term and low dose VVC treatment enhanced the exercise endurance in weight-loaded swimming mice, with an associated increase in ANT_{in} activity at a low dose of treatment. However, varied effects on plasma fuel molecules, plasma metabolites, glycogen levels in skeletal muscle and liver, as well as mitochondrial functional status were observed between the acute and long-term treatment, which may possibly be related to the differences in the dose and duration of VVC treatment.

5. Conclusion

In conclusion, both acute and long-term VVC treatments were found to enhance the exercise endurance in weight-loaded swimming mice. The enhancement in exercise endurance afforded by acute VVC treatment was associated with the increase in plasma fuel molecule, the amelioration of systemic oxidative stress, and the improvement in mitochondrial function of skeletal muscle. The ensemble of results suggests that VVC may offer a promising prospect for enhancing the exercise endurance and alleviating fatigue in humans.

References

[1] Rosenthal, T.C., Majeroni, B.A., Pretorius, R. and Malik, K. (2008) Fatigue: An Overview. *American Family Physician*, **78**, 1173-1179.

[2] Afari, N. and Buchwald, D. (2003) Chronic Fatigue Syndrome: A Review. *The American Journal of Psychiatry*, **160**, 221-236. http://dx.doi.org/10.1176/appi.ajp.160.2.221

[3] Plioplys, A.V. and Plioplys, S. (1995) Electron-Microscopic Investigation of Muscle Mitochondria in Chronic Fatigue Syndrome. *Neuropsychobiology*, **32**, 175-181. http://dx.doi.org/10.1159/000119233

[4] Myhill, S., Booth, N.E. and McLaren-Howard, J. (2009) Chronic Fatigue Syndrome and Mitochondrial Dysfunction. *International Journal of Clinical and Experimental Medicine*, **2**, 1-6.

[5] Vander Heiden, M.G., Chandel, N.S., Schumacker, P.T. and Thompson, C.B. (1999) Bcl-xL Prevents Cell Death Following Growth Factor Withdrawal by Facilitating Mitochondrial ATP/ADP Exchange. *Molecular Cell*, **3**, 159-167. http://dx.doi.org/10.1016/S1097-2765(00)80307-X

[6] Zhang, D. and Wu, X. (1991) Chapter 5 Qi, Blood, Body Fluid, Essence of Life and Spirit. In: Liu, Y., Ed., *The Basic Knowledge of Traditional Chinese Medicine*, Hai Feng Publishing Co., Hong Kong, 49-53.

[7] Wong, H.S., Chen, N., Leong, P.K. and Ko, K.M. (2013) β-Sitosterol Enhances Cellular Glutathione Redox Cycling by Reactive Oxygen Species Generated From Mitochondrial Respiration: Protection Against Oxidant Injury in H9c2 Cells

and Rat Hearts. *Phytotherapy Research*, **28**, 999-1006. http://dx.doi.org/10.1002/ptr.5087

[8] Chiu, P.Y. and Ko, K.M. (2003) Time-Dependent Enhancement in Mitochondrial Glutathione Status and ATP Generation Capacity by Schisandrin B Treatment Decreases the Susceptibility of Rat Hearts to Ischemia-Reperfusion Injury. *Biofactors*, **19**, 43-51. http://dx.doi.org/10.1002/biof.5520190106

[9] Su, K.Y., Yu, C.Y., Chen, Y.W., Huang, Y.T., Chen, C.T., Wu, H.F. and Chen, Y.L. (2014) Rutin, a Flavonoid and Principal Component of Saussurea Involucrata, Attenuates Physical Fatigue in a Forced Swimming Mouse Model. *International Journal of Medical Sciences*, **11**, 528-537. http://dx.doi.org/10.7150/ijms.8220

[10] Chen, J.C., Hsiang, C.Y., Lin, Y.C. and Ho, T.Y. (2014) Deer Antler Extract Improves Fatigue Effect through Altering the Expression of Genes Related to Muscle Strength in Skeletal Muscle of Mice. *Evidence-Based Complementary and Alternative Medicine*, **2014**, Article ID: 540580. http://dx.doi.org/10.1155/2014/540580

[11] Holloszy, J.O. and Kohrt, W.M. (1996) Regulation of Carbohydrate and Fat Metabolism during and after Exercise. *Annual Review of Nutrition*, **16**, 121-138. http://dx.doi.org/10.1146/annurev.nu.16.070196.001005

[12] Conley, K.E., Jubrias, S.A., Cress, M.E. and Esselman, P.C. (2013) Elevated Energy Coupling and Aerobic Capacity Improves Exercise Performance in Endurance-Trained Elderly Subjects. *Experimental Physiology*, **98**, 899-907. http://dx.doi.org/10.1113/expphysiol.2012.069633

[13] Leong, P.K., Leung, H.Y., Wong, H.S., Chen, J.H., Chan, W.M., Ma, C.W., Yang, Y.T. and Ko, K.M. (2014) Long-Term Treatment with an Herbal Formula MCC Ameliorates Obesity-Associated Metabolic Dysfunction in High Fat Diet-Induced Obese Mice: A Comparative Study among MCC and Various Combinations of Its Constituents. *Chinese Medicine*, **5**, 34-46. http://dx.doi.org/10.4236/cm.2014.51005

[14] Leong, P.K., Chen, N., Chiu, P.Y., Leung, H.Y., Ma, C.W., Tang, Q.T. and Ko, K.M. (2010) Long-Term Treatment with Shengmai San-Derived Herbal Supplement (Wei Kang Su) Enhances Antioxidant Response in Various Tissues of Rats with Protection against Carbon Tetrachloride Hepatotoxicity. *Journal of Medicinal Food*, **13**, 427-438. http://dx.doi.org/10.1089/jmf.2009.1296

[15] Huang, S.C., Lee, F.T., Kuo, T.Y., Yang, J.H. and Chien, C.T. (2009) Attenuation of Long-Term *Rhodiola rosea* Supplementation on Exhaustive Swimming-Evoked Oxidative Stress in the Rat. *Chinese Journal of Physiology*, **52**, 316-324. http://dx.doi.org/10.4077/CJP.2009.AMH029

[16] Lee, F.T., Kuo, T.Y., Liou, S.Y. and Chien, C.T. (2009) Chronic *Rhodiola rosea* Extract Supplementation Enforces Exhaustive Swimming Tolerance. *The American Journal of Chinese Medicine*, **37**, 557-572. http://dx.doi.org/10.1142/S0192415X09007053

[17] Kimura, Y. and Sumiyoshi, M. (2004) Effects of Various *Eleutherococcus senticosus* Cortex on Swimming Time, Natural Killer Activity and Corticosterone Level in Forced Swimming Stressed Mice. *Journal of Ethnopharmacology*, **95**, 447-453. http://dx.doi.org/10.1016/j.jep.2004.08.027

[18] Qi, B., Liu, L., Zhang, H., Zhou, G.X., Wang, S., Duan, X.Z., Bai, X.Y., Wang, S.M. and Zhao, D.Q. (2014) Anti-Fatigue Effects of Proteins Isolated from *Panax quinquefolium*. *Journal of Ethnopharmacology*, **153**, 430-434. http://dx.doi.org/10.1016/j.jep.2014.02.045

[19] Frayn, K.N. (2010) Fat as a Fuel: Emerging Understanding of the Adipose Tissue-Skeletal Muscle Axis. *Acta Physiologica*, **199**, 509-518. http://dx.doi.org/10.1111/j.1748-1716.2010.02128.x

[20] Jeppesen, J. and Kiens, B. (2012) Regulation and Limitations to Fatty Acid Oxidation during Exercise. *Journal of Physiology*, **590**, 1059-1068.

[21] Kato, M., Kurakane, S., Nishina, A., Park, J. and Chang H. (2013) The Blood Lactate Increase in High Intensity Exercise Is Depressed by *Acanthopanax sieboldianus*. *Nutrients*, **5**, 4134-4144. http://dx.doi.org/10.3390/nu5104134

[22] Green, H.J. (1997) Mechanisms of Muscle Fatigue in Intense Exercise. *Journal of Sports Sciences*, **15**, 247-256. http://dx.doi.org/10.1080/026404197367254

[23] Fitts, R.H. (1994) Cellular Mechanisms of Muscle Fatigue. *Physiological Reviews*, **74**, 49-94.

[24] Cady, E.B., Jones, D.A., Lynn, J. and Newham, D.J. (1989) Changes in Force and Intracellular Metabolites during Fatigue of Human Skeletal Muscle. *Journal of Physiology*, **418**, 311-325.

[25] Stary, C.M. and Hogan, M.C. (2005) Intracellular pH during Sequential, Fatiguing Contractile Periods in Isolated Single *Xenopus* Skeletal Muscle Fibers. *Journal of Applied Physiology*, **99**, 308-312. http://dx.doi.org/10.1152/japplphysiol.01361.2004

[26] Karlsson, J., Funderburk, C.F., Essen, B. and Lind, A.R. (1975) Constituents of Human Muscle in Isometric Fatigue. *Journal of Applied Physiology*, **38**, 208-211.

[27] Van Beekvelt, M.C., Drost, G., Rongen, G., Stegeman, D.F., Van Engelen, B.G. and Zwarts, M.J. (2006) Na^+-K^+-ATPase Is Not Involved in the Warming-Up Phenomenon in Generalized Myotonia. *Muscle & Nerve*, **33**, 514-523. http://dx.doi.org/10.1002/mus.20483

[28] Allen, D.G., Lamb, G.D. and Westerblad, H. (2008) Skeletal Muscle Fatigue: Cellular Mechanisms. *Physiological Reviews*, **88**, 287-332. http://dx.doi.org/10.1152/physrev.00015.2007

[29] Jacobs, R.A., Flück, D., Bonne, T.C., Bürgi, S., Christensen, P.M., Toigo, M. and Lundby C. (1985) Improvements in Exercise Performance with High-Intensity Interval Training Coincide with an Increase in Skeletal Muscle Mitochondrial Content and Function. *Journal of Applied Physiology*, **115**, 785-793. http://dx.doi.org/10.1152/japplphysiol.00445.2013

[30] Won, J.C., Park, J.Y., Kim, Y.M., Koh, E.H., Seol, S., Jeon, B.H., Han, J., Kim, J.R., Park, T.S., Choi, C.S., Lee, W.J., Kim, M.S., Lee, I.K., Youn, J.H. and Lee, K.U. (2010) Peroxisome Proliferator-Activated Receptor-γ Coactivator 1-α Overexpression Prevents Endothelial Apoptosis by Increasing ATP/ADP Translocase Activity. *Thrombosis, and Vascular Biology*, **30**, 290-297. http://dx.doi.org/10.1161/ATVBAHA.109.198721

List of Abbreviations

Adenine nucleotide translocase (ANT); Analysis of Variance (ANOVA); 2,2'-azino-bis(3-ethylbenzothiazoline-6-sulfonic acid) diammonium salt (ABST); Bovine serum albumin (BSA); tert-Butylhydroperoxide (t-BHP); N, N-dimethyl-p-phenylenediamine (DMPD); Non-esterified fatty acid (NEFA); Reactive oxygen metabolites (ROM); Reactive oxygen species (ROS); Sarcoplasmic reticulum (SR); V-vital capsule (VVC).

19

Expression Imbalance of Cholinergic M_2 and M_3 Receptors Contributes to the Motility Reduction of the Small Intestine in Spleen Qi Deficiency

Fan Zhao, Xudong Liu, Wenjun Liu, Jiyan Cai, Lingzhi Wang, Huaxin Yu, Lu Wang, Lide Zhang, Deshan Wang, Dehong Shan*

Liaoning University of Traditional Chinese Medicine, Shenyang, China
Email: *Dehongshan@lnutcm.edu.cn

Abstract

Objective: To study roles of cholinergic M_2 and M_3 receptors in the motility reduction of small intestine (SI) in spleen qi deficiency. Methods: 16 male SD rats were randomly divided in the control group and spleen qi deficiency group (model group)—8 rats each group; spleen qi deficiency model of the improper diet and overfatigue was established; the SI propelling rate (SIPR) was used to evaluate the SI motility; ELISA was used to measure concentrations of acetylcholine (ACh), cyclic adenosine monophosphate (cAMP) and protein kinase A (PKA) in the SI tissue; immohistochemistry was employed to detect expressions of cholinergic M_2 and M_3 receptors. Results: Compared with those in the control group, SIPR was reduced; expression of M_2 receptors was increased; and expression of M_3 receptors and concentrations of cAMP and PKA were decreased, significantly, in the model group. Conclusions: Expression imbalance of cholinergic M_2 and M_3 receptors might contribute to the motility reduction of the SI in spleen qi deficiency.

Keywords

Spleen Qi Deficiency, Small Intestine Motility, M_2 Receptor, M_3 Receptor

1. Introduction

Poor appetite and abdominal distension are common symptoms of spleen qi deficiency, and both of them relate

*Corresponding author.

to the reduction of gastrointestinal (GI) kinetics. Generally, smooth muscles (SM) of the GI tract are predominantly innervated by adrenergic and cholinergic nerves of the autonomic nervous system (ANS), and the latter was focused in the present study due to its excitatory effect. Acetylcholine (ACh) released by cholinergic nerves can activate muscarinic receptors to evoke the SM contraction [1]. Muscarinic receptors in the GI tract are primarily M_2 and M_3 subtypes. Although M_2 receptors outnumber M_3 receptors by up to 4:1, M_3 subtype is the primary receptor to evoke the SM contraction directly, whereas M_2 subtype is the conditional receptor, and inhibits the synthesis of cyclic adenosine monophosphate (cAMP) and protein kinase A (PKA), thereby abrogating the muscle relaxation [2].

Abnormal expressions of M_2 and M_3 subtypes contribute to GI diseases [3] [4]; however, it is still not known whether these two receptors involve in the pathology of spleen qi deficiency. In the present study, based on the rat spleen qi deficiency model of improper diet and overfatigue, the small intestine propelling rate (SIPR) and related cholinergic components were tested, attempting to reveal regulatory roles of M_2 and M_3 receptors in the SI motion of spleen qi deficiency.

2. Materials and Methods

2.1. Animals

Sixteen male SD rats weighing 220 ± 10 g (Liaoning Changsheng Biotechnology Co., Ltd (SCXK (Liao) 2010-0001) were used. Rats were randomly divided into 2 groups of 8 each, the control group and spleen qi deficiency model group (model group). Animals were group housed under the following laboratory condition: temperature 23˚C ± 1˚C, humidity 40% - 60%. Animal care procedures were carried out in accordance with the National Institutes of Health Guide for the Care and Use of Laboratory Animals, and every effort was made to minimize the animal suffering.

2.2. Establishment and Evaluation of the Spleen Qi Deficiency Model

Rats in the model group were treated according to the following protocol for 2 weeks: food and water were available *ad libitum* on odd days and fed only with cabbage on even days; forced to swim to fatigue in 35˚C - 37˚C water every day. Evaluation criterion for spleen qi deficiency is: 1) emaciation: the significant decrease of the body mass; 2) poor appetite: the significant reduction of food and water intake, detected in metabolic cages; 3) mental fatigue: the significant reduction of the motion distance and vertical times in the open field during 5 min, checked with the OFT-100 opening activity experiment system (Chengdu TME Technology Co, Ltd., Chengdu, China); 4) lack of strength: the significant decrease of the forelimb strength, checked with YLS-13A Grip Strength Meter for Rats and Mice (Jinan Yi Yan Technology Development Co., Ltd., Shandong, China).

2.3. Measurement of SIPR

Fasted without water deprivation for 24 h, rats were intragastric administration (1 ml/100g) of 10% carbon powder suspension (5% active carbon and 10% acacia gum), then anesthetized with 10% chloral hydrate (0.35 ml/100g) after 30 min. The SI from the pylorus to the ileocecal junction was carefully taken out, and SIPR was calculated as the following equation: (spreading distance of carbon power/the SI length) × 100%.

2.4. Concentration Measurement of ACh, cAMP and PKA in the SI Tissue

About 2 cm SI from the pylorus was taken out and cleaned with 4˚C saline, and the tissue homogenate was prepared for ELISA. Concentrations of ACh, cAMP and PKA (kits were purchased from Beijing Boosen Biological Technology Co., Ltd., Beijing, China) were determined by an auto analyzer (iMark, Bio-Rad, USA).

2.5. Expressions of M_2 and M_3 Receptors

Immunostaining of M_2 and M_3 receptors was performed using the polink-2 plus HRP detection system for rabbit primary antibody with commercially available kits (Beijing Boosen Biological Technology Co., Ltd., Beijing, China). Sections cut at 4 μm thickness from the SI tissue embedded in paraffin blocks were deparaffinized with xylene, hydrated in ethanol, incubated in 3% H_2O_2 for 10 min, washed 3 times for 2 min with PBS. Sections were incubated with anti-M_2 receptor (1:100) or anti-M_3 receptor (1:100) in PBS at 4˚C for 24 h, washed with

PBS 3 times for 2 min, and Reagent 1 was added at 37˚C for 10 - 20 min, washed with PBS 3 times for 2 min, followed with Reagent 2 in the same way. Sections were added with diaminobenzidine tetrahydrochloride for 5 min, counterstained with hematoxylin, dehydrated, and mounted. PBS was used to replace primary antibodies as the negative control. Mean optic density (MOD) was measured with BI-2000 system (Chengdu TME Technology Co, Ltd., Chengdu, China).

2.6. Statistical Analysis

The data were expressed as mean ± S.D., and statistical analysis was performed between groups by ANOVA using SPSS 16.0 software (SPSS Inc., Chicago, IL, USA). A value of $p < 0.05$ or less was considered to show statistical significance.

3. Results

3.1. Model Evaluation of Spleen Qi Deficiency

Table 1 showed that all items in the model group were significantly less than those in the control group. The reduced body mass meant "emaciation", decreases of food and water intake suggested "poor appetite", the reduction of the motion distance and vertical times in the open field implied "mental fatigue", and the decrease of forelimb strength represented "lack of strength". These results confirmed that spleen qi deficiency model of improper diet and overfatigue was established successfully.

3.2. Changes of SIPRs

SIPRs in the control and model group were 64.31% ± 5.31% and 46.75% ± 4.41%, respectively ($n = 8$, $p < 0.01$, **Figure 1**).

3.3. Changes of Related Cholinergic Components

Table 2 showed that, compared with those in the control, expression of M_2 receptor was increased significantly, expression of M_3 receptor and concentrations of cAMP and PKA were decreased markedly, but the ACh level remained unchanged, in the model group.

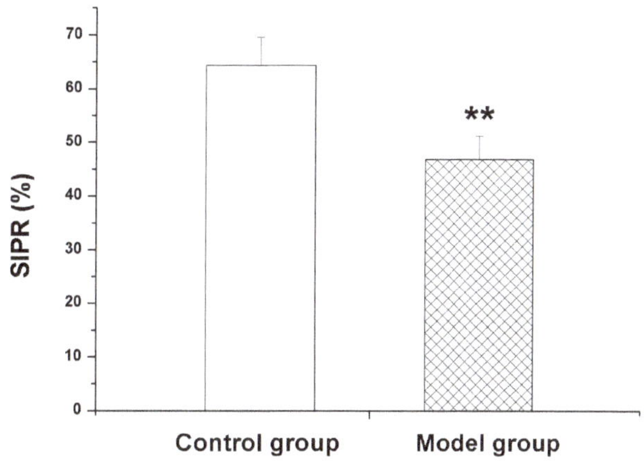

Figure 1. SIPRs of rats. Values are means ± S.D. ($n = 8$). $^{**}p < 0.01$ versus the control.

Table 1. Model evaluation of rat spleen qi deficiency.

Group	Body mass (g)	Food intake (g)	Water intake (ml)	Motion distance (cm)	Vertical times	Forelimb strength (g)
Control group	371.47 ± 22.46	32.31 ± 9.61	89.4 ± 24.0	9512.90 ± 1881.59	20.6 ± 5.9	1363.54 ± 105.83
Model group	239.78 ± 12.10**	21.05 ± 5.21*	59.3 ± 8.1**	4930.35 ± 1253.18**	15.3 ± 3.6*	1215.54 ± 127.72*

Values are means ± S.D. ($n = 8$). $^{*}p < 0.05$, $^{**}p < 0.01$ versus the control.

Table 2. Changes of related cholinergic components.

Group	Ach (μmol/mg)	Expression of M_2 receptors	Expression of M_3 receptors	cAMP (mmol/mg)	PKA (pg/ml)
Control group	3.42 ± 0.40	0.117 ± 0.004	0.181 ± 0.004	13.52 ± 0.60	0.463 ± 0.045
Model group	3.37 ± 0.51	0.215 ± 0.004**	0.130 ± 0.002**	10.63 ± 0.80*	0.320 ± 0.051*

Values are means ± S.D. (n = 8). $^{*}p < 0.05$, $^{**}p < 0.01$ versus the control.

4. Discussion

According to the basic theory of traditional Chinese medicine, spleen dominates the transformation and transportation, which includes the whole GI function and related regulatory mechanisms. As a matter of fact, the SI is one of the main performers of spleen qi. The SI can receive the chyme from the stomach and digest it into fine nutrients and waste, the former is sent upward, the latter is conveyed into the large intestine. Therefore, the SI motility plays an important role in spleen qi.

Spleen qi can be damaged by various causes, for example, improper diet, overfatigue, cold and dampness, etc. Patients with spleen qi deficiency exhibit poor appetite, abdominal distension, emaciation, mental fatigue and lack of strength, lack of qi and no desire to speak, yellowish complexion, and so on. The main pathology of spleen qi deficiency is the reduction of digestion and absorption, especially the hypofunction of the SI. In the present study, the rat model of spleen qi deficiency of improper diet and overfatigue was successfully established, and the SI motility was evaluated with SIPR. Results showed that SIPR was significantly reduced in the model group, suggesting the SI motility was decreased in spleen qi deficiency.

Among regulatory mechanisms of the SI motion, the cholinergic activity of ANS plays a classic excitatory role, which was focused in the present study. Cholinergic M_2 and M_3 receptors express widely in the GI tract, and they can bind with ACh to evoke the SM contraction. Although the number of M_2 receptors is much greater than that of M_3 receptors, the contractile response of SM to ACh is mediated extensively by the minor M_3 subtype. M_3 receptors stimulate phospholipase C via Gq/11-type G proteins, inducing the hydrolysis of phosphatidylinositol 4,5-bisphosphate and then liberates inositol 1,4,5-trisphosphate to release Ca^{2+} from intracellular stores [5], resulting in the SM contraction through activation of the contractile proteins. In contrast, M_2 receptors play a conditional role in concert with M_3 receptors to modulate contraction [2]. Activation of M_2 receptors inhibit the elevation of the adenylate cyclase activity to decrease synthesis of cAMP and PKA, thereby abrogating muscle relaxation, and opens non-selective cation channels to increase Na^+ influx, elevating the SM excitability [6] [7]. However, M_3 receptors exert a permissive role over the M_2 receptor mediated cation current [8]. Hence, it is thought that M_3 receptors directly evoke the SM contraction, whereas M_2 receptors play an indirect role in the SM contraction.

The imbalance of activities mediated by M_2 and M_3 subtypes occurs in various GI diseases, however, it is not clear that such an imbalance occurs in spleen qi deficiency. In the present study, it was found that ACh concentration in the SI tissue of model rats was unchanged, which suggested that excitability of cholinergic nerves might be not altered in spleen qi deficiency, but expression of M_2 receptors was increased and expression of M_3 receptors was decreased, indicating that the imbalance of activities mediated by M_2 and M_3 subtypes occurred in spleen qi deficiency. Such an imbalance might induce the abnormal response of SM to ACh, resulting in the reduction of the SI motility. As M_3 receptors evoke the SI contraction directly, the down-regulated expression of M_3 receptors contributed greatly to the motility reduction of the SI. In contrast, the up-regulated expression of M_2 receptors might enhance SM responses to ACh, for example, elevating the SM excitability, decreasing intracellular cAMP and PKA levels. Although these responses might compensate some loss of the SI motility, such activities were limited because the effect of M_2 receptors on the SM contraction is indirect and controlled by M_3 receptors.

5. Conclusion

In conclusion, expression imbalance of cholinergic M_2 and M_3 receptors contributed to the motility reduction of the SI in spleen qi deficiency.

Funding

Source of support: this work was supported by the National Program on Key Basic Research Project (973 Program, Grant No. 2013CB531702).

References

[1] Ganong, W.F. (2005) Review of Medical Physiology. 22nd Edition, McGraw-Hill Medical, New York.

[2] Unno, T., Matsuyama, H. and Komori, S. (2003) Interaction between the M_2- and M_3-Receptor Subtypes in Muscarinic Electrical and Mechanical Responses of Intestinal Smooth Muscles. *Neurophysiology*, **35**, 262-273. http://dx.doi.org/10.1023/B:NEPH.0000008787.19396.d4

[3] Ehlert, F.J. (2003) Pharmacological Analysis of the Contractile Role of M_2 and M_3 Muscarinic Receptors in Smooth Muscle. *Receptors and Channels*, **9**, 261-277. http://dx.doi.org/10.1080/10606820308265

[4] Matsui, M., Motomura, D., Fujikawa, T., Jiang, J., Takahashi, S., Manabe, T. and Taketo, M.M. (2002) Mice Lacking M_2 and M_3 Muscarinic Acetylcholine Receptors Are Devoid of Cholinergic Smooth Muscle Contractions But Still Viable. *Journal of Neuroscience*, **22**, 10627-10632.

[5] Haga, T. (2013) Molecular Properties of Muscarinic Acetylcholine Receptors. *Proceedings of the Japan Academy. Series B, Physical and Biological Sciences*, **89**, 226-256. http://dx.doi.org/10.2183/pjab.89.226

[6] Tobin, G., Giglio, D. and Lundgren, O. (2009) Muscarinic Receptor Subtypes in the Alimentary Tract. *Journal of Physiology and Pharmacology*, **60**, 3-21.

[7] Zholos, A.V., Tsvilovskyy, V.V. and Bolton, T.B. (2003) Muscarinic Cholinergic Excitation of Smooth Muscle: Signal Transduction and Single Cationic Channel Properties. *Neurophysiolfogy*, **35**, 283-301. http://dx.doi.org/10.1023/B:NEPH.0000008789.82582.42

[8] Griffin, M.T., Matsui, M., Ostromm, R.S. and Ehlert, F.J. (2009) The Guinea Pig Ileum Lacks the Direct, Highpotency, M_2-Muscarinic, Contractile Mechanism Characteristic of the Mouse Ileum. *Naunyn-Schmiedeberg's Archives of Pharmacology*, **380**, 327-335. http://dx.doi.org/10.1007/s00210-009-0434-8

20

Effects of Qing'E Formula on the Expression of Bone Metabolic Markers and VDR mRNA in Postmenopausal Osteoporosis Patients

Bo Shuai, Yanping Yang*, Lin Shen#, Hui Ke

Department of Integrated Traditional Chinese and Western Medicine, Union Hospital, Tongji Medical College, Huazhong University of Science and Technology, Wuhan, China

Email: #bobo3137@126.com

Abstract

Objectives: To study the partial mechanism of treating postmenopausal osteoporosis patients (POPs) using the ancient recipe of Qing'E Formula (QEF) by observing its effects on bone metabolic markers and VDR mRNA expression in primary POPs. Methods: Analysis was performed on 120 outpatient and inpatient POPs treated in our hospital between January and October 2013, where the patients were randomly divided into Qing'E group (QEF + Caltrate), Calcitriol group (Caltrate + Calcitriol soft capsules), and Compare group (Caltrate), each with a follow-up period of 1 year. Statistical analysis was then performed on bone mineral density, blood bone metabolic markers (β-CTX, N-MID, T-PINP) and changes in VDR mRNA expressions in the POPs before and after the treatments. Results: Prior to the treatments, bone mineral density and blood β-CTX, N-MID, T-PINP and VDR mRNA expression in the 3 groups of POPs exhibited no statistically significant differences, and the blood β-CTX, N-MID, T-PINP and VDR mRNA expression in the control group showed no statistically significant differences before and after the treatments. There were no significant differences in bone mineral density in the Qing'E group and the Calcitriol group before and after the treatments whereas the bone mineral density decreased in the control group after the treatments. As for blood β-CTX, N-MID, T-PINP and VDR mRNA expression, the measurements in POPs in the Qing'E group and the Calcitriol group were significantly higher than that of the control group. Conclusion: By adjusting the VDR mRNA expression, the QEF, a kidney-invigorating Chinese herbal formula, is capable of activating bone metabolism to prohibit further losses of bone mass, thereby preventing the deterioration of osteoporosis.

Keywords

Qing'E Formula, VDR mRNA, Osteoporosis, Bone Metabolism, Bone Density

*This author contributed equally to this work.

#Corresponding author.

1. Introduction

With the aging of population in our society, osteoporosis and other metabolic bone diseases and their complications have become one of the key factors affecting the healthy living of the elderly population and increasing the society's economic burdens. The QEF, a Chinese herbal formula, has the efficacy of "nourishing livers and kidneys", "increasing energy and blood" and "regenerating bone marrows". Preliminary studies by the research team showed that QEF could effectively raise $1,25(OH)_2D_3$ and mRNA expression in the blood of ovariectomized rats, thereby effectively controlling osteoporosis. This study proposes the further study on the partial mechanism of treating POPs using ancient recipe QEF by studying its effects on the special sequence of β collagen in blood markers of bone metabolism (β-Crosslaps, β-CTX), N-terminal osteocalcin (N-MID), total N-terminal propeptide of type I procollagen (T-PINP) and VDR mRNA expression in POPs.

2. Materials and Methods

2.1. Research Objects and Grouping

The research objects were 120 primary POPs, with an average age of 53 ± 6 years old. The subjects, comprising of either inpatient or outpatient patients of the hospital, were randomly segregated into three groups, *i.e.* the Qing'E group, who were given the treatment combination of Caltrate and QEF; the Calcitriol group, who were given the treatment combination of Caltrate and Calcitriol soft capsules; and the compare group, who were only given Caltrate treatments. The groups, consisting of 40 POPs each, were given treatments for the period of 1 year. The administering method of medicine is in the "Experiment Medicine" section. This study has been approved by the ethics committee of Wuhan Union Hospital Research Center, along with endorsement from all personnel participating in the study. The participating POPs had also refrained from taking any medicine that affects bone metabolism and coagulation functions two weeks prior to the determination.

2.2. Experiment Medicine

The making process of experiment medicine—ancient herbal formula QEF: The ingredients include the following: *Eucommia* (fried with salt) 480 g, Psoralen (fried with salt) 240 g, walnut (fried) 150 g, Salvia 240 g and garlic 120 g. Garlic was steamed, dried, crushed into fine powder with *Eucommia*, Salvia and Psoralen and then sifted. Walnut was then mashed and grinded with the above powder before the mixture was further sifted and mixed. For every 100 grams of the powder, 50 - 70 grams of refining honey was added for producing the Qing'E pill. The experiment objects were then allocated randomly and received treatments under the experiment medicine or the control medicine. QEF were administered three times daily with warm water whereas Calcitriol soft capsules were administered twice a day, with 1 pill for each intake. In addition to the experiment medicine, the experiment groups and the control group were also given 1 piece of Caltrate daily to ensure patients' compliance and facilitate better treatments. Any traditional Chinese medicine or modern western medicine that affects bone metabolism and coagulation functions were prohibited during the course of the observation period.

2.3. Experiment Methods

2.3.1. Information Collection and Bone Density Testing

Physical examination and survey results of all patients were recorded in detail before and after the treatments. The U.S. made Hologic 2000 Plus Dual-energy X-ray Bone Densitometer and conventional standard software were used to measure bone density at the lumbar spine, the proximal femur, Ward', and greater trochanter. Patients were placed in the position according to requirements, followed by analysis of the images and the results were reported with reference to the WHO diagnostic criteria (g/cm^2). The results were automatically printed and exported from the equipment's supporting printer. The bone density of all patients was measured by one single person using the same equipment to minimize variations in statistical analysis.

2.3.2. Measurement of Blood Bone Metabolic Markers in Patients

Blood samples were drawn from the cubital vein in patients at approximately 10 a.m. every day. Part of the collected blood sample was then centrifuged for 15 minutes (speed: 1000 ×g, temperature 2˚C - 8˚C) and stored in refrigerator at −70˚C while bone metabolic markers β-CTX, N-MID, T-PINP in blood were collected, all the blood were delivered to the same central biochemical lab for tests following the collection, and the tests were conducted strictly according to the instructions listed on the test kits.

2.3.4. Measurement of Blood Adiponectin mRNA in Patients

VDR mRNA expression was measured in the other portion of the blood samples, the VDR primer: under the role of reverse transcriptase M-MLV, the m RNA reverse transcribed into c-DNA molecules. The reaction system was as follows: H_2O 5.5 µl, Oligo (dT18) 1.0 µl, TRNA 6.0 µl, RNasin 0.5 µl, 5 × buffer 4.0 µl, 10 mM dNTP 2.0 µl, RTase 1.0 µl; the reaction conditions: 42 Celsius for 60 minutes, and 95 Celsius for 5 minutes. Quantitative PCR reaction system as follows: cDNA 1 µl, Buffer 10 × 5 µl, $MgCl_2$ (25 mM) 7 µl, dNTP 10 mM 1 µl, F (20 pmol/µl) 0.8 µl, R (20 pmol/µl) 0.8 µl, SYBR GreenI 1 µl, Taq enzyme (5 U/µl) 0.5 µl; the reaction conditions: 94 Celsius for 30 minutes, 53 Celsius for 30 minutes, and 72 degree for 30 minutes for 50 cycles. Ct values were calculated and analyzed: the sample relative value = $2^{-(\Delta Ct\beta\text{-actin} - \Delta Ct\ \text{test sample})}$, ΔCt = Ct negative control − Ct sample, ΔΔCt = ΔCt*β*-actin − ΔCt sample = Ct sample − Ct*β*-actin.

2.4. Statistical Methods

Statistical Methods: Test results were represented by $\bar{x} \pm S$, statistical methods such as analysis of variance, paired sample t test and t-test for independent samples were used for testing and analysis, $p < 0.05$ represented statistical significance and data was analyzed using the SPSS13.0 software.

3. Results

3.1. BMD Changes in the 3 Groups of Patients before and after Treatments

There was no statistically significant difference in BMD among the three groups of patients before the treatments. After the treatments, the Qing'E group of patients saw slight increases in the BMD in lumbar spine, femoral neck, ward and the greater trochanter when compared with the measurements before the treatment; however, the difference was not statistically significant. There was no difference in the BMD in lumbar spine, femoral neck, ward and the greater trochanter in the Calcitriol group before and after the treatments whilst the BMD in these same parts saw significant decrease in the control group. There was no difference in BMD in lumbar spine, femoral neck, ward and the greater trochanter between the Qing'E group and the Calcitriol group, whilst, the measurements in the control group were significantly lower than the above 2 groups (**Figure 1**).

3.2. Changes in Bone Metabolic Markers *β*-CTX, N-MID and T-PINP Expression in the 3 Groups of Patients before and after the Treatments

The *β*-CTX, N-MID and T-PINP expression in the blood of the 3 groups of patients had no statistical significance before the treatments. After the treatments, there was no difference in the content of *β*-CTX, N-MID and T-PINP between the Qing'E and Calcitriol groups, however, the post-treatment contents were lower after treatments in both groups. There was no statistically significant difference in *β*-CTX, N-MID and T-PINP in the control group before and after the treatments, and the content in this group were significantly higher than that of the Qing'E and Calcitriol groups (**Figure 2**).

3.3. Difference in VDR mRNA Expression in the 3 Groups of Patients before and after the Treatments

There was no significant difference in VDR mRNA expression among the 3 groups of patients before the treatments. The post-treatment VDR mRNA expression in the Qing'E and Calcitriol groups were higher after treatments, but there was no significant difference between the 2 groups. There was no difference in VDR mRNA expression in the control group before and after treatments (**Figures 3(a)-3(c)**).

4. Discussion

Due to the withering of ovary, older women experience sharp decrease in estrogen in the body, which leads to significant negative balance of bone metabolism where the rate of bone resorption becomes faster than bone formation, resulting in osteoporosis. Postmenopausal women experience significant reduction in estrogen, which

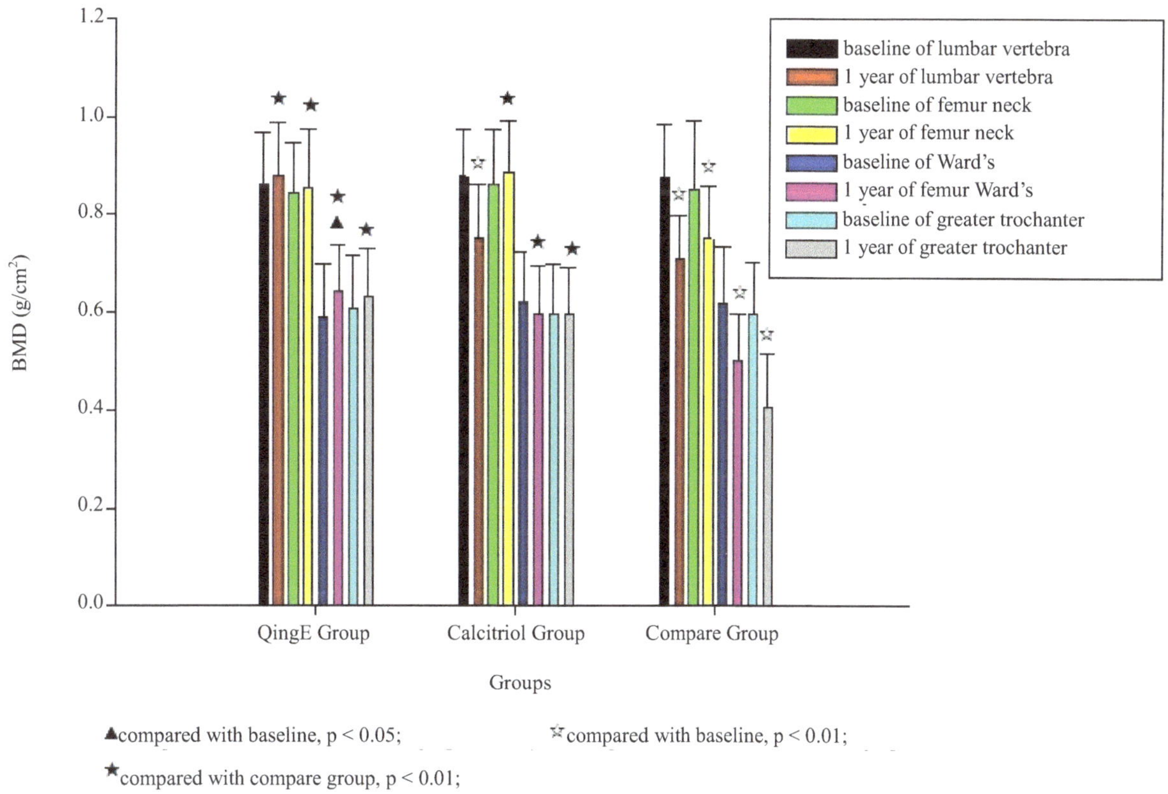

Figure 1. BMD changes in the 3 groups of patients before and after treatments.

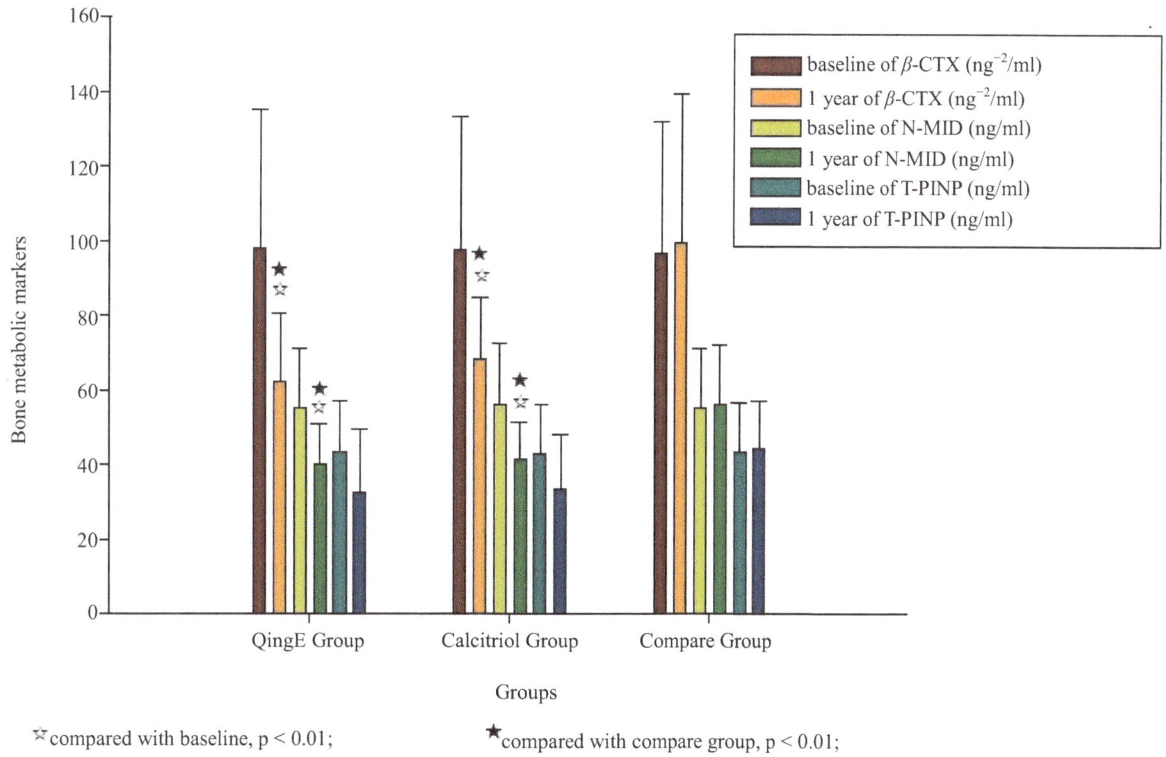

Figure 2. Changes in bone metabolic markers β-CTX, N-MID and T-PINP expression in the 3 groups of patients before and after the treatments.

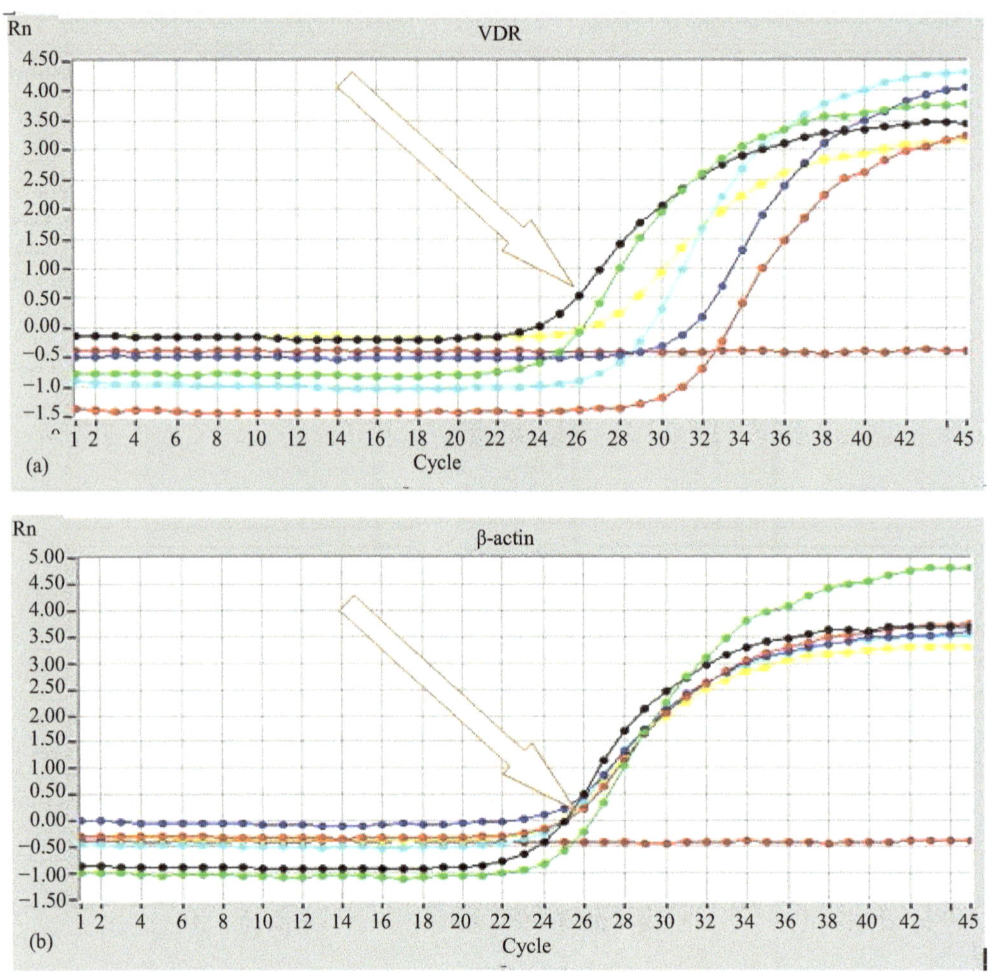

(a)

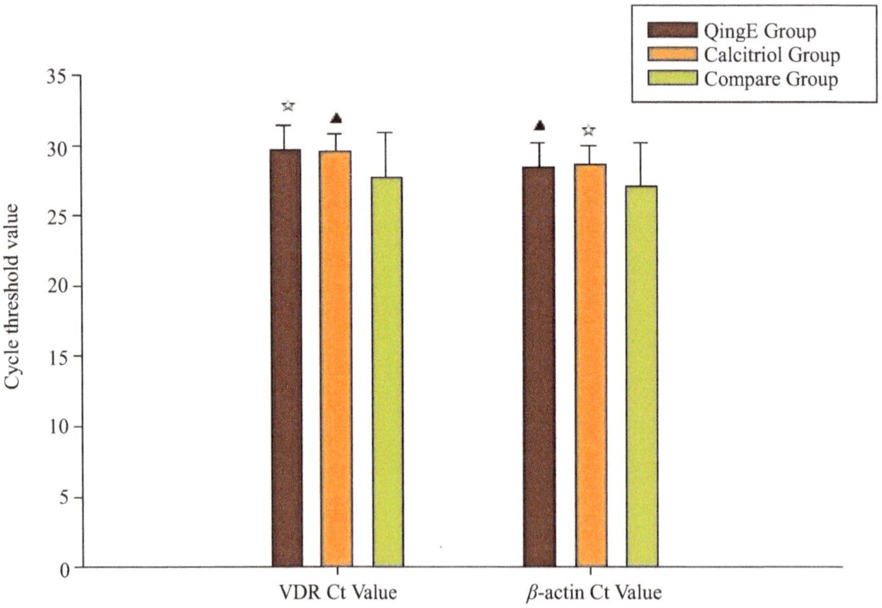

▲compared with compare group, $p < 0.05$; ☆compared with compare group, $p < 0.01$;

(b)

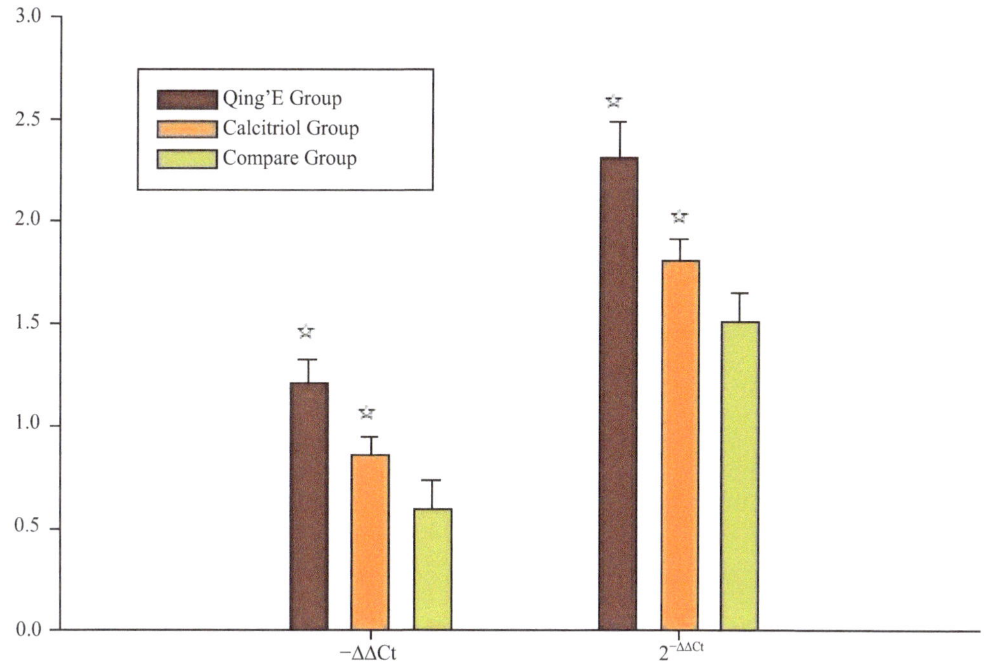

☆compared with compare group, $p < 0.01$;

(c)

Figure 3. Difference in VDR mRNA expression in the 3 groups of patients before and after the treatments.

inhibits the secretion of parathyroid hormone (PTH) and the reduction of PTH creates barriers to the activation of 1α-hydroxylase in livers, which would in turn lead to decrease in the synthesis of $1,25(OH)_2D_3$. Addition of active vitamin D_3 in the treatment for postmenopausal women could promote intestinal absorption of calcium and enhance the cellular activity of osteoclasts and osteoblasts, thereby promoting the mineralization of bones, bone formation and the absorption of the old bones. $1,25(OH)_2D_3$ is the active form of the most bioactive vitamin D in the body. The biological activity of vitamin D is mainly the result of the interaction of 1,25(OH) and the VDR of the nucleus in target organs. The combination of $1,25(OH)_2D_3$ and VDR forms a hormone-receptor complex, which would combine with the hormone response elements in the VDR gene to regulate VDR expression through the interaction with other regulatory factors [1] [2]. Researches have shown that vitamin D receptor gene polymorphism is closely associated with bone density of Han race in Guangxi, Beijing, Wuhan, Fujian and Guangzhou and other racial groups [3]-[5]. Preliminary studies by the research team showed that QEF could effectively suppress VDR mRNA expression in the kidney of ovariectomized rats to promote the expression of vitamin D and the absorption of calcium, thereby effectively controlling postmenopausal osteoporosis [6] [7]. Research has shown that the relative expression of VDR mRNA in the kidney of ovariectomized rats is significantly lower than the normal control group, which is consistent with the findings of this study [8]. VDR mRNA expression in the figure has significantly strengthened in the blood of active vitamin D_3 treatment group (Calcitriol group). This might be attributable to the direct supplement of active vitamin D_3, which has led to the significant increase in the content of "exogenous" $1,25(OH)_2D_3$ in the blood, which in turn leads to the increase in VDR mRNA expression. There is no significant difference in VDR mRNA between QEF and Calcitriol groups, suggesting the possibility of including "kidney essence", etc. in QEF to increase VDR mRNA expression, thereby achieving the same effects as Calcitriol soft capsules.

In "Qing'E Pill" prescription, *Eucommia ulmoides* oliv is warm-natured, with the effect of making kidney and bones strong, so in the book "Ben Cao Ji Yan", there was such a description, "*Eucommia ulmoides* oliv is only herb to strengthen lower energizer, remove pains of foots and legs, and fix knees and loins." Also in another ancient book named "Ben Cao Jing Shu", it was said "*Psoralea corylifolia* can warm the kidney, raise 'Yang' from 'Yin', raise 'fire' from 'soil', can cure kidney weakness and difficulties in sitting up." In "Ju Fang Qing'E Pill", it described that "*Juglans regia* can invigorate the kidney and promote blood circulation, garlic bulb can make the retention pass and dredge collaterals… The combination of these four kinds of herb is called 'Qing'E Pill', which can not only cure kidney weakness and difficulties in sitting up, but also strengthen bone and musculature, promote blood circulation, make hair dark, and bring a good look." After thousands years of clinical validation, Qing'E Pill was effective, safe and economical, however, there was a lack of specific mechanism research.

The β-CTX, N-MID and T-PINP are three types of bone metabolic markers recommended by the International Osteoporosis Foundation (IOF). The β-CTX is the organic component of bone matrix, of which 90% are type I collagen synthesized in bones, but are also decomposed into degradation products that are released into the blood. The β-CTX is a typical product of collagen degradation of type I collagen. The examination of β-CTX can be used for monitoring the anti-resorptive treatment for osteoporosis or other bone diseases, and the efficacy can be reflected within several weeks. The N-MID are produced by osteoblasts during bone synthesis. Both complete osteocalcin and large N-MID fragments are present in the blood; however, the former is unstable and may split and degrade into the latter. The N-MID osteocalcin is regarded as a marker of bone synthesis, which can be used in conjunction with β-CTX for monitoring the treatment of diseases such as osteoporosis. The determination of the concentration of total PINP in the blood is one of the test items of bone markers, which can be used for monitoring the treatment of osteoporosis in postmenopausal women clinically.

The biological activity of vitamin D is mainly the result of the interaction of 1,25(OH) and the VDR of the nucleus in target organs. Vitamin D can enhance osteoblast activity in bone metabolism and promote the formation of bone mineralization. In addition, it also has positive effects on relatively mature osteoblasts, such as increasing the expression of OC and ALP, promoting the mRNA expression of type I collagen of osteoblast in the late maturity stage and the secretion of type I collagen, promoting the synthesis and secretion of osteoblasts and the mineralization of bone matrix, as well as improving the quality and quantity of bones.

The results of this study show that QEF can reduce bone resorption through the adjustment of VDR mRNA expression. This experiment uses stable and effective active vitamin D_3 reported in literatures as the reference drug for the control study [9]-[11]. Data shows similar drug efficacy between QEF and active vitamin D_3, as both are able to increase VDR mRNA expression in the body in reducing bone resorption and strengthening the quality and quantity of bones. The results suggest that the ancient recipe QEF has comparable efficacy in the prevention and treatment of postmenopausal osteoporosis as appropriate supplement of active vitamin D_3.

Acknowledgements

The authors would like to thank LV Lin for his expertise and assistance in performing the blood collection, and Wang Quanshen for his technical assistance.

Research Support

Innovation Fund of Huazhong University of Science and Technology (Item Number: 2013QN235); National Natural Science Foundation of China (Project Number: 81273907 and 81072493).

References

[1] Fan, L.Y., Tu, X.Q., Zhu, Y., Zhou, L., Pfeiffer, T., Feltens, R., Stoecker, W. and Zhong, R. (2005) Genetic Association of Vitamin D Receptor Polymorphisms with Autoimmune Hepatitis and Primary Biliary Cirrhosis in the Chinese. *Journal of Gastroenterology and Hepatology*, **20**, 249-255. http://dx.doi.org/10.1111/j.1440-1746.2005.03532.x

[2] Van Etten, E. and Mathieu, C. (2005) Immunoregulation by 1,25-Dihydroxyvitamin D_3: Basic Concepts. *The Journal of Steroid Biochemistry and Molecular Biology*, **97**, 93-101. http://dx.doi.org/10.1016/j.jsbmb.2005.06.002

[3] Zhou, Y., Zhang H. and Cai D.H. (2005) Influence of Estrogen and Progesteron on Bone Metabolism and Renal Expression of 1,25-Dihydroxyvitamin D_3 Receptors mRNA in Ovariectomized Rats. *Academic Journal of Second Military Medical University*, **26**, 1270-1273.

[4] Municio, M.J. and Traba, M.L. (2004) Effects of 24, 25-$(OH)_2D_3$, 1,25-$(OH)_2D_3$ and 25(OH)D_3 on Alkaline and Tartrate-Resistant Acid Phosphatase Activities in Fetal Rat Calvaria. *Journal of Physiology and Biochemistry*, **60**, 219-224. http://dx.doi.org/10.1007/BF03167032

[5] Uchida, M., Shima, M., Chikazu, D., Fujieda, A., Obara, K., Suzuki, H., Nagai, Y., Yamato, H. and Kawaguchi, H. (2001) Transcriptional Induction of Matrix Metalloproteinase-13 (Collagenase-3) by 1 Alpha,25-Dihydroxyvitamin D_3 in Mouse Osteoblastic MC3T3-E1 Cells. *Journal of Bone and Mineral Research*, **16**, 221-230.

http://dx.doi.org/10.1359/jbmr.2001.16.2.221

[6] Shuai, B., Shen, L., Yang, Y.P., Xie, J., Zhou P.Q., Xu X.J., Li, C.G. and Wu, M.X. (2012) Effect of Bushenhuoxue Decoction on the Osteogenic Differentiation of Bone Marrow Stromal Cells in the Steroid Induced Osteonecrosis of the Femoral Head. *Research of Integrated Traditional Chinese and Western Medicine*, **4**, 297-301.

[7] Shuai, B., Shen, L., Yang, Y.P., Xie, J., Shou, Z.X. and Wei, B. (2010) Low Plasma Adiponectin as a Potential Biomarker for Osteonecrosis of the Femoral Head. *The Journal of Rheumatology*, **37**, 2151-2155. http://dx.doi.org/10.3899/jrheum.100342

[8] Guo, L.J., Luo, X.H., Xie, H., Zhou, H.D. and Liao, E.Y. (2005) The Effects of 1Alpha,25-Dihydroxyvitamin D_3 in Regulation Matrix Metalloproteinase and Tissue Metalloproteinase Inhibitors in Human Osteoblasts. *Zhonghua Nei Ke Za Zhi*, **44**, 125-128.

[9] Xue, Z.W., Shang, X.M., Lv, S.H., Xu, H., Zhang, Q. and Wang, C. (2013) Effects of Shenshao Decoction on the Inflammatory Response in The aorta of a Rat Atherosclerotic Model. *Chinese Journal of Integrative Medicine*, **19**, 347-352. http://dx.doi.org/10.1007/s11655-013-1457-z

[10] Yao, F.A., Dobs, A.S. and Brown, T.T. (2006) Alternative Therapies for Osteoporosis. *The American Journal of Chinese Medicine*, **34**, 721. http://dx.doi.org/10.1142/S0192415X06004235

[11] Ling, J.Y., Shen, L., Liu, Q., Xue, S., Ma, W., Wu, H., Li, Z.X. and Zhu, R. (2013) Changes in Platelet GPIbα and ADAM17 during the Acute Stage of Atherosclerotic Ischemic Stroke among Chinese. *Journal of Huazhong University of Science and Technology* (*Medical Sciences*), **33**, 438-442.

21

Effect of Ethanol Extract of Venenum Bufonis on Biofilm Formation of *Staphylococcus aureus*

Bing Yan[1], Man Guo[1], Liping Zhao[2*]

[1]School of Life Sciences and Technical, Mudanjiang Normal University, Mudanjiang, China
[2]School of Life Sciences, University of Science and Technology of China, Hefei, China
Email: [*]zhaolp@ustc.edu.cn

Abstract

Ethanol extract of Venenum Bufonis has shown many valuable bioactivities, but little is known about its effect on biofilm formation of *Staphylococcus aureus*. In this study, biofilm formation of *S. aureus* NCTC8325 with or without ethanol extract of Venenum Bufonis was tested using microtitre plate assay and Confocal Laser Scanning Microscope (CLSM) system. Results show that the biofilm formation of *S. aureus* with ethanol extract of Venenum Bufonis was significantly lower than that of the control group without ethanol extract of Venenum Bufonis. Meanwhile, the reduction degree was correlated to the concentration of ethanol extract of Venenum Bufonis positively. With CLSM system we can observe that looser and less biomass of the biofilm structure of the experimental group appeared than that of the control group. These results suggested that ethanol extract of Venenum Bufonis has inhibitory effect on biofilm formation of *S. aureus*.

Keywords

Ethanol Extract of Venenum Bufonis, *S. aureus*, Biofilm Formation

1. Introduction

Staphylococcus aureus, as an important opportunistic pathogen is a leading cause of human bacterial infection worldwide and is endemic in both hospital and community, which can cause potentially life-threatening nosocomial and community-acquired infections, such as osteomyelitis and endocarditis [1] [2]. *S. aureus* has the ability to adhere to many tissues and implants in humans to form biofilms, which enables it to survive in antimicrobial stress and immune responses causing refractory chronic infections. Novel strategies that target biofilm-

[*]Corresponding author.

associated infections caused by *S. aureus* will be considered as future therapies [3]-[5].

Venenum Bufonis, a traditional Chinese medicine used as a topical anesthetic and cardiac medication, is extracted from the dried white secretion of auricular glands and skin glands of Chinese toad (*Bufo melanostictus* Schneider or *Bufo bufo gargarzinas* Gantor). Ethanol extract of Venenum Bufonis has shown strong pharmacological activity, including the effects on antiproliferative [6] and on anti-osteosarcoma [7], killing various cancer cells by inducing their apoptosis [8] [9]. However, to date, the effect of ethanol extract of Venenum Bufonis on *S. aureus* biofilm formation has not been reported. In this study, we investigated the effects of ethanol extract of Venenum Bufonis against biofilm formation of *S. aureus in vitro*, and concluded that ethanol extract of Venenum Bufonis has inhibitory effect on biofilm formation of *S. aureus*.

2. Materials and Methods

2.1. Bacterial Strains and Growth Conditions

The bacterial strains used in this study including *S. aureus* NCTC8325, and *S. aureus* NCTC8325pGFP carrying the fluorescent protein were provided by University of Science & Technology China. They were grown at 37˚C in tryptic soy broth (TSB) medium (BD) or TSB with chloramphenicol (15 μg/mL). Medium was supplemented with 3% sodium chloride or 0.5% glucose when necessary.

2.2. Production of Ethanol Extracts of Venenum Bufonis

Venenum Bufonis was purchased in China toad Venenum Bufonis industry. It was ground into powder and was suspended in 10 mL 80% ethanol solution each 0.5 g and extracted two times at 70˚C water bath for 90 min. The solvent of the extract was removed in a rotary evaporator under vacuum. The resulting residue was dissolved in 80% ethanol at 50 mg/mL extract concentration and was diluted with 80% ethanol to 25 mg/mL, 12.5 mg/mL, 6.25 mg/mL, and 3.125 mg/mL concentration.

2.3. Antimicrobial Activity

Overnight cultures of *S. aureus* NCTC8325 were initiated by touching a sterile wire loop to three individual colonies on every plate and inoculating into 2 mL of TSB medium. The inoculum was cultured to a final concentration of 10^6 CFU/mL in fresh TSB and was dispensed into 96-well plates (Corning, Steuben, NY) containing serial dilutions of ethanol extracts of Venenum Bufonis (2.5 mg/mL, 1.25 mg/mL, 0.625 mg/mL, 0.3125 mg/mL, 0 mg/mL). At the same time 1 μg/mL vancomycin was used as standard antibiotic control. Plates were incubated at 37˚C for 12 h and then ten-fold serial dilutions of cultures were performed by successive transfer (0.1 mL) through seven microfuge tubes containing 0.9 mL of TSB. Four appropriate dilutions were dropped on LB agar plates and viable colonies were counted after incubation at 37˚C for 24 h. Experiments were repeated three times with four parallels.

2.4. Biofilm Formation in Microtitre Plate Assay

Biofilm formation under static conditions was determined by the microtitre plate assay based on the method described previously [10]. Briefly, the overnight cultures were made at a 1:100 dilution using fresh TSB containing 3% NaCl or 0.5% glucose. The diluted cell suspension was inoculated into flat-bottom 96-well polystyrene plates (Costar 3599, Corning Inc., Corning, NY), 200 μl each well containing serial dilutions of ethanol extract of Venenum Bufonis (2.5 mg/mL, 1.25 mg/mL, 0.625 mg/mL, 0.3125 mg/mL, 0 mg/mL). The plates were incubated at 37˚C for 12 h and wells were rinsed gently with water five times to remove non-adherent cells. Subsequently, the plates were stained with 0.5% crystal violet for 15 min, and then rinsed again with water to remove unbound stain. After that, the plates were dried, and the optical density at 560 nm (OD560) was determined with an enzyme-linked immunosorbent assay reader (biotek Elx800, USA) in a 5 × 5 scan model.

2.5. Observation of Biofilm Formation in Laser Scanning Confocal Microscope System (CLSM)

Overnight cultures of *S. aureus* NCTC8325pGFP, which was transformed with the GFP plasmid for fluorescence detection from *S. aureus* NCTC8325, was inoculated at a 1:100 dilution in fresh TSB containing 3% NaCl and 15 μg/mL chloramphenicol to maintain plasmid selection into glass bottom culture dishes (35 mm petri dish, 10 mm microcell, MatTek, USA), 1 mL each dish. The experimental group contained 1.25 mg/mL ethanol extracts of Venenum Bufonis. Dishes were incubated at 37°C for 12 h and were rinsed gently with water five times to remove non-adherent cells. CLSM was performed on a Zeiss LSM710 collected at 1 μm intervals. Selected confocal images stood for similar areas of interest and each confocal experiment was repeated four times. The confocal images were acquired from Zeiss ZEN 2010 software package (Carl Zeiss, Jena, Germany) and the three-dimensional biofilm images were rendered with Imaris 7.0 (Bitplane, Zurich, Switzerland).

2.6. Statistical Analysis

The paired *t* test was used for statistical comparisons between groups. The level of statistical significance was set at a P value of ≤0.05.

3. Results and Discussion

3.1. Inhibitory Effect of Ethanol Extract of Venenum Bufonis on *S. aureus*

Figure 1 shows the viable counts of *S. aureus* NCTC8325 after exposure to TSB with or without the extract from Venenum Bufonis for 12 h at 37°C. Compared with the control group without the extract of Venenum Bufonis, the viable counts of bacteria of the experimental group containing ethanol extract of Venenum Bufonis were decreased significantly, and the reducing extent was positively correlated with the concentration of ethanol extract of Venenum Bufonis. Viable counts were almost 100 times lower in the presence of 0.3125 mg/mL ethanol extract of Venenum Bufonis, 1000 times lower in the presence of 0.625 mg/mL ethanol extract of Venenum Bufonis and 10,000 times lower in the presence of 2.5 mg/mL ethanol extract of Venenum Bufonis compared with the control group. These data show that certain concentrations of ethanol extract of Venenum Bufonis can inhibit the growth of *S. aureus*, but the increase of ethanol extract of Venenum Bufonis concentration cannot completely kill the bacteria. However, there were no viable bacteria in the standard antibiotic control that contains 1 μg/mL vancomycin (data not shown).

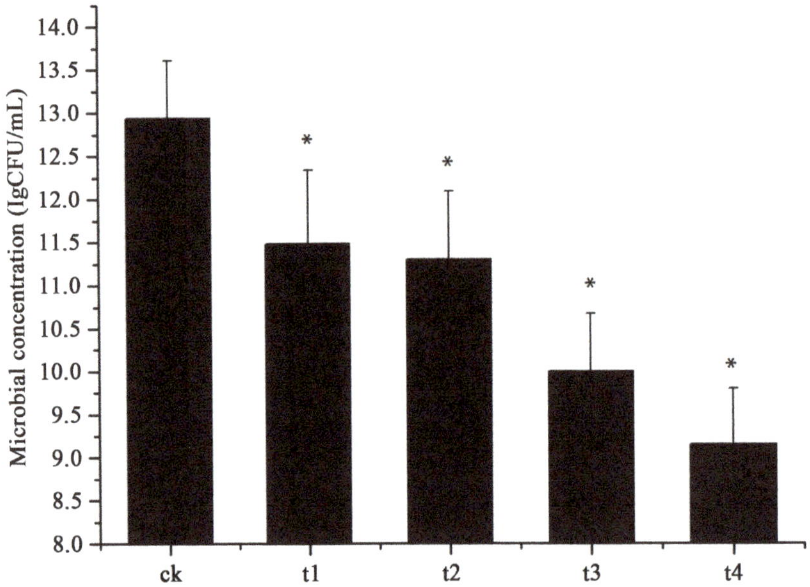

Figure 1. Colony counts (lgCFU/mL) of *S. aureus* NCTC8325 following 12 h of incubation at 37°C with or without ethanol extract of Venenum Bufonis. ck: control group no ethanol extract of Venenum Bufonis, t1: 0.3125 mg/mL ethanol extract of Venenum Bufonis, t2: 0.625 mg/mL ethanol extract of Venenum Bufonis, t3: 1.25 mg/mL ethanol extract of Venenum Bufonis, t4: 2.5 mg/mL ethanol extract of Venenum Bufonis. *Significantly different from no Venenum Bufonis control ($P < 0.05$).

3.2. Inhibitory Effect of Ethanol Extract of Venenum Bufonis on Biofilm Formation of *S. aureus*

To investigate whether ethanol extract of Venenum Bufonis affects biofilm formation of *S. aureus*, we monitored the biofilm formation of *S. aureus* NCTC8325 using a microtitre plate assay. As shown in **Figure 2**, strains of the control group without ethanol extract of Venenum Bufonis formed strong biofilm after 12 h incubation at 37˚C. However, strains of the experimental groups with different concentrations of ethanol extract of Venenum Bufonis formed weaker biofilm as measured by quantitative spectrophotometric analysis based on OD560 after crystal violet staining. Moreover, this discrepancy was increasing with the increase of ethanol extract of Venenum Bufonis concentration when cultivated in TSB containing 3% NaCl (**Figure 2(a)**). When cultivated in TSB containing 0.5% glucose, stains of *S. aureus* with 0.625 mg/mL ethanol extract of Venenum Bufonis formed biofilm significantly more weakly than the control group (**Figure 2(b)**).

In order to directly observe the effect of ethanol extract of Venenum Bufonis on biofilm formation of *S. aureus*, we used CLSM system and strains that can constitutively express green fluorescent protein GFP. After 12 h incubation at 37˚C in TSB containing 3% NaCL, strains of the control group without ethanol extract of Venenum Bufonis produced intact and rough biofilms as monitored by CLSM. In contrast, biofilms produced by strains of the experimental group with 1.25 mg/mL ethanol extract of Venenum Bufonis were undetectable (**Figure 3**).

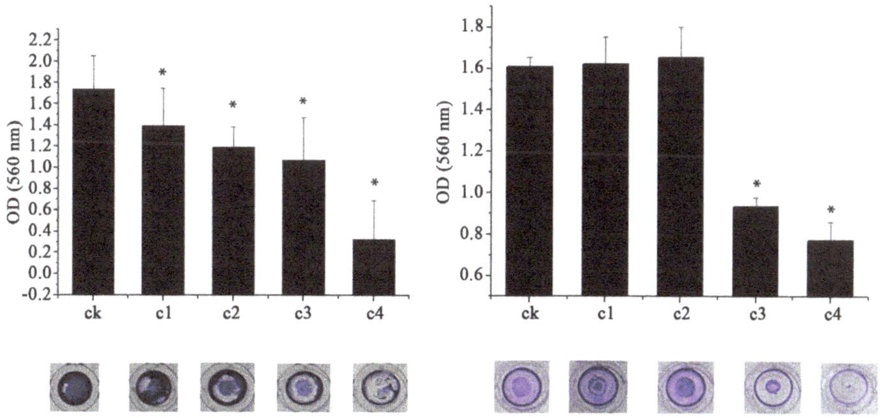

(a) (b)

Figure 2. Biofilm formation of *S. aureus* NCTC8325 when cultivated in TSB containing 3% NaCL (a) or TSB containing 0.5% glucose (b) in 96-well plates for 12 h at 37˚C with or without ethanol extract of Venenum Bufonis. The cells that adhered to the plate after staining with crystal violet were measured by OD560. ck: control group no ethanol extract of Venenum Bufonis, c1: 0.15625 mg/mL ethanol extract of Venenum Bufonis, c2: 0.3125 mg/mL ethanol extract of Venenum Bufonis, c3: 0.625 mg/mL ethanol extract of Venenum Bufonis, c4: 1.25 mg/mL ethanol extract of Venenum Bufonis. *Significantly different from no Venenum Bufonis control ($P < 0.05$).

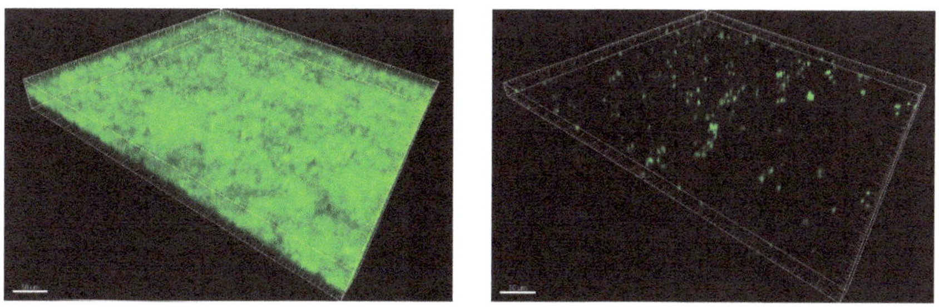

(a) (b)

Figure 3. Observation of biofilm formation of *S. aureus* NCTC8325pGFP when cultivated in TSB containing 3% NaCL and 15 μg/mL chloramphenicol in glass bottom culture dishes for 12 h at 37˚C without (a) or with 1.25 mg/mL ethanol extract of Venenum Bufonis (b). Biofilm integrity and GFP fluorescence were monitored by CLSM and the three-dimensional images were rendered with Imaris 7.0.

Biofilm formation of *S. aureus* plays an important role in catheter-related infections, which is difficult to control and brings serious threat to human health. Searching for new drugs to inhibit the biofilm formation of *S. aureus* has become a new strategy for clinical infection treatment. Here, we provide evidence that ethanol extract of Venenum Bufonis has inhibitory effect on biofilm formation of *S. aureus*, suggesting a potential clue for therapy in *S. aureus* biofilm-associated infection.

However, the biofilm formation of *S. aureus* is a complex process, which involves a variety of factors, including quorum sensing systems, two component and other signal systems from a network to regulate. This study is only a preliminary detection to the effect of ethanol extract of Venenum Bufonis on biofilm formation of *S. aureus*. More specific mechanism involved in this process remains to be further studied in detail.

On the other hand, the component of Venenum Bufonis is complex. Through separation and identification, it was proved to contain many toad toxins, bufalin ligands, bufalin tryptamines and other compounds such as morphine and epinephrine. The effective components of Venenum Bufonis in general are fat soluble, which can be extracted by 80% ethanol. The active ingredient of Venenum Bufonis that inhibits the growth and the biofilm formation of *S. aureus* can be bufadienolides and telocinobufagin; however the specific mechanism needs further study.

4. Conclusion

This study provided evidence that the ethanol extract of Venenum Bufonis, which is a traditional Chinese medicine, could inhibit the biofilm formation of *S. aureus*. The results suggested a potential clue for therapy in *S. aureus* biofilm-associated infection.

Acknowledgements

We thank Professor Baolin Sun in School of Life Sciences, University of Science and Technology of China for providing the strains. This work was supported by the provincial key research project of Heilongjiang Province in Mudanjiang Normal College (sy 201230).

References

[1] Lowy, F.D. (1998) *Staphylococcus aureus* Infections. *New England Journal of Medicine*, **339**, 520-532. http://dx.doi.org/10.1056/NEJM199808203390806

[2] Otto, A., van Dijl, J.M., Hecker, M. and Becher, D. (2014) The *Staphylococcus aureus* Proteome. *International Journal of Medical Microbiology*, **304**, 110-120. http://dx.doi.org/10.1016/j.ijmm.2013.11.007

[3] Costerton, J.W., Montanaro, L. and Arciola, C.R. (2005) Biofilm in Implant Infections: Its Production and Regulation. *The International Journal of Artificial Organs*, **28**, 1062-1068.

[4] Del Pozo, J.L. and Patel, R. (2007) The Challenge of Treating Biofilm-Associated Bacterial Infections. *Clinical Pharmacology and Therapeutics*, **82**, 204-209. http://dx.doi.org/10.1038/sj.clpt.6100247

[5] Archer, N.K., Mazaitis, M.J., Costerton, J.W., Leid, J.G., Powers, M.E. and Shirtliff, M.E. (2011) *Staphylococcus aureus* Biofilms: Properties, Regulation, and Roles in Human Disease. *Virulence*, **2**, 445-459. http://dx.doi.org/10.4161/viru.2.5.17724

[6] Wang, S.H., Wang, Y.C., Nie, Y.L., Hai, Y.N., Sun, H.F., Yuan, Z.L. and Nan, K.J. (2013) Antiproliferative Activity of the Chinese Medicinal Compound, Delisheng, Compared with Rg3 and Gemcitabine in HepG2 Cells. *Indian Journal of Pharmaceutical Sciences*, **75**, 578-584.

[7] Chen, G., Jiang, X., Li, J., Duan, G., Yang, L., Zhang, Y. and Wang, F. (2014). Study on Anti-Osteosarcoma Activity of Ethanol Extract of Venenum Bufonis *in Vitro*. *African Journal of Traditional, Complementary, and Alternative Medicines. African Networks on Ethnomedicines*, **11**, 73-77.

[8] Zhang, D.M., Liu, J.S., Tang, M.K., Yiu, A., Cao, H.H., Jiang, L., Chan, J.Y., Tian, H.Y., Fung, K.P. and Ye, W.C. (2012) Bufotalin from Venenum Bufonis Inhibits Growth of Multidrug Resistant HepG2 Cells through G2/M Cell Cycle Arrest and Apoptosis. *European Journal of Pharmacology*, **692**, 19-28. http://dx.doi.org/10.1016/j.ejphar.2012.06.045

[9] Li, M., Yu, X., Guo, H., Sun, L., Wang, A., Liu, Q., Wang, X. and Li, J. (2014) Bufalin Exerts Antitumor Effects by Inducing Cell Cycle Arrest and Triggering Apoptosis in Pancreatic Cancer Cells. *Tumour Biology*, **35**, 2461-2471. http://dx.doi.org/10.1007/s13277-013-1326-6

[10] Beenken, K.E., Blevins, J.S. and Smeltzer, M.S. (2003) Mutation of sarA in *Staphylococcus aureus* Limits Biofilm Formation. *Infection and Immunity*, **71**, 4206-4211. http://dx.doi.org/10.1128/IAI.71.7.4206-4211.2003

22

The Effect of Electroacupuncture on Neuronal Apoptosis and Related Functions in Rats with Acute Spinal Cord Injury

Liang Zhang[1], Changming Li[1], Renfu Quan[2*], Shangju Xie[1]

[1]Research Institute of Orthopedics, Zhejiang Chinese Medical University, Hangzhou, China
[2]Department of Orthopedics, Xiaoshan Traditional Chinese Medical Hospital, Hangzhou, China
Email: [*]quanrenfu@126.com

Abstract

Objective: **To investigate the effect and significance of electroacupuncture (EA) on neuronal apoptosis and hindlimb motor and bladder functional improvement in rats with acute spinal cord injury (SCI).** ***Methods***: **Sixty healthy Sprague Dawley rats were randomly assigned to sham, model, EA, and EA control groups (n = 15 each). EA group rats received EA treatment at Zhibian and Shuidao acupoints seven times daily, whereas EA control group rats received EA at two points, 0.5 cm away from Zhibian and Shuidao, respectively. Histomorphological changes in spinal cord tissue were examined using hematoxylin-eosin staining. Neuronal apoptosis was detected by TUNEL assay. Bcl-2, Bax, and Bad protein levels were detected using immunohistochemistry. Additionally, hindlimb motor function, residual urine volume and maximum bladder capacity were measured.** ***Results***: **HE staining revealed a morphologically and structurally intact spinal cord in the EA group, and the tissue contained scattered blood cells without edema. In the EA control group, there were small morphological defects in the spinal cord, and the tissue contained fewer blood cells with local edema. Compared with the EA control and model groups, Bax and Bad levels were significantly decreased in the EA group and Bcl-2 expression was increased ($P < 0.05$). After SCI, hindlimb function scores, residual urine volume, and maximum bladder capacity in rats of the EA group significantly differed from those of the EA control group ($P < 0.05$).** ***Conclusion***: **EA may induce SCI-induced improvements in hindlimb motor and bladder functions by affecting neuronal apoptosis and relevant gene expression changes.**

[#]Corresponding author.

Keywords

Electroacupuncture, Spinal Cord Injury, Neuronal Apoptosis, Molecular Mechanism

1. Introduction

Spinal cord injury (SCI) is a serious threat to human health. It often causes paraplegia and quadriplegia, leading to a series of serious complications and sequelae, such as urinary tract infection, respiratory tract infection, renal function impairment, and bedsores [1] [2]. SCI can substantially affect quality of life and family life situations, making it an urgent, worldwide problem to be addressed in the field of medicine. In recent years, there have been an increasing number of studies focused on the treatment, rehabilitation, and mechanisms of acute SCI. It is currently believed that mechanical injury to the spinal cord itself destroys its continuity and integrity. Following primary injury, the body initiates secondary injury to the spinal cord, leading to changes in the microenvironment, such as ischemia and hypoxia, inflammation, intracellular and extracellular calcium imbalance, excessive production of free radicals, excitatory amino acid changes, cytotoxic substances, and apoptosis, which are counterproductive to spinal cord functional recovery.

Electroacupuncture (EA) is an important part of traditional Chinese medicine, with a dual therapeutic effect of acupuncture and electrostimulation. EA stimulation at certain acupoints promotes Qi and blood circulation *via* meridian vessels to help regulate yin and yang and strengthen resistance to pathogenic factors. Previous acupuncture studies have focused on the analgesic, antispastic, and antidepressant effects [3]. Apoptosis is an important biological process, which involves a series of gene-regulated, initiative, cell death processes. Apoptosis exists in a number of diseases, such as Alzheimer's disease, Parkinson's disease, and traumatic injury [4] [5]. However, abnormal apoptosis can cause drastic deterioration in a variety of neurodegenerative diseases. Previous studies have documented the role of neuronal apoptosis and apoptotic gene expression in SCI [6]. In addition, Bcl-2 family proteins are key regulators of apoptosis, among which the proportion of Bcl-2, Bad, and Bax expression is the "molecular switch" to initiate apoptosis [7] [8]. It has been shown that down-regulation of Bcl-2 expression and up-regulation of Bax expression are non-conducive to the survival of hippocampal neurons [9]. A number of reports document that EA has a curative effect on neurodegenerative diseases, such as SCI [10] [11], although the underlying mechanisms remain unclear. The present study investigated the effect of EA treatment at Zhibian and Shuidao acupoints on neuronal apoptosis in rats with SCI. We further examined relevant changes in Bad, Bax and Bcl-2 expression to explore the possible molecular mechanisms of EA for promoting neuronal functional improvement after SCI.

2. Materials and Methods

2.1. Experimental Animals and Grouping

A total of 60 healthy, adult, male Sprague Dawley (SD) rats (220 - 250 g body weight) were purchased from the Experimental Animal Center of Xiamen University, Fujian Province, China (License No.: SYXK (Fujian) 2013-0006). After 1 week of adaptive feeding, the rats were randomly assigned to the sham, model, EA, and EA control groups (n = 15 each). Animals were sacrificed at 7 d post-surgery, and a 0.5-cm-long tissue sample was taken from above and below the injured spinal cord segment for further testing.

2.2. Reagents and Instruments

Bcl-2, Bax, and Bad were purchased from Bioworld (Louis Park, MN, USA). The TUNEL kit was purchased from Beijing Zhongshan Reagent Company (Beijing, China). Disposable Hwato acupuncture needles and an electroacupuncture device were purchased from Suzhou Medical Appliance Factory (Jiangsu Province, China). The fixative was prepared with 4% paraformaldehyde in phosphate-buffered saline (PBS).

2.3. Animal Model Establishment

An SD rat model with moderate SCI was established using a modified Allen's method [12] [13]. Rats were fasted for 8 h, and individual rats then underwent surgery in a random order. All groups were anesthetized via an intraperitoneal injection of 10% chloral hydrate (0.3 mL/100mg) and then fixed in a prone position. An approximately 2.5-cm-long, median, chest-back incision was aseptically made, through which the skin and subcutaneous tissues were dissected layer by layer to expose one vertebral body in the upper and lower positions, respectively. The T9-T10 spinous processes and complete vertebral plate were gouged to expose the 0.8-mm-wide spinal dura mater. A 10-g Kirschner wire was allowed to freely fall along a scaled catheter from a height of 60 mm, which hit a 4-mm-diameter, 2-mm-wide semicircle of thin, plastic material. The object was immediately removed, thereby inducing moderate injury to the posterior horn of the spinal cord. The surrounding tissues and skin were sutured layer by layer postoperatively using 4-0 silk. The entire surgery was performed at 37˚C ± 0.5˚C. Animals were intraperitoneally administered 800 million U/d penicillin postoperatively daily to prevent infection. Individuals were fed in separate cages at a room temperature of 20˚C - 25˚C and supplied with adequate food and water. The bladder was massaged twice daily using Crede's method [14] [15] to help void urine until the reestablishment of reflex bladder emptying. Specific criteria were assigned for the success of model establishment: following initial injury, the injured spinal cord segment showed bleeding and edema; the rat exhibited a tail-wagging reflex with retraction-like fluttering of both lower extremities and the body; and there was flaccid paralysis in both lower extremities upon return of consciousness after anesthesia.

2.4. Intervention Strategy

After successful model construction, the model and sham groups remained untreated. The EA group underwent EA treatment upon return of consciousness after anesthesia. The rat was fixed within a custom-made rat bag. Acupoints were chosen according to international standard acupoints developed by the World Health Organization. Zhibian (BL54) was located in the lower hip, *i.e.*, at the joint of outer and middle 1/3 intervals of the connection between the greater trochanter and sacral vertebra-coccygeal vertebra junction. Shuidao (ST28) was located in the abdomen, approximately 2 cm away from the third equal interval above the pubic symphysis on the midline between pubic symphysis and xiphosternal symphysis (divided into 13 equal parts) (**Figure 1**). Skin at the acupoints was prepared and disinfected. Stainless steel 0.25-mm-diameter acupuncture needles were used to punctuate the acupoints to 4 - 5 mm deep, followed by 1 min of twirling and 15 min of retaining. The ipsilateral Zhibian and Shuidao points were connected to a JL2B electrical pulse stimulator to form a loop, and 2/100 Hz frequency and 1 mA current were applied for 15 min of stimulation. The EA treatment alternated left and right daily. For the EA control group, treatment was performed as described for the EA group at two points 0.5 cm away for Zhibian and Shuidao, respectively.

2.5. Evaluation Indices and Methods

2.5.1. Behavioral and Motor Function Scoring

Following model establishment, the motor function in rats of different groups was scored using the Basso, Beattie, and Bresnahan locomotor rating scale (BBB scale). SCI rats were allowed free activity in an open space. Because of limited hindlimb mobility, the rat was unable to support its body, and the hindlimbs and buttocks dragged on the ground. Rats scoring >2 points were considered to be failed model establishment and were subsequently excluded from the experimental group. Rats were later supplemented to these groups. BBB scoring was performed prior to model establishment, as well as immediately and 7 d after model establishment to ex-

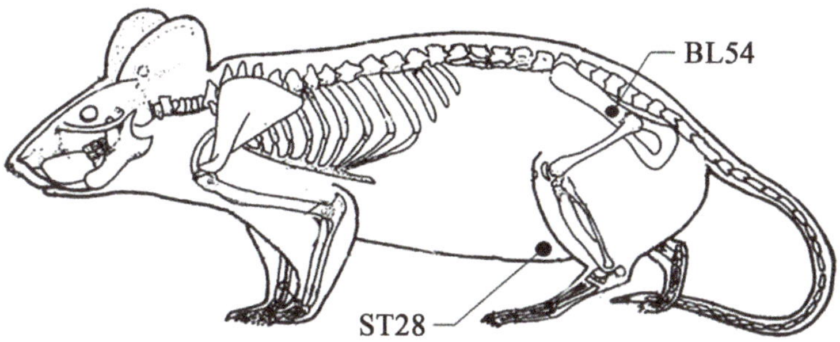

Figure 1. Schematic showing the Zhibian and Shuidao acupoints in the rat.

amine hindlimb motor functional recovery following acute SCI. Scoring criteria included the number of movable hindlimb joints, motor coordination, and fine motor joint function. Scores were divided into 21 grades. The higher the score, the better the recovery of motor function.

2.5.2. Residual Urine Volume Measurement

At 1 and 7 d post-surgery, residual urine volume was measured by manual expression of the bladder. When held in an upright position, rats often exhibited automatic micturition. After the rat supported itself and voided urine, forefingers of both hands were used to squeeze three times from the abdomen to the pelvis. During this process, pre-weighed absorbent papers were placed underneath. Following manual expression, the absorbent papers were weighed again. Increase in the weight of papers (g) was taken as the residual urine volume (mL), because the density of urine is close to that of water, $\rho \approx 1$.

2.5.3. Maximum Bladder Capacity Measurement

Maximum bladder capacity was measured at 1 and 7 d post-surgery. The rat was fixed in a supine position on a custom-made board. Iodophor was used to disinfect the external urethral orifice and anus. Two catheters were filled with sterile saline to remove the contained gas prior to use. Following lubrication with paraffin oil, one sterilized F3 urinary catheter was slowly inserted into the urethra and bladder (4.0 - 5.0 cm depth) via the external urethral orifice. The second F3 catheter was then lubricated with paraffin oil and slowly inserted along the end of the first catheter to the deeper depth. Crede's method was used to void urine. Once the residual urine was completely voided from the bladder through the catheter, sterile saline was slowly injected into the bladder perfusion catheter with a 1-mL syringe. The other discharger catheter placed on the rat board was subjected to close observation, and perfusion was stopped when liquid overflowed. The total volume of injected saline solution was recorded as the bladder's maximum functional capacity.

2.5.4. Spinal Cord Tissue Sampling

At 7 d after model establishment, the rats were anesthetized via intraperitoneal injection with 10% chloral hydrate (0.3 mL/100g). After thoracotomy, intubation was performed from the left ventricle to the aorta, and the right atrial appendage was then cut. The tissue was perfused with 150 mL 9% normal saline and then fixed with 250 mL 40 g/L paraformaldehyde. After 2 h, a 0.5-cm-long spinal cord tissue was taken from above and below the injured segment, respectively. The specimens were fixed in the same fixative for another 24 h, followed by conventional paraffin embedding. Serial sections (~6 μm thick) were prepared for hematoxylin-eosin (HE) staining, terminal deoxyribonucleotidyl transferase-mediated dUTP nick-end labeling (TUNEL) assay, and immunohistochemical (IHC) analysis.

2.5.5. HE Staining

HE staining was performed on three tissue sections randomly selected from each rat in different groups. After dewaxing, the sections were rinsed with double-distilled water for 1 min and stained with hematoxylin for 10 min. Excess dye was removed with double-distilled water, and specimens were immersed in 1% hydrochloric alcohol for 1 min of color separation (to avoid over-separation). Following treatment with an alkaline pro-blue solution, the sections were rinsed with flowing water and then counterstained with eosin for 2 min, dehydrated with graded ethanol (50%, 70%, 80%, 90%, and 100%), clarified using xylene, and mounted with neutral gum. Changes in the structure and morphology of spinal cord tissues were examined under an Olympus optical microscope.

2.5.6. TUNEL Detection of Apoptotic Cells

Three tissue sections from each rat were dewaxed and digested with proteinase K (0.02% mass fraction) for 30 min. The sections were fixed in 40 g/L paraformaldehyde and then incubated with drops of horseradish peroxidase at 37°C for 30 min. Finally, diaminobenzine (DAB) was used for coloration, followed by counterstaining with lighter hematoxylin, dehydration, and mounting. The number of positive cells was quantified, and the apoptotic index (AI) = number of apoptotic nuclei/total number of nuclei.

2.5.7. IHC Staining

Three tissue sections from each rat were used to detect Bcl-2, Bad, and Bax expression with an SP kit following the manufacturer's instructions. After conventional dewaxing, the sections were processed with 3% hydrogen peroxide, followed by high-temperature restoration and serum blocking. The sections were incubated with drops of primary antibody (dilution factor 1:150) at 4˚C overnight. The negative control was prepared with PBS substituting the primary antibody. On the following day, secondary antibody was dropped onto the sections and incubated for 20 min, followed by incubation with strept avidin-biotin complex (SABC) at 37˚C for 20 min. Thereafter, DAB was added for coloration and the color development background was examined by microscopy. Between the above steps, sections were rinsed three times with 0.01 mol/L PBS for 5 min each. Finally, the sections were dehydrated with gradient alcohol, clarified with xylene, and mounted with neutral resin. Morphological changes in spinal cord tissue were examined under a light microscope.

2.6. Statistical Analysis

Data are presented as mean ± standard deviation ($\bar{x}$ ± s). For normally distributed data with equal variances, comparison of group means was performed using one-way analysis of variance with the LSD and SNK methods. For normally distributed data with unequal variances, the Tamhane T2 and Dunnett T3 methods were used for variance test and pairwise comparison. Data that did not follow a normal distribution were analyzed using the rank-sum test. Statistical analysis was performed using SPSS13.0 (SPSS, Chicago, IL, USA).

3. Results

3.1. Behavioral Observations and BBB Scores

Prior to surgery, all groups had normal BBB scores. Immediately post-surgery, only the sham group had a BBC score of 21, whereas the remaining three groups had the same BBC score of 0, indicating successful model establishment. Compared with the model group, the EA and EA control groups had no significant difference in BBC score immediately or 1 d post-surgery ($P > 0.05$). However, BBC scores were significantly greater in the latter two groups than in the model group at 3 and 7 d post-surgery ($P < 0.05$). Compared with the EA control group, the EA group had significantly increased BBC scores at 7 d post-surgery ($P < 0.05$) (**Table 1**).

3.2. Residual Urine Volume

Residual urine volume was measured in rats at 1 d post-surgery and remeasured after 7 d of treatment. Compared with the model group, the EA and EA control groups had no significant difference in residual urine volume at 1 d post-surgery ($P > 0.05$). However, the residual urine volume of rats was significantly less in the EA group compared with the model group at 7 d post-surgery ($P < 0.05$). The decrease in residual urine volume of the EA group was more significant when compared with the EA control group at 7 d post-surgery ($P < 0.05$) (**Table 2**).

3.3. Maximum Bladder Capacity

Maximum bladder capacity was measured in rats at 1 d post-surgery and remeasured after 7 d of treatment. There was no significant difference in maximum bladder capacity of rats in the EA and EA control groups compared with the model group at 1 d post-surgery ($P > 0.05$). However, maximum bladder capacity was significantly less in the EA group compared with the model group at 7 d post-surgery ($P < 0.05$). The decrease in maximum bladder capacity was more significant in the EA group compared with the EA control group at 7 d post-surgery ($P < 0.05$) (**Table 3**).

Table 1. Comparison of BBB scores at different time points after spinal cord injury in different groups of rats ($\bar{x}$ ± s).

Group	BBB score			
	Immediately post-surgery	1 d post-surgery	3 d post-surgery	7 d post-surgery
Model	0 ± 0	0.6 ± 0.52	1.9 ± 0.74	3.9 ± 1.20
EA	0 ± 0	0.7 ± 0.53	2.9 ± 1.10■■	7.5 ± 1.58■■◆◆
EA control	0 ± 0	0.8 ± 0.52	2.7 ± 0.95■■	5.3 ± 1.95■■
Sham	21 ± 0	21 ± 0	21 ± 0	21 ± 0

Note: EA, electroacupuncture; 3 and 7 d post-surgery, compared with the model group, ■■$P < 0.05$; and 7 d post-surgery, compared with the EA control group, ◆◆$P < 0.05$.

Table 2. Comparison of residual urine volume at different time points after spinal cord injury in different groups of rats ($\bar{x} \pm s$).

Group	Number of rats	Residual urine volume (mL)	
		1 d post-surgery	7 d post-surgery
Model	15	2.02 ± 0.20	1.41 ± 0.07
EA	15	1.99 ± 0.15	1.14 ± 0.09■■◆◆
EA control	15	2.00 ± 0.16	1.23 ± 0.06■■

Note: EA, electroacupuncture; 7 d post-surgery, compared with the model group, ■■$P < 0.05$; and 7 d post-surgery, compared with the EA control group, ◆◆$P < 0.05$.

Table 3. Comparison of maximum bladder capacity at different time points after spinal cord injury in different groups of rats ($\bar{x} \pm s$).

Group	Number of rats	Maximum bladder capacity (mL)	
		1 d post-surgery	7 d post-surgery
Sham	15	0.93 ± 0.06	0.94 ± 0.09
Model	15	3.16 ± 0.14	1.67 ± 0.07■■
EA	15	2.95 ± 0.11	2.79 ± 0.12■■◆◆
EA control	15	2.89 ± 0.13	2.65 ± 0.11■■

Note: EA, electroacupuncture; 7 d post-surgery, compared with the model group, ■■$P < 0.05$; and compared with the EA control group, ◆◆$P < 0.05$.

3.4. HE Staining

Light microscopy revealed histological changes in rat spinal cord tissue specimens of different groups. In the sham group (**Figure 2(A)**), the spinal cord displayed intact morphology and structure; gray matter neurons exhibited normal morphology and uniform distribution, with normal cell membrane, nucleus, and interstitial spaces; and white matter fibers were evenly distributed, with intact myelin sheath in an orderly arrangement.

In the model group (**Figure 2(B)**), the spinal cord appeared incomplete with defects of nerve tissue; the tissue presented with severe bleeding in the presence of a large number of blood cells; tissue was loose and had edema, while cells exhibited vacuolar degeneration with some karyopyknosis; nerve fibers were dissolved and missing; there was a decreased number of gray matter neurons, with neuronal swelling, karyorrhexis; the extracellular matrix exhibited a vacuolated pattern; and white matter fibers were decreased, unevenly distributed, and demyelinated, showing incomplete morphology with mutual integration.

In the EA group (**Figure 2(C)**), the morphology and structure of the spinal cord were generally intact, and the tissue contained scattered blood cells without edema; gray matter neurons exhibited normal morphology and vacuolar degeneration was alleviated; vacuolar degeneration still existed in some cells and the nuclei showed no significant pyknosis; and white matter fibers were evenly distributed and appeared morphologically intact without demyelination.

In the EA control group (**Figure 2(D)**), the spinal cord had a small amount of defects and the tissue contained fewer blood cells, with local edema; there were slightly less gray matter neurons, some of which still presented with vacuolar degeneration and karyopyknosis; and white matter fibers were slightly decreased and unevenly distributed, some of which were demyelinated (**Figure 2**).

3.5. TUNEL Data

TUNEL data showed that apoptosis was widely present in the spinal cord tissues. The number of TUNEL-positive cells was significantly increased in the model group. By comparison, EA treatment substantially reduced the number of TUNEL-positive cells ($P < 0.01$). The reduction in TUNEL-positive cell number was significant in the EA group compared with the EA control group ($P < 0.05$), indicating that EA treatment at Zhibian and Shuidao significantly reduced neuronal apoptosis in the spinal cord after injury (**Table 4**, **Figure 3**).

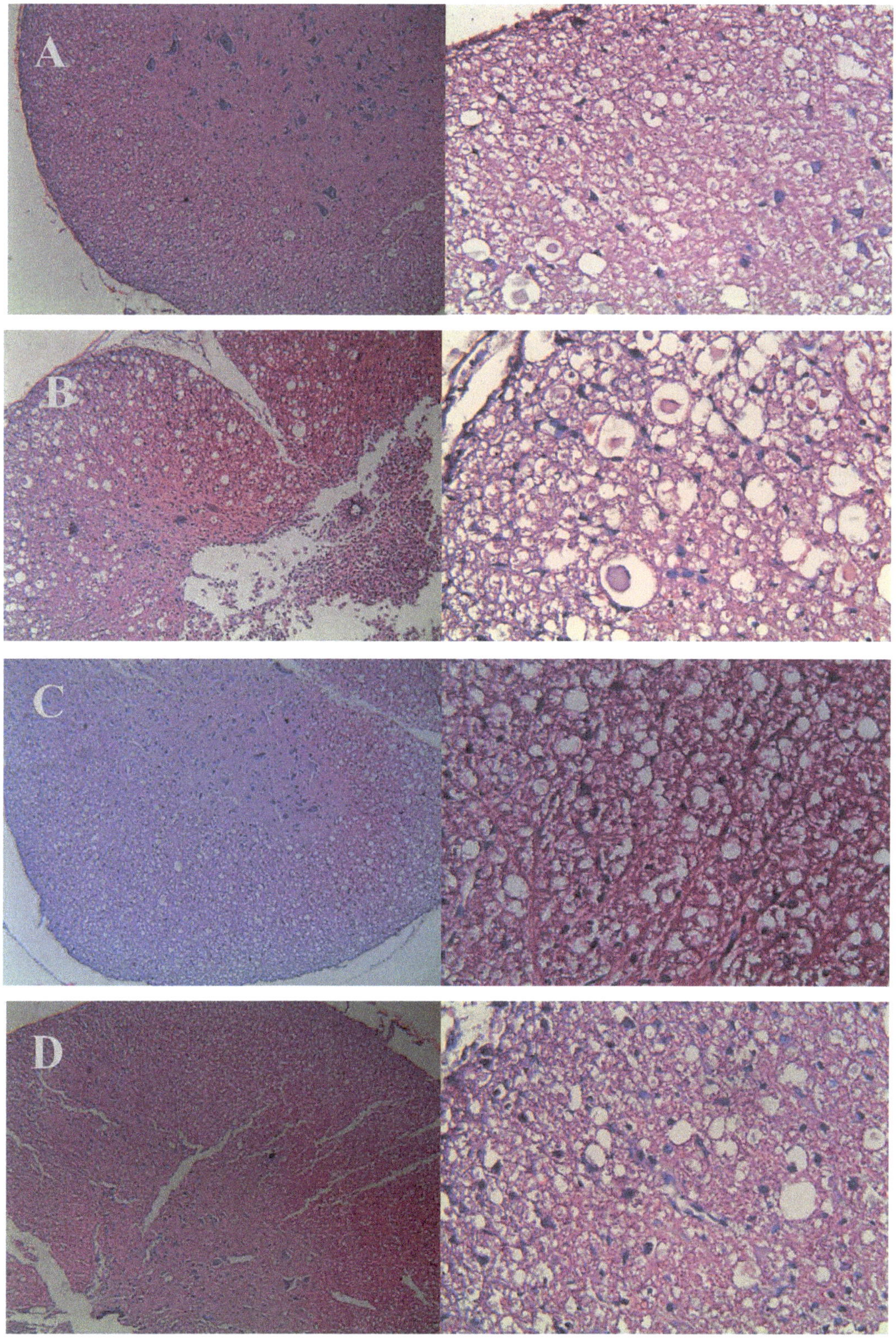

Figure 2. Microscopic observations of HE staining in injured spinal cord tissue specimens from rats of different groups at 7 d post-surgery (left, ×100, and right, ×400 for each group). (A) Sham group; (B) Model group; (C) Electroacupuncture (EA) group; and (D) EA control group. After spinal cord injury, the spinal cord showed incomplete morphology, with nervous tissue defects. After EA treatment, the spinal cord displayed intact morphology and structure, significantly better than those in the model and EA control groups.

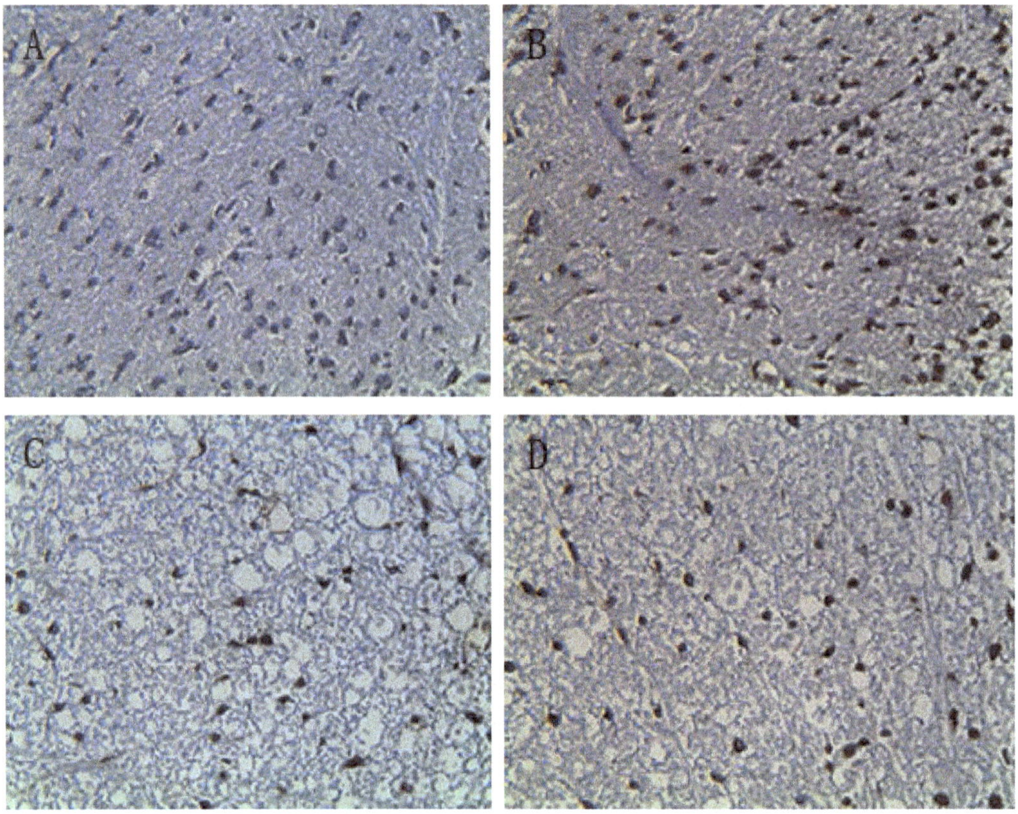

Figure 3. Microscopic observations of TUNEL staining in injured spinal cord tissue specimens from rats of different groups at 7 d post-surgery (×100). (A) Sham group; (B) Model group; (C) Electroacupuncture (EA) group; and (D) EA control group. After spinal cord injury, spinal cord neurons showed different degrees of apoptosis, as well as proliferating gliocytes. The EA group had fewer apoptotic neurons, indicating that EA treatment inhibited apoptosis and promoted spinal cord injury repair. There were more apoptotic neurons in the spinal cord tissue of the EA control group, indicating that EA treatment at Zhibian and Shuidao acupoints was more effective.

Table 4. The results of TUNEL assay on injured spinal cord tissue at 7 d post-surgery in different groups of rats ($\bar{x} \pm s$).

Group	Number of rats	Apoptotic index
Sham	15	0.161 ± 0.11
Model	15	0.953 ± 0.02
EA	15	$0.691 \pm 0.06^{\star\star\blacklozenge\blacklozenge}$
EA control	15	$0.838 \pm 0.04^{\bullet\bullet}$

Note: EA, electroacupuncture; compared with the model group, $^{\star\star}P < 0.05$, $^{\bullet\bullet}P < 0.05$; and compared with the EA control group, $^{\blacklozenge\blacklozenge}P < 0.05$.

3.6. IHC Staining

Positive IHC staining presented as a brown color. At 7 d after SCI, the number of Bcl-2-positive cells significantly decreased, but the number of Bax- and Bad-positive cells increased. After Zhibian and Shuidao EA treatment, the number of Bcl-2-positive cells significantly increased, while the number of Bax- and Bad-positive cells significantly decreased. These quantitative changes were statistically significant between the EA and EA control groups ($P < 0.05$), indicating that EA treatment at both acupoints and non-acupoints promoted Bcl-2 expression and inhibited Bax and Bad expression, but the regulatory effect was more significant in the EA group (**Table 5**, **Figure 4**).

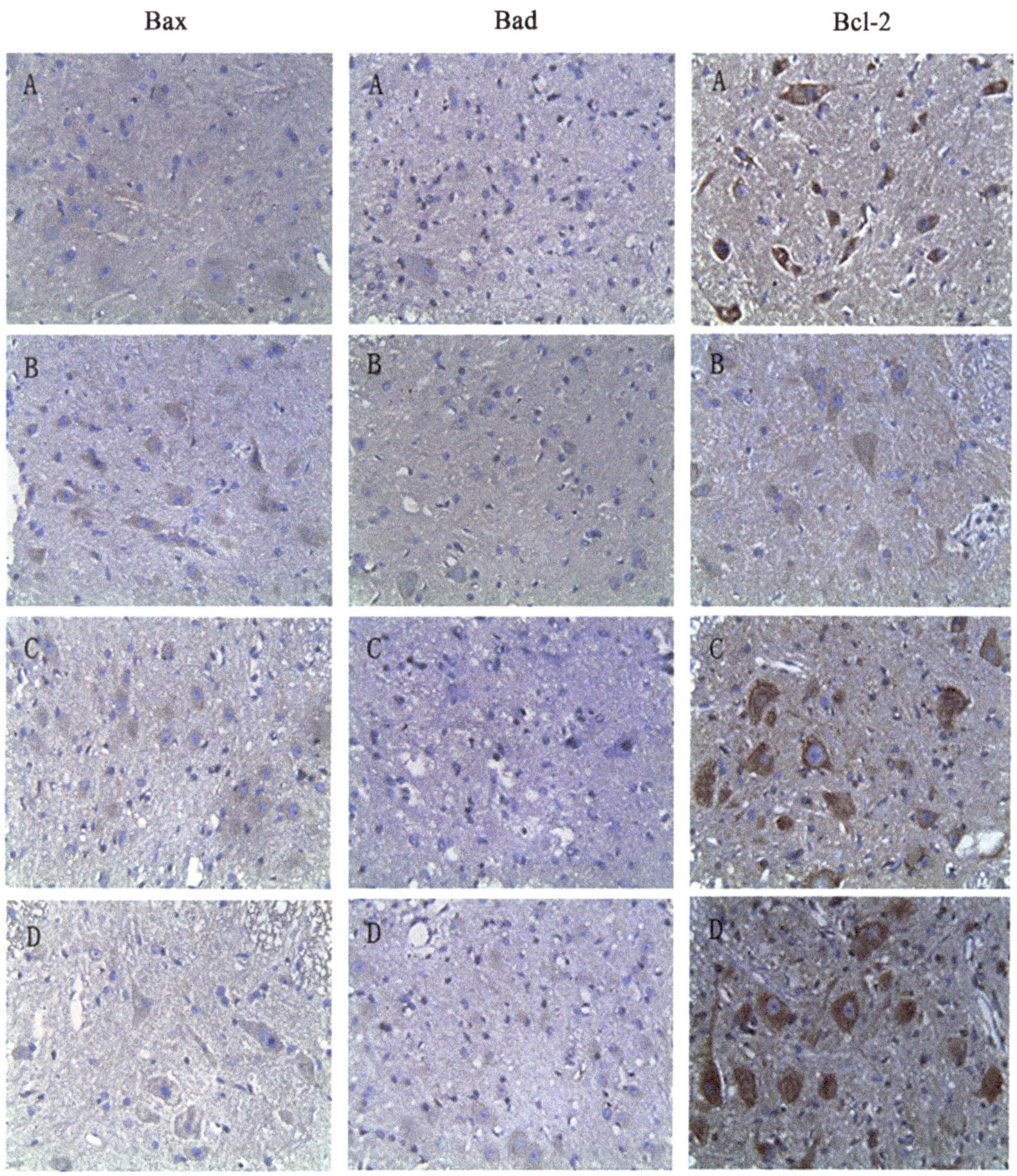

Figure 4. Microscopic observations of Bad, Bax, and Bcl-2 expression in injured spinal cord tissue specimens from rats of different groups at 7 d post-surgery (×100). (A) Sham group; (B) Model group; (C) Electroacupuncture (EA) group; and (D) EA control group. After spinal cord injury, Bad and Bax expression increased, while Bcl-2 expression decreased. EA treatment significantly promoted Bcl-2 expression, but inhibited Bad and Bax expression.

Table 5. The results of immunohistochemical analysis of Bax, Bad, and Bcl-2 in injured spinal cord tissue at 7 d post-surgery in different groups of rats ($\bar{x} \pm s$).

Group	Bad	Bax	Bcl-2
Sham	0.06895 ± 0.012	0.027039 ± 0.004	0.187429 ± 0.006
Model	0.128251 ± 0.021	0.150294 ± 0.003	0.103892 ± 0.014
EA	0.054116 ± 0.009★★■■	0.078775 ± 0.007★★■■	0.173388 ± 0.004★★■■
EA control	0.071302 ± 0.004●●	0.117657 ± 0.018●●	0.145866 ± 0.005●●

Note: EA, electroacupuncture; compared with the model group, ★★$P < 0.01$, ●●$P < 0.05$; and compared with EA control group, ■■$P < 0.05$.

4. Discussion

Presently, SCI is characterized by high mortality, high disability rate, difficult rehabilitation, longer course, and high cost of treatment. SCI prevention, treatment, and rehabilitation have attracted increasing attention in the field of medicine and there is a great need for a simple and efficient means of treatment for this disease. Acupuncture is well known for its simple operation. It is also free of toxic side effects, has a low price, and has proven efficacy. Research shows that acupuncture plays a positive role in neurodegenerative diseases. It can stimulate the release of substances from the central nervous system, such as endorphins, calcitonin gene-related peptides, and neuropeptide Y [16] [17]. Additionally, acupuncture regulates enzyme activity to maintain neuronal self-protective mechanisms [18]. Moreover, it can promote proliferation and differentiation of endogenous neural stem cells in the central nervous system [19]. The present study found that motor nerve function in rats after EA treatment was significantly better than in the model and EA control groups. Additionally, bladder capacity tended to stabilize, with no significant trend towards a decrease in the EA group. These results indicated that the early application of EA stimulation promoted restoration of motor function in rats. However, the protective mechanism of EA for SCI and relevant complications is still unclear. Further studies are needed to better understand the role EA plays in neuronal apoptosis.

Traumatic brain injury, SCI, and stroke are all associated with the occurrence of apoptosis [20]. Crowe *et al.* [21] first found that the occurrence of apoptosis after SCI caused motor and sensory dysfunction. There is a sequential process of primary and secondary injuries after SCI, and the ultimate extent of the injury is mainly determined by secondary injury initiated by a variety of factors. Apoptosis is an important secondary injury factor that mainly involves the death receptor pathway and mitochondrial signaling pathway. The mitochondrial signaling pathway is the primary pathway for disease development and progression, whereas the Bcl-2 family plays a key role in regulating the execution phase of apoptosis. Common apoptotic genes include Bcl-2, Bax, Bcl-xl, and Bad, among which Bax and Bcl-2 are antagonistic to each other, whereby the Bcl-2/Bax ratio determines the extent of apoptosis [22]. The anti-apoptotic factor Bcl-2 is mainly localized in the mitochondrial outer membrane, endoplasmic reticulum, and nuclear membrane. When cells receive apoptotic stimuli, Bcl-2 and Bcl-xL form heterodimers with the anti-apoptotic protein of the Bcl-2 family through the BH3 domain. This mechanism maintains the localization of pro-apoptotic proteins within the cell and protects cells from undergoing the apoptosis process. Bax and Bad are both pro-apoptotic genes. Increased Bax expression initiates apoptosis possibly through two mechanisms: on one hand, Bax forms a heterodimer with Bcl-2, thereby inhibiting the anti-apoptotic effects of Bcl-2. On the other hand, Bax itself forms a heterodimer to exert a pro-apoptotic effect. Bad is normally localized in the cytoplasm, and when cells are subject to apoptotic stimuli, Bad rapidly dephosphorylates and migrates to the mitochondria, thereby inducing apoptosis [23].

In the present study, a large number of apoptotic neurons were present in spinal cord tissue of the model and treatment groups after SCI. Following EA treatment for 7 d, the number of apoptotic cells in the EA group significantly decreased compared with the model and EA control groups. Additionally, Bcl-2 expression was relatively low after SCI, but significantly increased after 7 d of EA treatment compared with the model and EA control groups. These results coincided with previous studies [24] [25] and showed that Bax and Bad expression substantially increased after SCI, but decreased after EA intervention. As the key anti-apoptotic and pro-apoptotic factors, increased Bcl-2 expression and drastically reduced Bax and Bad expression may be related to positive and negative regulation of Bcl-2 and Bax. After EA stimulation, Bcl-2 competitively binds to the Bax protein to form a stable Bax/Bcl-2 heterodimer, counteracting Bax/Bax-induced apoptosis. Bad can bind to Bcl-2 and Bcl-xl to form heterodimers. However, after EA stimulation, p-Bad can bind to the chaperone protein 14-3-3 and thus interfere with the binding of Bad to Bcl-2 and Bcl-xl, further inhibiting apoptosis. Therefore, mutual regulation of Bcl-2, Bax, and Bad proteins can inhibit neuronal apoptosis after SCI, whereas EA treatment promotes Bcl-2 expression and reduces Bax and Bad expression. This may be one of the reasons why EA inhibits injured spinal cord apoptosis and promotes spinal cord repair.

5. Conclusion

In conclusion, this study demonstrated that EA treatment at the Zhibian and Shuidao acupoints significantly improved relevant functions after SCI. One of the possible mechanisms is that EA treatment inhibits expression of pro-apoptotic genes Bax and Bad, but promotes expression of anti-apoptotic gene Bcl-2. However, the occurrence of apoptosis is a complex regulatory process. It includes three stages of gene regulation, signal transduction, and apoptotic execution, respectively, ultimately eliminating unnecessary or abnormal cells. Activation of the signal transduction pathway during the early stages of apoptosis is a necessary precondition for the occurrence of apoptosis and has been increasingly used in studies of neurological diseases in recent years. Nevertheless, further studies are needed to determine the exact mechanism underlying the promotion of spinal cord injury repair by EA treatment.

Acknowledgements

This study was supported by the Zhejiang Chinese Medical Science Research Foundation (No. 2008CB067).

References

[1] Xia, L.P., Fan, F., Tang, A.L. and Ye, W.Q. (2014) Effects of Electroacupuncture Combined with Bladder Training on the Bladder Function of Patients with Neurogenic Bladder after Spinal Cord Injury. *International Journal of Clinical and Experimental Medicine*, **7**, 1344-1348.

[2] Fischer, M.J., Krishnamoorthi, V.R., Smith, B.M., Evans, C.T., St Andre, J.R., Ganesh, S., *et al.* (2012) Prevalence of Chronic Kidney Disease in Patients with Spinal Cord Injuries/Disorders. *American Journal of Nephrology*, **36**, 542-548. http://dx.doi.org/10.1159/000345460

[3] Xing, G.G., Liu, F.Y., Qu, X.X., Han, J.S. and Wan, Y. (2007) Long-Term Synaptic Plasticity in the Spinal Dorsal Horn and Its Modulation by Electroacupuncture in Rats with Neuropathic Pain. *Experimental Neurology*, **208**, 323-332. http://dx.doi.org/10.1016/j.expneurol.2007.09.004

[4] Hwang, L., Choi, I.Y., Kim, S.E., Ko, I.G., Shin, M.S., Kim, C.J., *et al.* (2013) Dexmedetomidine Ameliorates Intracerebral Hemorrhage-Induced Memory Impairment by Inhibiting Apoptosis Andenhancing Brain-Derived Neurotrophic Factor Expression in the Rat Hippocampus. *International Journal of Molecular Medicine*, **31**, 1047-1056.

[5] Sung, Y.H., Kim, S.C., Hong, H.P., Park, C.Y., Shin, M.S., Kim, C.J., *et al.* (2012) Treadmill Exercise Ameliorates Dopaminergic Neuronal Loss through Suppressing Microglial Activation in Parkinson's Disease Mice. *Life Sciences*, **91**, 1309-1316. http://dx.doi.org/10.1016/j.lfs.2012.10.003

[6] Okuno, S., Saito, A., Hayashi, T. and Chan, P.H. (2004) The c-Jun N-Terminal Protein Kinase Signaling Pathway Mediates Bax Activation and Subsequent Neuronal Apoptosis through Interaction with Bim after Transient Focal Cerebral Ischemia. *Journal of Neuroscience*, **24**, 7879-7887. http://dx.doi.org/10.1523/JNEUROSCI.1745-04.2004

[7] Chen, M.H., Ren, Q.X., Yang, W.F., Chen, X.L., Lu, C. and Sun, J. (2013) Influences of HIF-1α on Bax/Bcl-2 and VEGF Expressions in Rats with Spinal Cord Injury. *International Journal of Clinical and Experimental Pathology*, **6**, 2312-2322.

[8] Li, Y., Gu, J., Liu, Y., Long, H., Wang, G., Yin, G., *et al.* (2013) iNOS Participates in Apoptosis of Spinal Cord Neurons via p-BAD Dephosphorylation Following Ischemia/Reperfusion (I/R) Injury in Rat Spinal Cord. *Neuroscience Letters*, **545**, 117-122. http://dx.doi.org/10.1016/j.neulet.2013.04.043

[9] Sun, W., Winseck, A., Vinsant, S., Park, O.H., Kim, H. and Oppenheim, R.W. (2004) Programmed Cell Death of Adult-Generated Hippocampal Neurons Is Mediated by the Proapoptotic Gene Bax. *Journal of Neuroscience*, **24**, 11205-11213. http://dx.doi.org/10.1523/JNEUROSCI.1436-04.2004

[10] Norrbrink, C. and Lundeberg, T. (2011) Acupuncture and Massage Therapy for Neuropathic Pain Following Spinal Cord Injury: An Exploratory Study. *Acupuncture in Medicine*, **29**, 108-115. http://dx.doi.org/10.1136/aim.2010.003269

[11] Pei, J., Sun, L., Chen, R., Zhu, T., Qian, Y. and Yuan, D. (2001) The Effect of Electro-Acupuncture on Motor Function Recovery in Patients with Acute Cerebral Infarction: A Randomly Controlled Trial. *Journal of Traditional Chinese Medicine*, **21**, 270-272.

[12] Lin, H.S., Ji, Z.S., Zheng, L.H., Guo, G.Q., Chen, B., Zhang, G.W. and Wu, H. (2012) Effect of Methylprednisolone on the Activities of Caspase-3, -6, -8 and -9 in Rabbits with Acute Spinal Cord Injury. *Experimental and Therapeutic Medicine*, **4**, 49-54.

[13] Zhou, Y., Liu, X.H., Qu, S.D., Yang, J., Wang, Z.W., Gao, C.J., *et al.* (2013) Hyperbaric Oxygen Intervention on Expression of Hypoxia-Inducible Factor-1α and Vascular Endothelial Growth Factor in Spinal Cord Injury Models in Rats. *Chinese Medical Journal* (*English*), **126**, 3897-3903.

[14] Rajan, R.K., Juler, G. and Eltorai, I.M. (2000) Sigmoid Colon Rupture Secondary to Credé's Method in a Patient with Spinal Cord Injury. *The Journal of Spinal Cord Medicine*, **23**, 90-91.

[15] Nomura, S., Ishido, T., Teranishi, J. and Makiyama, K. (2000) Long-Term Analysis of Suprapubic Cystostomy Drainage in Patients with Neurogenic Bladder. *Urologia Internationalis*, **65**, 185-189. http://dx.doi.org/10.1159/000064873

[16] Feng, X.D., Yang, S.L., Liu, J., Huang, J., Peng, J., Lin, J.M., *et al.* (2013) Electroacupuncture Ameliorates Cognitive

Impairment through Inhibition of NF-κB-Mediated Neuronal Cell Apoptosis in Cerebral Ischemia-Reperfusion Injured Rats. *Molecular Medicine Reports*, **7**, 1516-1522.

[17] Lee, B., Sur, B., Shim, J., Hahm, D.H. and Lee, H. (2014) Acupuncture Stimulation Improves Scopolamine-Induced Cognitive Impairment via Activation of Cholinergic System and Regulation of BDNF and CREB Expressions in Rats. *BMC Complementary and Alternative Medicine*, **14**, 338.

[18] Cha, M.H., Bai, S.J., Lee, K.H., Cho, Z.H., Kim, Y.B., Lee, H.J., *et al.* (2010) Acute Electroacupuncture Inhibits Nitric oxide Synthase Expression in the Spinal Cord of Neuropathic Rats. *Neurological Research*, **32**, 96-100. http://dx.doi.org/10.1179/016164109X12537002794363

[19] Liu, Z., Ding, Y. and Zeng, Y.S. (2011) A New Combined Therapeutic Strategy of Governor Vessel Electro-Acupuncture and Adult Stem Cell Transplantation Promotes the Recovery of Injured Spinal Cord. *Current Medicinal Chemistry*, **18**, 5165-5171. http://dx.doi.org/10.2174/092986711797636144

[20] Kim, D.H., Ko, I.G., Kim, B.K., Kim, T.W., Kim, S.E., Shin, M.S., *et al.* (2010) Treadmill Exercise Inhibits Traumatic Brain Injury-Induced Hippocampal Apoptosis. *Physiology & Behavior*, **101**, 660-665. http://dx.doi.org/10.1016/j.physbeh.2010.09.021

[21] Crowe, M.J., Bresnahan, J.C., Shuman, S.L., Masters, J.N. and Beattie, M.S. (1997) Apoptosis and Delayed Degeneration after Spinal Cord Injury in Rats and Monkeys. *Nature Medicine*, **3**, 73-76.

[22] Hou, Q., Cymbalyuk, E., Hsu, S.C., Xu, M. and Hsu, Y.T. (2003) Apoptosis Modulatory Activities of Transiently Expressed Bcl-2: Roles in Cytochrome *c* Release and Bax Regulation. *Apoptosis*, **8**, 617-629. http://dx.doi.org/10.1023/A:1026187526113

[23] Zhang, X.H., Chen, S.Y., Tang, L., Shen, Y.Z., Luo, L., Xu, C.W., *et al.* (2013) Myricetin Induces Apoptosis in HepG2 Cells through Akt/p70S6K/Bad Signaling and Mitochondrial Apoptotic Pathway. *Anti-Cancer Agents in Medicinal Chemistry*, **13**, 1575-1581. http://dx.doi.org/10.2174/1871520613666131125123059

[24] Bleicken, S., Wagner, C. and Garcia-Saez, A.J. (2013) Mechanistic Differences in the Membrane Activity of Bax and Bcl-xL Correlate with Their Opposing Roles in Apoptosis. *Biophysical Journal*, **104**, 421-431. http://dx.doi.org/10.1016/j.bpj.2012.12.010

[25] Wang, T., Liu, C.Z., Yu, J.C., Jiang, W. and Han, J.X. (2009) Acupuncture Protected Cerebral Multi-Infarction Rats from Memory Impairment by Regulating the Expression of Apoptosis Related Genes Bcl-2 and Bax in Hippocampus. *Physiology & Behavior*, **96**, 155-161. http://dx.doi.org/10.1016/j.physbeh.2008.09.024

23

Molecular Identification of Chinese Materia Medica and Its Adulterants Using ITS2 and *psbA-trnH* Barcodes: A Case Study on Rhizoma Menispermi

Pei Yang[1*], Xiwen Li[1,2*], Hong Zhou[1], Hao Hu[3], Hui Zhang[4], Wei Sun[2], Yitao Wang[3], Hui Yao[1#]

[1]Institute of Medicinal Plant Development, Chinese Academy of Medical Sciences and Peking Union Medical College, Beijing, China
[2]Institute of Chinese Materia Medica, China Academy of Chinese Medical Sciences, Beijing, China
[3]State Key Laboratory of Quality Research in Chinese Medicine, Institute of Chinese Medical Sciences, University of Macau, Macau, China
[4]Development Center of Traditional Chinese Medicine and Bioengineering, Changchun University of Chinese Medicine, Changchun, China
Email: [#]scauyaoh@sina.com

Abstract

Rhizoma Menispermi, derived from the rhizoma of *Menispermum dauricum* DC., is one of the most popular Chinese medicines. However Rhizoma Menispermi is often illegally mixed with other species in the herbal market, including *Aristolochia mollissimae* Hance, which is toxic to the kidneys and potentially carcinogenic. The use of DNA barcoding to authenticate herbs has improved the management and safety of traditional medicines. In this paper, 49 samples belonging to five species, including 34 samples of *M. dauricum*, from different locations and herb markets in China were collected and identified using DNA barcoding. The sequences of all 34 samples of Rhizoma Menispermi are highly consistent, with only one site variation in internal transcribed spacer 2 (ITS2) of nuclear ribosomal DNA and no variations in the *psbA-trnH* region. The intra-specific genetic distance is much smaller than inter-specific one. Phylogenetic analysis shows that both sequences allow the successful identification of all species. Nearest distance and BLAST1 methods for the ITS2 and *psbA-trnH* regions indicate 100% identification efficiency. Our research shows that DNA barcoding can effectively distinguish Rhizoma Menispermi from its adulterants from both commercial and original samples, which provides a new and reliable way to monitor com-

[*]These two authors contributed equally to this work.
[#]Corresponding author.

mercial herbs and to manage the modern medicine market.

Keywords

Rhizoma Menispermi, *Menispermum dauricum* DC., ITS2, *psbA-trnH*, Identification, Adulterants

1. Introduction

Rhizoma Menispermi (Beidougen) is a commonly used traditional Chinese herbal medicine recorded in Chinese Pharmacopoeia as an analgesic and antipyretic drug. Rhizoma Menispermi is derived from the rhizoma of the plant *Menispermum dauricum* DC. (Menispermaceae), which is widely distributed in North China. Recent studies have shown that the alkaloids from *M. dauricum* have various bioactivities, which include anti-arrhythmic and anti-tumor effects [1]. Zhao *et al.* stated that the phenolic alkaloids in the rhizome of *M. dauricum* could protect against brain ischemia injury [2]. In addition, the water-soluble polysaccharides extracted from Rhizoma Menispermi significantly inhibit cell proliferation and DNA synthesis in human ovarian carcinoma SKOV3 cells [3]. Rhizoma Menispermi has become a focus of research because of its newly discovered medicinal properties.

Medication safety is currently a research hot spot, which has become necessary with the increase in market demand for medicinal plants. The rhizome of *Aristolochia mollissimae* Hance (Aristolochiaceae), an adulterant of Rhizoma Menispermi, shows profound nephrotoxicity and carcinogenicity [4]. Radix et Rhizoma Sophorae Tonkinensis (Shandougen), the root and the rhizome of *Sophora tonkinensis* Gagnep., is the most common adulterant in the herb market. Several studies have explored traditional methods to distinguish these two medicinal species [5]. In China, *M. dauricum* is the only species in the genus *Menispermum*; however, medicinal plants in the same family, such as *Stephania tetrandra* S. Moore and *Cocculus orbiculatus* (L.) DC, are commonly interchanged because of their similar morphological characteristics. An accurate identification of these medicinal plants is essential to ensuring the purity and safety of medicines for consumers.

The traditional identification of herbal medicines is mainly based on the morphological characteristics of the source plants, microscopic observations, and the physical form or chemical compositions. These parameters are subjective and can be affected by the external environment, leading to inaccurate classification of herbal authenticity. DNA barcoding has emerged as a cost-effective standard for species identification and has brought a renaissance to the study of taxonomy [6]. DNA barcoding has been proven highly effective in identifying medicinal herbs with high accuracy and reproducibility. The internal transcribed spacer 2 (ITS2) of nuclear ribosomal DNA has been validated as a novel DNA barcode to identify medicinal plant species [7] and is now recommended as the universal DNA barcode for plants [8]. In addition, the China Plant Barcode of Life Group [9] has confirmed that ITS/ITS2 should be incorporated into the core barcode set for seed plants. The chloroplast intergenic spacer, *psbA-trnH*, has been suggested as a candidate barcode sequence after a large-scale study found high variability and efficiency of detection across a broad range of flowering plants [10]. This region is one of the most variable non-coding regions of the plastid genome in angiosperms [11]. In this study, the ITS2 and *psbA-trnH* regions were used to distinguish Rhizoma Menispermi from its adulterants. The extraction of DNA from different tissues of herb species may be hampered by different chemical compositions and growing environments. Leaves and other fresh tissues are generally used in published literatures, whereas roots, which have high polysaccharides and polyphenols content, are rarely used. In this study, *M. dauricum* rhizomas were used to verify the use of DNA barcoding in the identification of *M. dauricum* and its adulterants. Commercial materials were included to evaluate the prospective application of the DNA barcoding method in monitoring crude drugs in the market.

2. Material and Method

2.1. Taxon Sampling

Forty-nine samples of various herbal species were collected from different locations and markets in China (**Table 1**). A total of 4 original plant samples and 30 rhizoma samples of *M. dauricum* were collected from main

Table 1. Detailed information of experimental samples in this study.

Taxon	Sampling part	Voucher No.	Location	GenBank Accession NO.	
				ITS2	*psbA-trnH*
Menispermum dauricum	Rhizoma	YC0146MT01	Chengde, Hebei	KC902480	KC902468
M. dauricum	Rhizoma	YC0146MT02	Chengde, Hebei	KC902481	/
M. dauricum	Leaf	YC0146MT03	Songfengshan, Heilongjiang	KC902482	KC902460
M. dauricum	Rhizoma	YC0146MT04	Songfengshan, Heilongjiang	KC902483	KC902467
M. dauricum	Rhizoma	YC0146MT05	Songfengshan, Heilongjiang	KC902484	KC902466
M. dauricum	Leaf	YC0146MT06	Chifeng, Inner Mongolia	KC902485	KC902465
M. dauricum	Rhizoma	YC0146MT07	Xiaoxinganling, Heilongjiang	KC902486	KC902464
M. dauricum	Rhizoma	YC0146MT08	Fushun, Liaoning	KC902487	KC902463
M. dauricum	Rhizoma	YC0146MT09	Wangqing, Jilin	KC902488	KC902459
M. dauricum	Rhizoma	YC0146MT10	Wangqing, Jilin	KC902489	/
M. dauricum	Rhizoma	YC0146MT11	Fengcheng, Liaoning	KC902490	KC902462
M. dauricum	Rhizoma	YC0146MT12	Fengcheng, Liaoning	KC902491	KC902461
M. dauricum	Leaf	YC0146MT13	Yichun, Heilongjiang	KC902492	KC902458
M. dauricum	Rhizoma	YC0146MT14	Fushun, Liaoning	KC902493	KC902476
M. dauricum	Rhizoma	YC0146MT15	Xiaoxinganling, Heilongjiang	KC902494	KC902475
M. dauricum	Rhizoma	YC0146MT16	Chifeng, Inner Mongolia	KC902495	KC902474
M. dauricum	Rhizoma	YC0146MT18	Qingdao, Shandong	KC902496	KC902473
M. dauricum	Rhizoma	YC0146MT19	Qingdao, Shandong	KC902497	KC902472
M. dauricum	Rhizoma	YC0146MT20	Shangluo, Shaanxi	KC902498	KC902471
M. dauricum	Rhizoma	YC0146MT21	Shangluo, Shaanxi	KC902499	KC902470
M. dauricum	Rhizoma	YC0146MT22	Ziyang, Sichuan	KC902500	KC902469
M. dauricum	Rhizoma	YC0146MT23	Anguo Medicine Market, Hebei	KC902501	KC902479
M. dauricum	Rhizoma	YC0146MT25	Bozhou Medicine Market, Anhui	KC902502	KC902477
M. dauricum	Rhizoma	YC0146MT26	Bozhou Medicine Market, Anhui	KC902503	/
M. dauricum	Rhizoma	YC0146MT28	Drug Store I, Beijing	KC902504	/
M. dauricum	Rhizoma	YC0146MT29	Drug Store I, Beijing	KC902505	/
M. dauricum	Rhizoma	YC0146MT31	Drug Store II, Beijing	KC902506	KC902457
M. dauricum	Rhizoma	YC0146MT32	Drug Store II, Beijing	KC902507	KC902456
M. dauricum	Rhizoma	YC0146MT33	Drug Store III, Beijing	KC902508	KC902455
M. dauricum	Rhizoma	YC0146MT34	Drug Store III, Beijing	KC902509	/
M. dauricum	Rhizoma	YC0146MT35	Drug Store IV, Beijing	KC902510	KC902454
M. dauricum	Rhizoma	YC0146MT36	Drug Store IV, Beijing	KC902511	KC902453
M. dauricum	Rhizoma	YC0146MT37	Drug Store V, Beijing	KC902512	/
M. dauricum	Leaf	PS0345MT01	IMPLAD, Beijing	GQ434390	/

Continued

Sophora tonkinensis	Root	YC0104MT01	Drug Store II, Beijing	KC902514	KC902515
So. tonkinensis	Root	YC0104MT02	Drug Store III, Beijing	KJ766117	KJ766122
So. tonkinensis	Root	YC0104MT03	Tianlin County, Guangxi	KJ766116	KJ766123
So. tonkinensis	Root	YC0104MT04	Meilin County, Guangxi	KJ766118	KJ766124
So. tonkinensis	Leaf	PS0228MT01	Nanning, Guangxi	GQ434351	GQ434960
Aristolochia mollissima	Leaf	YC0514MT01	Nanyang, Henan	KJ766113	KJ766119
A. mollissima	Leaf	YC0514MT02	Nanyang, Henan	KJ766114	KJ766120
A. mollissima	Leaf	YC0514MT03	South China Botanical Garden, Guangdong	KJ766115	KJ766121
Stephania tetrandra	Leaf	PS0348MT01	Danfeng, Shaanxi	/	GQ434988
St. tetrandra	Leaf	PS0348MT02	Xuancheng, Anhui	/	GQ434989
St. tetrandra	Root	YC0200MT01	Anguo Medicine Market, Hebei	/	KJ766125
St. tetrandra	Root	YC0200MT02	Anguo Medicine Market, Hebei	/	KJ766126
Cocculus orbiculatus	Leaf	PS0353MT02	Xuancheng, Anhui	GQ434395	GQ434990
C. orbiculatus	Leaf	PS0353MT03	Chengdu, Sichuan	GQ434396	GQ434991
C. orbiculatus	Leaf	PS0353MT04	Putian, Fujian	GQ434397	GQ434992

"/" means the sample failed to obtain the sequence.

producing areas and different drug stores and markets. Additional 15 samples of species, which were often confused as *M. dauricum*, were also obtained. All samples were identified by Professor Yulin Lin of Institute of Medicinal Plant Development (IMPLAD), Chinese Academy of Medical Sciences, Peking Union Medical College. The samples were deposited in the herbarium of the institute.

2.2. DNA Extraction, Amplification and Sequencing

The surface of the rhizoma samples was first wiped with 75% ethanol, and the outer epidermis was scraped off. Approximately 40 mg for rhizoma samples and 20 mg for the leaves were used to extract genomic DNA using Bioteke DNA Exaction Kit (Bioteke Co., Beijing). For the rhizome samples, 1% PVP (Polyvinylpyrrolidone) was mixed before they were crushed. Then the crushed samples with lysate were heated to 56˚C by water bath for 8 h - 12 h. The succeeding steps were consistent with those used for the leaf samples. The primers and Polymerase Chain Reaction (PCR) conditions were previously described [7] [12]. All amplified products were bi-directionally sequenced. Data analysis was conducted according to the methods used in previous study [8].

2.3. Sequence Alignment, Genetic Analysis and Species Identification

Intra- and inter-specific genetic distances were computed with MEGA 5.0 [13] on the basis of the Kimura 2-Parameter (K2P) model. The sequence lengths and GC contents are listed in **Table 2**. Phylogenetic trees were constructed according to ITS2 and *psbA-trnH* regions with the use of the neighbor-joining (NJ) method, with 1000 bootstraps, in MEGA 5.0. Finally, BLAST1 and Nearest Distance methods were applied to species identification, as described in previous studies [7] [14].

3. Results

3.1. PCR, Sequencing Efficiency and Sequence Characteristics

Most genomic DNA samples showed smearing on agarose gel electrophoresis, which indicated DNA degradation. However, most of the samples were successfully amplified except the ITS2 sequence of *S. tetrandra*, suggesting that amplification of both ITS2 and *psbA-trnH* was not affected by the degradation of genomic DNA.

Table 2. Sequence characteristics of ITS2 and *psbA-trnH* of *M. dauricum* and its adulterants.

	ITS2	*psbA-trnH*
Amplification efficiency of *M. dauricum* (%)	100	100
Sequencing efficiency of *M. dauricum* (%)	100	76.5
Length of *M. dauricum* (bp)	203	315
Amplification efficiency of all taxa (%)	91.8	100
Sequencing efficiency of all taxa (%)	91.8	83.7
Length of all taxa (bp)	181 - 277	215 - 656
Aligned length (bp)	331	743
GC content range in *M. dauricum* (%)	52.7	24.4
GC content range (mean) in all taxa (%)	49.3 - 74.4 (62.8)	23.6 - 41.4 (26.6)
Number (and %) of variable sites in all taxa	163 (49.2)	319 (42.9)

The amplification efficiency of *psbA-trnH* was 100%, whereas the sequencing efficiency of *psbA-trnH* was 76.5% (**Table 2**). We failed to obtain the ITS2 sequence for *S. tetrandra* by using the universal ITS2 primer pairs described by Chen *et al.* [6]. However, the *psbA-trnH* region was obtained from all the samples of this species.

The sequence length of ITS2 in *M. dauricum* was 203 bp, with only one variable site observed in 34 sequences. The result of inter-specific sequence alignment showed that the length of ITS2 was 331 bp with 163 bp variable sites (49.2%). The sequence length of *psbA-trnH* in all *M. dauricum* samples was 315 bp, which indicated high consistency. The length of *psbA-trnH* sequences alignment was 743 bp with high variability (42.9%) across taxa. The GC contents of ITS2 and *psbA-trnH* of *M. dauricum* were 52.7% and 24.4%, which averaged 62.8% and 26.6%, respectively across all taxa (**Table 2**). One of the adulterants, *A. mollissima*, had the highest GC content with 74.4% in the ITS2 locus.

3.2. Intra- and Inter-Specific Genetic Distances and Species Identification

The intra- and inter-specific K2P distances of ITS2 and *psbA-trnH* of *M. dauricum* and its adulterants are presented in **Table 3**. All the experimental samples of *M. dauricum* were highly conserved in ITS2 and *psbA-trnH* regions. The maximum intra-specific distance (0.005 in ITS2) was due to a single C-A variation at the 82 bp site. The inter-specific K2P distances of the two sequences were expectedly higher, with an average of 0.457 and 0.428 for ITS2 and *psbA-trnH* respectively. NJ trees indicated that both sequences allowed the successful identification of all species; with each separate species grouped into distinct clades (**Figure 1** and **Figure 2**). All the sequences were examined by the Nearest Distance and BLAST1 methods. The successful identification rates of the two regions were 100% with the two methods.

4. Discussion

Fresh leaves have been traditionally used as the raw material for DNA barcoding. Currently, DNA barcoding is used to identify traditional Chinese medicines derived from other source tissues such as Rhizoma et Radix Notopterygii [15], Radix Gentianae Macrophyllae [16], Herba Ephedrae [17], and Flos Lonicerae Japonicae [18]. Chiou *et al.* [19] described that DNA extracted from various medicinal tissues and processed materials was usually degraded and even contaminated by microorganisms. For root and rhizome medicinal materials, the accumulation of secondary metabolites, such as polysaccharides and polyphenols, can affect the quantity and purity of the extracted DNA and the success of downstream applications, including PCR. The general approaches to improve the quality and quantity of DNA extracted from medicinal parts include extending the water bath time to 8 h - 12 h at 56˚C, increasing the amount of the sample, and simultaneously increasing the use of beta-mercaptoethanol and PVP. In addition, extracting the crushed samples by buffer for two to three times [20] will help to remove the polysaccharides and polyphenols in the medicinal parts of crude drugs. In this study, 36 rhizoma samples were collected, including 16 dried and long-stored rhizoma samples of commercial materials, and successfully

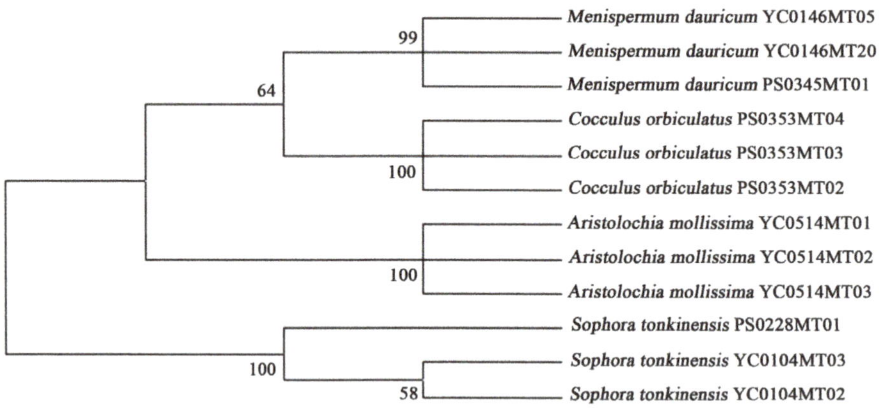

Figure 1. Phylogenetic tree of Rhizoma Menispermi and its adulterants constructed with the representative ITS2 sequences using NJ method. The bootstrap scores (1000 replicates) are shown (≥50%) for each branch.

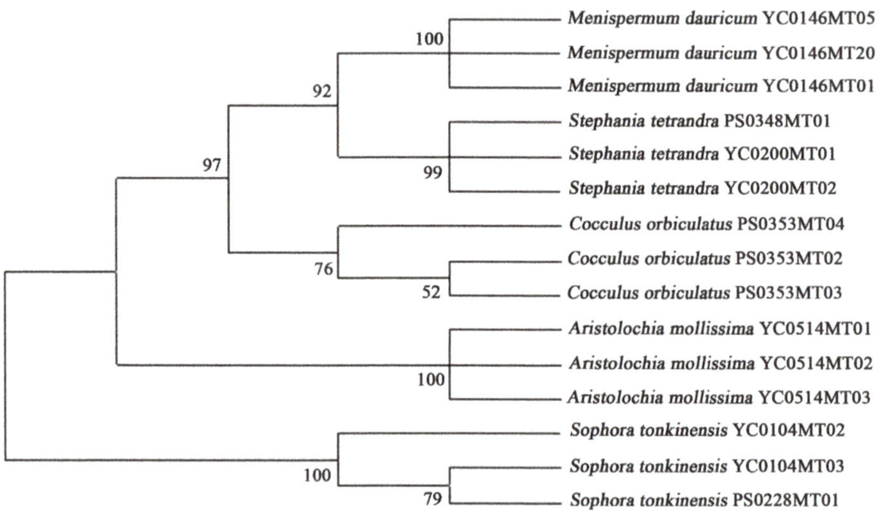

Figure 2. Phylogenetic tree of Rhizoma Menispermi and its adulterants constructed with the representative *psbA-trnH* sequences using NJ method. The bootstrap scores (1000 replicates) are shown (≥50%) for each branch.

Table 3. The K2P genetic distances of ITS2 and *psbA-trnH* sequences of Rhizoma Menispermi and its adulterants.

K2P genetic distances	Range of genetic distances (mean)	
	ITS2	*psbA-trnH*
Intra-specific distances of *M. dauricum*	0 - 0.005 (0.000)	0 (0.000)
Inter-specific distances between Rhizoma Menispermi and its adulterants	0.035 - 0.509 (0.457)	0.033 - 0.624 (0.428)

amplified by PCR. The result showed that the primers used were universal, and the ITS2 and *psbA-trnH* loci were easy to amplify. Wiping with 75% ethanol and scraping the outer epidermis helped prevent the risk of soil fungal contamination to a certain extent. No fungal sequence interference was observed during the experiments. Xu *et al.* [21] verified the operability of ITS2 locus between *S. tonkinensis* and its adulterants, including *M. dauricum*, using sequences downloaded from GenBank and several plant materials. DNA barcoding could identify fresh original plant samples of *S. tonkinensis* and its adulterants. However, no medicinal material samples were included. In this study, we focused on testing the applicability of DNA barcoding to distinguish medicinal materials.

New technology contributes to the success of identification methods. In the 2010 edition of *Chinese Pharmacopoeia*, allele-specific diagnostic PCR was recorded as a new method of identifying *Zaocys dhumnades* (Cantor). DNA barcoding technology uses universal primers and the same PCR reaction conditions across samples to construct a reference database. These factors increase the value of such a method in practical applications. The Food and Drug Administration approved DNA barcoding for seafood identification [22]. In the contemporary medicine market, this technology will help stop the spread of fake and adulterant materials with similar appearance to true medicines. Kool *et al.* [23] used root samples sold by herbalists in Marrakech, Morocco, to determine the applicability of DNA barcoding to modern drug markets. The results of their study showed that *rpoC*1, *psbA-trnH*, and ITS had high sequencing success rates, and combining all three loci allowed the identification of the majority of the market samples up to the genus level. DNA barcoding was used to successfully detect substitution and contamination in herbal products in North America [24]. These two previous studies indicated that DNA barcoding can be applied to the identification of commercial herbs. In the current study, we collected 16 commercial medicinal materials, including Rhizoma Menispermi, Radix et Rhizome Sophorae Tonkinensis, and Radix Stephaniae Tetrandrae. DNA is expected to show increasing degradation with an increase in storage time in dried commercial root drugs. We show that all the commercial materials were effectively identified, and the results were consistent with the information indicated on the medicinal drug labels. Sequence conservation in commercial medicinal materials and original samples from a single species indicated that DNA barcoding can consistently identify commercialized medicinal plants.

The *psbA-trnH* region is among the most variable non-coding regions in the chloroplast genome, and this variation means that this intergenic spacer can offer high levels of species discrimination [11]. However, Chase *et al.* [25] stated that a high rate of insertion/deletion may hamper application to barcoding. Agarose gel electrophoresis demonstrated that both ITS2 and *psbA-trnH* had high amplification efficiency. However, the sequencing efficiency of *psbA-trnH* sequences was almost 10% lower than that of the ITS2 sequences, even if bi-directional sequencing was used. This result was likely due to poly-A and poly-T structures in the *psbA-trnH* intergenic spacer. When a continuous repeated A or T structure emerges, the quality of the followed sequence will decrease, so the determination of the complete intergenic spacer is limited. The sequencing efficiency caused a 23.5% decline compared with the amplification efficiency in *M. dauricum*. In all samples used in this study, we also observed continuous repeated nucleotide structures belonging to Menispermaceae and *S. tonkinensis* (Leguminosae).

DNA barcoding technology has contributed to the development of taxonomy [6] and authentication, especially in traditional Chinese herbal medicine. A stable and accurate method is urgently needed for the circulation and standard management of traditional Chinese herbal medicines. This study is the first to use DNA barcoding to authenticate Rhizoma Menispermi (particularly commercial variants) and its adulterants. The stability and accuracy of the two regions (ITS2 and *psbA-trnH*) were examined. The intra-specific genetic distances and sequence alignment indicated that *M. dauricum* from different production areas had few variable sites in ITS2 and *psbA-trnH* sequences. The existence of multiple copies of the ITS2 region in plants may affect the stability of the obtained sequences. However, Song *et al.* [26] showed that despite multiple intra-genomic variants, the use of the major variants alone was sufficient for phylogenetic construction and species determination in most cases. The ITS2 sequences of *M. dauricum* were highly consistent; intra-specific variations were nearly absent. Multi-copies of ITS2 did not affect sequence amplification, sequencing, and analysis in *M. dauricum*. The high conservation of the ITS2 region was also discovered in *Panax ginseng* and *Panax quinquefolius* [27].

5. Conclusion

In conclusion, both ITS2 and *psbA-trnH* can be successfully amplified from commercial and natural samples of the important traditional Chinese medicine, Rhizoma Menispermi and its adulterants. As a result, accurate species identification and validation of product authenticity are facilitated. Compared with the ITS2 regions, the *psbA-trnH* sequence should not be the first choice for the DNA barcoding of Menispermaceae species on the basis of high poly-N structures and reduced sequencing efficiency. However, in consideration of the results for *S. tetrandra*, *psbA-trnH* can still be used as a complementary barcode for ITS2 in species identification.

Acknowledgements

We thank Dr. Jingyuan Song from Institute of Medicinal Plant Development, Chinese Academy of Medical

Sciences for revising an earlier version of this manuscript. This work was supported by the Program for Changjiang Scholars and Innovative Research Team (No. IRT1150), and National Natural Science Foundation of China (No. 81073001, 81373922).

References

[1] Shan, B.E., Ren, F.Z., Liang, W.J., Zhang, J., Li, Q.X. and Zeng, Y.P. (2006) Isolation and Purification of Antitumor Component in Rhizoma Menispermi and Analysis of Its Activity. *Carcinogenesis, Teratogenesis & Mutagenesis*, **3**, No. 007.

[2] Zhao, B., Chen, Y., Sun, X., Zhou, M., Ding, J., Zhan, J.J. and Guo, L.J. (2012) Phenolic Alkaloids from *Menispermum dauricum* Rhizome Protect against Brain Ischemia Injury via Regulation of GLT-1, EAAC1 and ROS Generation. *Molecules*, **17**, 2725-2737. http://dx.doi.org/10.3390/molecules17032725

[3] Lin, M., Xia, B., Yang, M., Gao, S., Huo, Y. and Lou, G. (2013) Characterization and Antitumor Activities of a Polysaccharide from the Rhizoma of *Menispermum dauricum. International Journal of Biological Macromolecules*, **53**, 72-76. http://dx.doi.org/10.1016/j.ijbiomac.2012.11.012

[4] Hoang, M.L., Chen, C.H., Sidorenko, V.S., He, J., Dickman, K.G., Yun, B.H., Moriya, M., Niknafs, N., Douville, C., Karchin, R., Turesky, R.J., Pu, Y.S., Vogelstein, B. and Papadopoulos, N. (2013) Mutational Signature of Aristolochic Acid Exposure as Revealed by Whole-Exome Sequencing. *Science Translational Medicine*, **5**, 197ra102.

[5] Chen, H. (2010) The Difference and the Reasonable Application of *Menispermum dauricum* and *Sophorae tonkinensis. Chinese Medicine Modern Distance Education of China*, **8**, 60-61.

[6] Miller, S.E. (2007) DNA Barcoding and the Renaissance of Taxonomy. *Proceedings of the National Academy of Sciences of the United States of America*, **104**, 4775-4776. http://dx.doi.org/10.1073/pnas.0700466104

[7] Chen, S.L., Yao, H., Han, J.P., Liu, C., Song, J.Y., Shi, L.C., Zhu, Y.J., Ma, X.Y., Gao, T., Pang, X.H., Luo, K., Li, Y., Li, X.W., Jia, X.C., Lin, Y.L. and Leon, C. (2010) Validation of the ITS2 Region as a Novel DNA Barcode for Identifying Medicinal Plant Species. *PLoS One*, **5**, e8613. http://dx.doi.org/10.1371/journal.pone.0008613

[8] Yao, H., Song, J., Liu, C., Luo, K., Han, J.P., Li, Y., Pang, X.H., Xu, H.X., Zhu, Y.J., Xiao, P.G. and Chen, S.L. (2010) Use of ITS2 Region as the Universal DNA Barcode for Plants and Animals. *PLoS One*, **5**, 13102. http://dx.doi.org/10.1371/journal.pone.0013102

[9] Li, D.Z., Gao, L.M., Li, H.T., Wang, H., Ge, X.J., Liu, J.Q., Chen, Z.D., Zhou, S.L., Chen, S.L., Yang, J.B., Fu, C.X., Zeng, C.X., Yan, H.F., Zhu, Y.J., Sun, Y.S., Chen, S.Y., Zhao, L., Wang, K., Yang, T. and Duan, G.W. (2011) Comparative Analysis of a Large Dataset Indicates That Internal Transcribed Spacer (ITS) Should Be Incorporated into the Core Barcode for Seed Plants. *Proceedings of the National Academy of Sciences of the United States of America*, **108**, 19641-19646. http://dx.doi.org/10.1073/pnas.1104551108

[10] Kress, W.J., Wurdack, K.J., Zimmer, E.A., Weigt, L.A. and Janzen, D.H. (2005) Use of DNA Barcodes to Identify Flowering Plants. *Proceedings of the National Academy of Sciences of the United States of America*, **102**, 8369-8374. http://dx.doi.org/10.1073/pnas.0503123102

[11] Shaw, J., Lickey, E.B., Schilling, E.E. and Small, R.L. (2007) Comparison of Whole Chloroplast Genome Sequences to Choose Noncoding Regions for Phylogenetic Studies in Angiosperms: The Tortoise and the Hare III. *American Journal of Botany*, **94**, 275-288. http://dx.doi.org/10.3732/ajb.94.3.275

[12] White, T.J. (1990) Amplification and Direct Sequencing of Fungal Ribosomal RNA Genes for Phylogenetics. In: *PCR Protocols, a Guide to Methods and Applications*, 315-322.

[13] Tamura, K., Peterson, D., Peterson, N., Stecher, G., Nei, M. and Kumar, S. (2011) MEGA5: Molecular Evolutionary Genetics Analysis Using Maximum Likelihood, Evolutionary Distance, and Maximum Parsimony Methods. *Molecular Biology and Evolution*, **28**, 2731-2739. http://dx.doi.org/10.1093/molbev/msr121

[14] Ross, H.A., Murugan, S. and Li, W.L. (2008) Testing the Reliability of Genetic Methods of Species Identification via Simulation. *Systematic Biology*, **57**, 216-230. http://dx.doi.org/10.1080/10635150802032990

[15] Xin, T.Y., Yao, H., Luo, K., Xiang, L., Ma, X.C., Han, J.P., Lin, Y.L., Song, J.Y. and Chen, S.L. (2012) Stability and Accuracy of the Identification of Notopterygii Rhizoma et Radix Using the ITS/ITS2 Barcodes. *Yao Xue Xue Bao*, **47**, 1098-1105.

[16] Luo, K., Ma, P., Yao, H., Xin, T.Y., Hu, Y., Zhen, S.H., Huang, L.F., Liu, J. and Song, J.Y. (2012) Identification of Gentianae Macrophyllae Radix Using the ITS2 Barcodes. *Yao Xue Xue Bao*, **47**, 1710-1717.

[17] Pang, X.H., Song, J.Y., Xu, H.B. and Yao, H. (2012) Using ITS2 Barcode to Identify Ephedraeherba. *China Journal of Chinese Materia Medica*, **37**, 1118-1121.

[18] Hou, D.Y., Song, J.Y., Shi, L.C., Ma, X.C., Xin, T.Y., Han, J.P., Xiao, W., Sun, Z.Y., Cheng, R.Y. and Yao, H. (2013) Stability and Accuracy Assessment of Identification of Traditional Chinese Materia Medica Using DNA Barcoding: A

Case Study on Flos Lonicerae Japonicae. *BioMed Research International*, **2013**, Article ID: 549037.

[19] Chiou, S.J., Yen, J.H., Fang, C.L., Chen, H.L. and Lin, T.Y. (2007) Authentication of Medicinal Herbs Using PCR-Amplified ITS2 with Specific Primers. *Planta Medica*, **73**, 1421-1426. http://dx.doi.org/10.1055/s-2007-990227

[20] Li, J.L., Wang, S., Yu, J., Wang, L. and Zhou, S.L. (2013) A Modified CTAB Protocol for Plant DNA Extraction. *Chinese Bulletin of Botany*, **48**, 72-78. http://dx.doi.org/10.3724/SP.J.1259.2013.00072

[21] Xu, X.L., Shi, L.C., Song, J.Y., Han, J.P., Yao, H., Chen, S.L., *et al.* (2012) Molecular Identification of Sophorae Tonkinensis Radix et Rhizoma Original Plant and Its Adulterants Based on ITS2 DNA Barcode. *World Science and Technology/Modernization of Traditional Chinese Medicine and Materia Medica*, **14**, 1147-1152.

[22] Yancy, H.F., Zemlak, T.S., Mason, J.A., Washington, J.D., Tenge, B.J. and Nguen, N.T. (2008) Potential Use of DNA Barcodes in Regulatory Science: Applications of the Regulatory Fish Encyclopedia. *Journal of Food Protection*, **71**, 210-217.

[23] Kool, A., Boer, H.J., Kruger, A., Rydberg, A., Abbad, A., Bjork, L. and Martin, G. (2012) Molecular Identification of Commercialized Medicinal Plants in Southern Morocco. *PLoS One*, **7**, e39459. http://dx.doi.org/10.1371/journal.pone.0039459

[24] Newmaster, S.G., Grguric, M., Shanmughanandhan, D., Ramalingam, S. and Ragupathy, S. (2013) DNA Barcoding Detects Contamination and Substitution in North American Herbal Products. *BMC Medicine*, **11**, 222. http://dx.doi.org/10.1186/1741-7015-11-222

[25] Chase, M.W., Cowan, R.S., Hollingsworth, P.M., Berg van den, C., Madrinan, S., Petersen, G. and Seberg, O. (2007) A Proposal for a Standardised Protocol to Barcode All Land Plants. *Taxon*, **56**, 295-299.

[26] Song, J.Y., Shi, L.C., Li, D.Z., Sun, Y.Z., Niu, Y.Y., Chen, Z.D., Luo, H.M., Pang, X.H., Sun, Z.Y., Liu, C., Lv, A.P., Deng, Y.P., Larson-Rabin, Z., Wilkinson, M. and Chen, S.L. (2012) Extensive Pyrosequencing Reveals Frequent Intra-Genomic Variations of Internal Transcribed Spacer Regions of Nuclear Ribosomal DNA. *PLoS One*, **7**, e43971. http://dx.doi.org/10.1371/journal.pone.0043971

[27] Chen, X.C., Liao, B.S., Song, J.Y., Pang, X.H., Han, J.P. and Chen, S.L. (2013) A Fast SNP Identification and Analysis of Intraspecific Variation in the Medicinal Panax Species Based on DNA Barcoding. *Gene*, **530**, 39-43. http://dx.doi.org/10.1016/j.gene.2013.07.097

24

Evaluation of Acute and Repeated Dose Toxicity of the Polyherbal Formulation Linkus Syrup in Experimental Animals

Allah Nawaz[1,2], Saira Bano[1], Zeeshan Ahmed Sheikh[1], Khan Usmanghani[1,3*], Iqbal Ahmad[4], Syed Faisal Zaidi[5], Aqib Zahoor[1], Irshad Ahmad[6,7]

[1]Research and Development Department, Herbion Pakistan (Pvt.) Limited, Karachi, Pakistan
[2]First Department of Internal Medicine, Faculty of Medicine, Graduate School of Medical & Pharmaceutical Sciences, University of Toyama, Toyama, Japan
[3]Jinnah University for Women, Karachi, Pakisntan
[4]Baqai Institute of Pharmaceutical Sciences, Baqai Medical University, Karachi, Pakistan
[5]Department of Basic Medical Sciences, College of Medicine, King Saud bin Abdulaziz University of Health Sciences, Jeddah, KSA
[6]Department of Pharmacy, The Islamia University of Bahawalpur, Bahawalpur, Pakistan
[7]Clinical Pharmacy and Health Care, Jinnah University for Women, Karachi, Pakistan
Email: *usman.ghani@herbion.com, *ugk_2005@yahoo.com

Abstract

The objective of the present study was to evaluate the pre-clinical efficacy and toxicity of polyherbal cough syrup Linkus. Method: Animals (healthy Wistar albino rats; (150 - 250 g) of either sex) were housed under standard environmental conditions; *i.e.* 25°C ± 1°C and 12 h dark/light cycle. Food and water were available *at libitum*. The rats were treated orally with the recommended doses of the test drug (Linkus). After 15 minutes, they were individually placed in a closed Plexiglas chamber (20 × 10 × 10 cm) and exposed to citric acid (0.1 g/ml) inhalation for 7 minutes. The cough reflexes were produced and counted for the last 5 minutes and compared with those of the control animals. The following studies were conducted to evaluate the toxicity of the test drug in healthy Wistar albino rats: lethal dose$_{50}$ (LD_{50}); rats of either sex (n = 10/sex) were treated orally with doses (1 or 5 g/kg) of the test drug. Mortality and behavioral changes were observed for 1 week. Repeated dose toxicity on the healthy Wistar albino rats of both sexes (n = 5/dose/sex) was treated orally with doses of 20 mg/kg (adult human dose = ~1400 mg), 500 mg/kg (adult human dose = ~35,000 mg) and 1000 mg/kg (adult human dose = ~70,000 mg) of test drug (Linkus) for 14

*Corresponding author.

days. Additionally, the control animals were treated orally with water for 14 days. Results: In female rats, the test drug (Linkus) at the dose of 300 mg/kg caused significant (p < 0.01) reduction in the cough reflexes as compared to the control. However, in male rats, a significant reduction was observed at the tested dose of 200 mg/kg (p < 0.05) and 300 mg/kg (p < 0.01). The test product did not cause mortality in rats at the given doses of 1 or 5 g/kg. Other signs of toxicity like hair loss and weight reduction were not observed. In female and male rats, the test drug (Linkus) at different doses did not show any abnormal effects on complete blood count profile of rats. Serum enzyme markers, *i.e.* alanine aminotransferase (ALT), alakaline phosphatase, gamma glutamyle transferase (GGT), direct bilirubin, creatinine, and proteins were also observed and found that the test drug at a higher dose did not cause any of the abnormality and had shown significant p value as compared to the control. Conclusion: The test drug (Linkus) could be an effective and safe cough syrup because it did not show any of the side effects or toxicity on experimental animals.

Keywords

Cough Expectorant, Alanine Amino Transferase (ALT), Polyherbal, Gamma Glutamyl Transferase (GGT), Toxicity

1. Introduction

Cough is defined as the process by which foreign material and mucus from the lungs and upper airway passage are removed. The expelled out mucus during cough is called as phlegm or sputum. It is a most common problem for which the person or patients seeks medical attention; if medical treatment is not started at an earlier stage, it may progress intensely so as to disturb the quality of life. If left untreated, it may lead to vomiting, miscarriage, fever, abdominal pain, headache, seizure, and chest pain etc. [1]. In the social life coughing condition generally causes the embarrassment and self-consciousness and those suffering feeling difficulty in speaking or to speak loud [2]. It has been cited in the literature that the herbal medicines are frequently utilized to cure cough mlaise. In the developed and developing countries there has been expanded use of the medicinal plants and their parts in the complementary and alternative medicine for the treatment of different cough ailments because of their safety, accessibility and efficacy [3] [4]. A major concern regarding the use of herbal medicines is the lack of the preclinical studies for safety evaluation [5]. Many medicinal plants such as *Ocimum sanctum* [6], *Passiflora incarnate* [7], *Adhatoda vasica* [8], *Glycyrrhiza glabra* [9], *Zingiber officinale* [10], *Asparagus racemosus* [11], *Trichodesma indicum* [12], *Asparagus racemosus* [13] and *Emblica officinalis* [14] have been cited in the literature for their antitussive activity. Previous work *in vitro* in experimental model has been done by Keter and coworkers on combination of herbal components on Wister rats for antitussive activity and the result demonstrated significant activity [15]. In another study Gupta and associates tested antitussive activity of combination of herbal drugs formulation and induced cough model in mice and formulation proved to be useful in alleviating cough [16]. In general concept it is commonly observed that many of the well-known herbal or eastern and natural supplements have not been thoroughly evaluated as western medicine to confirm their safety and efficacy. On the other hand, the text of associated products and food supplements had a chronic delusion. There is diversity found in the same brand of medicine claims on label, but from past 12 to 14 years the clinical and pharmacological interests in the efficacy and safety of herbal remedies were started but we found very rare complete study on mixture of herbs for alleviating the cough in experimental animals and to evaluate acute toxicity as well. Many people who frequently use the herbal medicine as self-medication were driven by the realization that, particularly complementary and alternative medicine offers a failure to treat chronic disease as cancer, diabetes, autoimmune disease, and persistent infection [17] [18]. It is worthwhile importance that these medicines cure the different ailments as claimed by different manufacturers and also physician practicing herbal or natural medicine for management of various disorders at their clinic but there is lack of evidence behind their theory to prove their efficacy and safety in scientific logic basis. It is a general concept from many centuries that herbal medicine is considered safe because these originated from natural sources but scientist and researchers have proven that many of the herbal medicinal plants are very toxic even at minor dose; for example toxic herbal product is the leaves of *Atropa belladonna*, *Aconitum* and *Digitalis pursuer* [19] which cause severe toxicities if taken without precautionary measures. In the current study, we followed the acute oral toxicity test in evaluating the toxicity and efficacy of the Linkus syrup. We conducted this study in two parts: first was to administer the Linkus syrup with different doses to evaluate acute and repeated does toxicity and in second we administered this test drug to animals for efficacy study by observing cough reflexes in comparison with control and Hydryllin (**Hydryllin** (Searle): [Aminophylline Plus Compound Syrup] + Active Ingredients: Aminophylline 32 mg, Ammonium chloride 30 mg, Diphenylhydramine 8 mg, Menthol 0.98 mg). Indications: productive cough, smokers' cough, cough associated with asthma and cough due to bronchitis and due to other respiratory diseases. Contraindication Hydryllin should not be given to patients with active peptic ulcers or acute myocardial infarction. It should not be used in patients with hypersensitivity to its components. Because of its diphenhydramine component, Hydryllin should be used in caution and in consultation with physician in asthmatic patients.

The tested animals were then monitored for 16 days for any sign of pathologic and behavioral toxicities detailed are given in methodology section. In market few combined Aherbal formulation study on antitussive activity so far reported. So in this scenario the dosage form design of Linkus consists of some of these herbal drugs but as such to the best of our knowledge no such work on the stated poly herbal as antitussive herbs is reported. Linkus syrup is a polyherbal formulation used for treating patients having complaints of cough in Pakistan and abroad. The Linkus syrup comprises of the following *Adhatoda vasica* (AV)—Bansa, *Piper longum* L. (PL)—Filfil Daraz, *Cordia latifolia* Roxb. (CL)—Sapistan, *Glycyrrhiza glabra* L. (GG)—Mulathi, *Hyssopus officinalis* L. (HO)—Zufa, *Alpinia galangal* Willd. (AG)—Khulanjan, *Viola odorata* L. (VO)—Banafsha, *Althea officinalis* L. (AO)—Khatmi, *Zizyphus vulgaris* Lam. (ZV)—Unnab, *Onosma bracteatum* Wall. (OB)—Gaozaban and excipients. Although herbal supplements may be considered to be safe, some are known to be toxic at high doses and others may have potentially adverse effects after prolonged use. The pre-clinical toxicological studies are necessary to be conducted on these herbal medicines to assess their efficacy and find out side or adverse effects. This product was developed in research and development department, Herbion Pakistan Private Limited, and it is intended to be used as remedy for alleviating cough symptoms.

2. Material and Method

2.1. Preparation of Linkus Extract and Syrup

The medicinal plants in test drug (Linkus) were purchased from Insaf Karyana Store Jodia Bazar, Karachi and authenticity of the samples was kindly carried out by Pro. Dr. Iqbal Azhar, Department of Pharmacognosy University of Karachi. The voucher specimens were deposited in Quality Control Herbarium Sections with identities as AV = B18, PL = F1, CL = S9, GG = M4, HO = Z1, AG = K2, VO = B2, AO = K3, ZV = U3, OB = B13.

Linkus syrup batch manufacturing size was of 2500.0 liters and the finished packs realized in 20,833 units, whereas pack size was of 120 ml in primary packaging in amber colored glass bottle. The details of Linkus ingredients and process of extraction are given in the **Table 1**.

The detailed method of preparation of Linkus syrup is given as under:

STEP I:

Grinding

Individual herbs were taken into the grinder according to the quantities mentioned above and were sieved through 60 # mesh to get the desired particle size.

STEP II:

Extraction

a) Individual grinded herbs were taken into extractor and water as solvent was added to the grinded herbs in the ratio of 1:10 with herb:solvent;
b) The extractors were heated with steam for 2 - 3 hours to get the desired extract in the form of decoction (individual liquid extract);
c) The decoctions were than filtered and transferred to evaporators to remove the extra solvent and to get the desired moisture content *i.e.* not more than 25%. The individual extracts were stored in the form of thick extracts;

Table 1. The herbs, extraction solvent and extraction yield of Linkus syrup.

Herb			Quality of Raw Herb (kg)	Solvent	Herb/Solvent Ratio	Extract Obtained (kg)
Botanical Name	**Vernacular Name**	**English Name**				
Adhatoda vasica	Bansa	Malabar Nut	150	Water	1.10	20
Glycyrrhiza glabra	Mulaithi	Licorice	100	Water	1.10	15
Piper longum	Filfil Draz	Lomg Papper	25	Water	1.10	5
Coredia latifolia	Sapistan	Sabestan	25	Water	1.10	5
Althea officinalis	Khatmi	Marshmello	25	Water	1.10	5
Zizyphus vulgaris	Unnab	Jujube	25	Water	1.10	5
Borago officinalis	Gaozaban	Sedge	25	Water	1.10	5
Hyssopus officinalis	Zufa	Hyssopus	12.50	Water	1.10	250
Alpinia galangal	Khulanjan	Galangal	12.50	Water	1.10	250
Viola odorata	Banafsha	Sweet Violet	6.250	Water	1.10	125

Excipients

Ingredients	Functions
Sugar	Sweetening and Bulking Agent
Citric Acid	Buffering (pH Maintaining) Agent
Sodium Benzoate	Anti-Microbial Preservative
Potassium Sorbate	Anti-Microbial Preservative
Glycerin	Humectant
Pippermint Oil	Flavoring Agent
Purified Water	Bulking Agent

d) Quality Control (QC) sampling was done of all the individual extracts to check the quality of the extracts. The following tests, such as pH, density, volume variations, and microbiological purity along with qualitative and quantitative estimations of polysaccharides, tanning agents, ascorbic acid and total alkaloides have been carried out.

STEP III:

Syrup manufacturing

a) Water as vehicle and bulking agent was added in a syrup manufacturing tank and heated to boil;
b) Sugar was then added in portions with continuous stirring;
c) Individual thick extracts were then added to the above one-by-one with continuous stirring;
d) Glycerin was then added to the above with continuous stirring;
e) Anti-microbial preservatives were then added by first dissolving and filtering in warm water and then added to the above with continuous stirring;
f) The syrup was then allowed to cool to reach the room temperature through chilled water circulation;
g) Flavor was then added to the syrup to get the bulk product;
h) Final filtration was done;
i) QC sampling was done to check the quality of the product.

STEP IV:

Syrup packaging

a) After QC release, the product was transferred to packaging hall through S.S. water pumps;
b) Syrup was filled automatically into 120 ml amber colored glass bottle;
c) Bottles were automatically labeled, punt into unit cartons along with leaf inserts;

d) QC sampling was done to check the quality of the finished product;
e) After QC release, the bottles were packed in master carton and finally to the pallets to shift them to finished goods store.

2.2. Experimental Animals

Healthy Wistar albino rats of both sexes weighing from 150 g to 250 g, were obtained from Animal Laboratory of Herbion Pakistan (Pvt.) Limited. They were housed in a cross-ventilated room and kept under standard environmental conditions, *i.e.* 25˚C ± 1˚C and 12/12 h dark/light cycle. Food and water were available *ad libitum*. They were divided into four groups of 10 rats per group. Each group comprised of five male and five female rats respectively. They were individually placed in a closed plexiglass chamber (20 × 10 × 10 cm) fed with standard rat pellet and water *ad libitum*. They were allowed to adaptation for 7 days to the laboratory conditions before the experiment. The experiments were performed in accordance with the ICH and FDA guidelines [20] [21].

2.2.1. Acute Toxicity Test (Lethal Dose$_{50}$ (LD$_{50}$))

Healthy Wistar albino rats of either sex (n = 5/sex) weighing between 150 - 250 g were treated orally with doses (1 or 5 g/kg) of the test product, maintained under standard laboratory conditions and used for the acute toxicity test. A total of 10 animals of equal numbers of male and female rats were used and each received a single oral-dose of 1000 mg/kg body weight of the test drug (Linkus). Animals were kept overnight fasting prior to the drug administration by oral gavage. After administration of the drug sample, food was withheld for further 3 - 4 h. Animals were observed individually at least once during the first 30 min after dosing, periodically during the first 24 h (with special attention during the first 4 h) and daily, thereafter, for a period of 7 days. Mortality and behavioral changes were observed for 1 week. Daily observations on the changes in skin and fur, eyes and mucus membrane (nasal), respiratory rate, circulatory signs (heart rate and blood pressure), autonomic effects (salivation, lacrimation, perspiration, piloerection, urinary incontinence and defecation) and central nervous system (ptosis, drowsiness, gait, tremors and convulsion) were noted.

2.2.2. Repeated Dose Toxicity

Healthy Wistar albino rats of both sexes (n = 5/dose/sex) were treated orally with doses of 20 mg/kg (adult human dose = ~1400 mg), 500 mg/kg (adult human dose = ~35,000 mg) and 1000 mg/kg (adult human dose = ~70,000 mg) of the test drug for 14 days. Additionally, the control animals were treated orally with water for 14 days.

3. Efficacy Study

The following animal model of cough was used to investigate the antitussive potential of Linkus:

3.1. Citric Acid Induced Cough

Healthy Wistar albino rats were treated orally with the recommended doses of Linkus. After 15 minutes, they were individually placed in a closed plexiglass chamber (20 × 10 × 10 cm) and exposed to citric acid inhalation (0.1 g/ml) for 7 minutes. The cough reflexes were counted for the last 5 minutes and compared with those of the control animals.

3.2. Measurement of Body Weight

The body weights of the treated animals were evaluated at 0, 7 and 14 day of the doses before analysing the tests.

3.3. Specimen Collection

At the last day of treatment all the treated rats were individually housed in metabolic cages for 24 h to collect the urine sample. On 15th day, *i.e.* 24 h after the last treatment, the urine sample was collected and following parameters were noted in the urine using urine analyzer (Uriscan) with the aid of urine-strips, *i.e.* glucose, blood cells, pH, protein, specific gravity and volume. For hematological analysis the blood was collected from the aforementioned control and the treated animals on the last day of treatment and then the samples were transferred to vacutainers and sent to the diagnostic facility of Dr. Panjwani Center for Molecular Medicine & Drug Research (PCMD), Karachi, for Complete Blood Count (CBC) testing. On 15th day, *i.e.* 24 h after the last treatment, the blood was collected from the treated animals and transferred to the test tubes. The heparinized blood was centrifuged within 5 min of the collection at 3000 rpm for 10 minutes. After centrifugation the serum has collected in ependdorf tubes and was used to observe any changes in the blood chemistry. The following parameters (prioritized parameters mentioned in Red Book updated 2007, FDA) were measured using chemical analyzer (Microlab, Merck) with the aid of commercially available kits *i.e.* alanine aminotransferases (ALT), alkaline phosphatase, gamma-glutamyl transpeptidase, total bilirubin, direct bilirubin, glucose, protein (total), urea and creatinine.

4. Statistical Analysis

The experimental results were subjected to were presented as mean ±Standard Error Mean (SEM). Differences between various means were evaluated by one way ANOVA followed by Least Significant Difference (LSD), by using SPSS version 18.0.

5. Results

The test product (Linkus) did not cause any mortality in Wistar albino rats at the given doses of 1 or 5 g/kg. Other signs of toxicity like hair loss and weight reduction were also not observed. In the female and male rats, the test drug at doses of 20, 500 and 1000 mg/kg did not cause any change on complete blood count and gave significant p value as compared to the control (**Table 2**).

The ALT levels were observed to be within the normal range at the administered dose of 1000 mg/kg. In the male rats, a significant reduction in ALP ($p < 0.05$).

In female rats, the creatinine level was significantly declined at the 20 mg/kg (**Table 3**) as compared to the control, protein ($p < 0.005$), urea ($p < 0.005$) and creatinine ($p < 0.05$) was noted at the three different doses *i.e.* 20, 500, 1000 mg/kg (**Table 4**).

In female rats, none of the tested parameters for urine analysis was significantly altered as compared to the control (**Table 4**). In male rats, at 20 mg/kg, the WBC ($p < 0.005$), ketones ($p < 0.05$) and protein ($p < 0.05$) were significantly reduced as compared to the control. At 1000 mg/kg, a significant increase in pH ($p < 0.05$) and specific gravity ($p < 0.05$), where as reduction in ketones ($p < 0.05$) and protein ($p < 0.05$) were observed. By comparing the test drug efficacy with the control drug (ADM), it was observed that in both male and female rats, the test drug at a dose of 300 mg/kg caused significant ($p < 0.01$) reduction in cough reflexes as compared to the control. The standard or control antitussive drug (Hydryllin syrup) also significantly reduced (500 mg/kg, $p < 0.05$) the cough reflexes as compared to the control as shown in **Table 5(a)** and **Table 5(b)** and **Figure 1**.

Table 2. Complete blood count of rats at different doses of Linkus syrup.

Rats	Dose (mg/kg)	Complete Blood Count							
		Hb (g/dl)	RBC (Million/μL)	Hct/Pev (%)	MCV (fl)	MCH (pg|)	MCHC (g/dl)	WBC (10^9/L)	Platelets Count
Female	Control	13 ± 0.1	7 ± 0.1	39 ± 0.4	57 ± 1	19 ± 0.3	33 ± 0.2	6 ± 1	873 ± 31
	20	12 ± 0.8	7 ± 0.2	38 ± 0.7	60 ± 1	20 ± 1.4	33 ± 1.7	4 ± 1	871 ± 50
	500	13 ± 0.5	7 ± 0.2	38 ± 0.4	56 ± 1	19 ± 1	34 ± 0.5	4 ± 1	829 ± 6
	1000	13 ± 1	7 ± 0.1	38 ± 0.2	57 ± 1	18 ± 0.2	31 ± 0.3	4 ± 1	892 ± 44
Male	Control	14 ± 0.2	8 ± 0.2	44 ± 0.5	57 ± 13	19 ± 0.5	32 ± 0.3	8 ± 1	960 ± 67
	20	14 ± 0.2	8 ± 0.2	43 ± 0.8	57 ± 0.5	17 ± 0.2	33 ± 0.1	7 ± 1	911 ± 39
	500	15 ± 0.2	8 ± 0.7	46 ± 0.4	58 ± 2	19 ± 0.07	32 ± 0.4	8 ± 1	853 ± 28
	1000	14 ± 0.2	8 ± 0.1	45 ± 0.8	57 ± 1	18 ± 0.3	32 ± 0.2	6 ± 1	834 ± 48

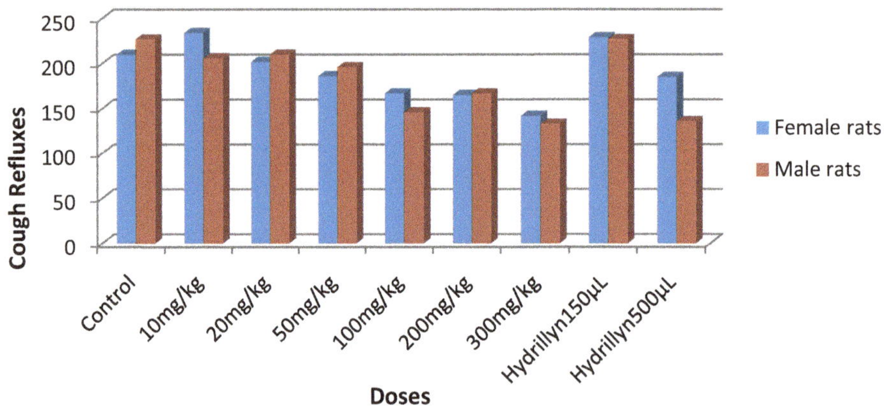

Figure 1. Cough reflexes of rats with test and control drugs.

Table 3. Urine analysis of rats at different doses of Linkus syrup.

Rats	Dose (mg/kg)	Urine Detail Report									
		pH	Gluc	SPG	RBC	WBC	Nit	Bili	Urobil	Ket	Prot
Female	Control	8 ± 0.4	15 ± 0	1 ± 0.001	20 ± 0	18 ± 0	13 ± 2	20 ± 0	25 ± 0	18 ± 0	76 ± 16
	20	8 ± 0.2	15 ± 0	1 ± 0.001	20 ± 0	25 ± 4	11 ± 2	20 ± 0	28 ± 3	21 ± 3	83 ± 8
	500	7 ± 0.3	15 ± 0	1 ± 0.002	20 ± 0	14 ± 2	13 ± 2	20 ± 0	25 ± 0	21 ± 3	51 ± 4
	1000	8 ± 0.3	15 ± 0	1 ± 0.002	20 ± 0	23 ± 8	11 ± 2	20 ± 0	25 ± 0	20 ± 2	92 ± 20
Male	Control	6 ± 0.2	15 ± 0	1 ± 0.001	20 ± 0	43 ± 5	10 ± 0	20 ± 0	28 ± 3	25 ± 9	130 ± 0
	20	6 ± 0.2	15 ± 0	1 ± 0.001	20 ± 2	40 ± 3	12 ± 1	20 ± 0	25 ± 0	27 ± 4	125 ± 25
	500	6 ± 0.3	15 ± 0	1 ± 0.002	20 ± 0	39 ± 4	10 ± 0	20 ± 0	25 ± 0	31 ± 4	130 ± 0
	1000	7 ± 0.5	15 ± 0	1.1 ± 0.002	20 ± 0	35 ± 0	12 ± 1	23 ± 3	32 ± 7	33 ± 3	79 ± 21

Table 4. Blood chemistry of rats at different doses of Linkus syrup.

Rats	Dose (mg/kg)	Blood Chemistry							
		ALT	ALP	GGT	T-bilib	D-bilib	Prot	Urea	Creat
Female	Control	38 ± 5	213 ± 9	1.4 ± 1	0.2 ± 0.03	0.6 ± 0.1	4 ± 0.4	26 ± 6	1.1 ± 0.1
	20	35 ± 6	127 ± 4	1 ± 1	0.3 ± 0.04	0.4 ± 0.01	4 ± 0.3	22 ± 2	0.7 ± 1
	500	40 ± 5	261 ± 57	1.2 ± 0.5	0.4 ± 0.03	0.3 ± 0.04	5 ± 0.5	30 ± 4	1.1 ± 0.1
	1000	33 ± 6	192 ± 22	1.2 ± 0.2	0.4 ± 0.2	0.4 ± 0.03	4 ± 0.04	28 ± 3	1.1 ± 0.01
Male	Control	46 ± 5	238 ± 24	2 ± 1	0.2 ± 0.04	0.5 ± 0.2	5.7 ± 0.8	28 ± 4	0.7 ± 0.1
	20	47 ± 4	217 ± 17	1 ± 0.2	0.4 ± 0.03	0.6 ± 0.2	4.6 ± 0.2	30 ± 3	0.5 ± 0.1
	500	49 ± 4	180 ± 10	2.4 ± 0.4	0.3 ± 0.04	0.6 ± 0.1	4.7 ± 0.4	30 ± 4	0.6 ± 0.1
	1000	45 ± 13	241 ± 14	1 ± 0.4	0.4 ± 0.1	0.3 ± 0.2	5.17 ± 2	28 ± 3	0.7 ± 0.1

Table 5. (a) Cough reflexes of rats with test drug; (b) Cough reflexes of rats with control drugs.

(a)

Rats	Cough Reflexes/5min						
	Control	10 mg/kg	20 mg/kg	50 mg/kg	100 mg/kg	200 mg/kg	300 mg/kg
Female	210 ± 23	234 ± 24	202 ± 28	186 ± 60	167 ± 6	165 ± 11	142 ± 13**
Male	227 ± 25	206 ± 31	210 ± 22	196 ± 18	146 ± 11	167 ± 5*	133 ± 19***

(b)

Treatment	Cough Reflexes/5min		
	Control	190.5 mg/kg	635.3 mg/kg
Hydrillin	211 ± 23	227 ± 18	136 ± 14

6. Discussion

The different studies on cough have been carried out to evaluate antitussive activity by utilizing the medicinal plants. In one of the citation the experiments have been conducted on *Glycyrrhiza glabra* and *Adhatoda vasica by* using a cough model induced by sulphur dioxide gas in mice. The effect of the ethanol extracts of *Glycyrrhiza glabra* and *Adhatoda vasica* on SO_2 gas induced cough in experimental animals have very significant effects at the level of $p < 0.01$ in inhibiting the cough reflex at a dose of 800 mg/kg and 200 mg/kg body wt p.o., in comparison with the control group. Mice showed an inhibition of 35.62%, in cough on treatment with *Glycyrrhiza glabra* and 43.02% inhibition on treatment with *Adhatoda vasica* within 60 min of the experiment. The antitussive activity of the extract was comparable to that of codeine sulphate (10, 15, 20 mg/kg body wt), a standard antitussive agent. Codeine sulphate, as a standard drug for suppression of cough, produced 24.80%, 32.98%, and 45.73% inhibition in cough at a dose of 10 mg/kg, 15 mg/kg and 20 mg/kg respectively, whereas, codeine sulphate (20 mg/kg) showed maximum 45.73% ($p < 0.001$) inhibition at 60 min of the experiment [22]. Polysaccharide fraction of *Althaea officinalis* mimics the intensity and frequency of cough by aqueous extract of its root and the anti-tussive activity is more effective than prenoxdiazine [23].

Marshmallow root extract and isolated mucilage polysaccharide were tested for antitussive activity in un-anaesthetized cats of both sexes at oral doses of 50 to 100 mg/kg body weight, in a cough induced by mechanical stimulation, in comparison with the cough-suppressing effects of Althaea syrup (1000 mg/kg), prenoxdiazine (30 mg/kg), dropropizine (100 mg/kg) and codeine (10 mg/kg). Both the extract and isolated polysaccharide significantly reduced the intensity and the number of cough efforts from laryngopharyngeal and tracheobronchial areas. The root extract was less effective than the isolated polysaccharide. The antitussive activity was found to be lower than that of codeine, but higher than those of prenoxdiazine and dropropizine. Polysaccharides of Marshmallow exhibited statistically significant cough-suppressing activity, which was noticeably higher than that of the non-narcotic drug used in clinical practice to treat coughing. By testing many plants, the most expressive antitussive activity was observed with the polysaccharide from marshmallow, containing the highest proportion of the uronic acid constituent. In a double blind clinical study, Rouhi and Ganji used *Althaea officinalis* in patients with hypertension who had been developed cough during taking of angiotensin converting enzyme inhibitors. The patients received 40 mg of *Althaea officinalis* three times daily as 20 drops for four weeks. The mean scores of the severity of the cough in the group which have been treated by *Althaea officinalis* had a significant change from the score of 2/66 + 0.958 (to) 1/23 + 1.006. Eight patients in the *Althaea officinalis* group showed almost complete cough abolition [24].

The cough in guinea pigs was induced by 0.3 M Citric Acid (CA) aerosol for 3 min interval, in which total number of cough efforts (sudden enhancement of expiratory flow accompanied by cough movement and sound) was counted. Specific airway resistance and its changes induced by citric acid aerosol were considered as an indicator of the *in vivo* reactivity changes. The results showed 1) *Althaea officinalis* polysaccharide rhamnogalacturonan dose-dependently inhibits cough reflex in unsensitized guinea pigs. Simultaneously, plant polysaccharide shortened the duration of antitussive effect when it was been tested in inflammatory conditions. 2) Rhamnogalacturonan did not influence airways reactivity *in vivo* conditions expressed as specific resistance values neither sensitized nor unsensitized groups of animals. 3) The antitussive activity of codeine (dose 10 mg/kg (−1) b.w. orally) tested under the same condition was comparable to higher dose of rhamnogalacturonan in unsensitized animals. 4) The characteristic cellular pattern of allergic airways inflammation was confirmed by histopathological investigations. Rhamnogalacturonan isolated from *Althaea officinalis* mucilage possesses very high cough suppressive effect in guinea pigs test system, which is shortened in conditions of experimentally induced air ways allergic inflammation [25].

The pre-clinical study was conducted on both the test (Linkus) and the control (Hydryllin) drugs on healthy albino rats. Generally, there was no test drug related mortality observed at the highest tested dose of 5 g/kg (2001). It was found that no acute toxicity observed in all the treated rats and according to statement that any of the tested substance with LD_{50} determined that dose greater than 1000 mg/kg could be considered as safe and low toxic [26]. In the light of this view the test drug at a higher dose of 5 g/kg did not show toxicity and mortality, hence considered safe. It was suggested that LD_{50} may not be considered as a biological constant due to the difference from one animal species to the other species, strains, gender, cage environment and the duration of treatment [27]. The data so generated on the efficacy and toxicity (lethal dose (LD_{50})), and the repeated toxicity dose was analyzed by using SPSS version 18.0. The test drug did not show any toxicity even at a dose of 1 or 5 g/kg as compared to the control. In repeated dose toxicity determination, the test drug was given at three different doses *i.e.* 20, 500 and 1000 mg/kg and the parameters assessed, included CBC, blood chemistry and urine analysis. The test product did not show any of the abnormality and pathology observed by assessing these parameters at a maximum dose of 1000 mg/kg. At higher doses no change in CBC profile of rats and blood chemistry and urine analysis were observed. The ALT levels were normal at the administered dose of 1000 mg/kg. In the male rats, a comparing the test drug efficacy with the control drug (Hydryllin), it was observed that in both male and female rats, the test drug at a dose of 300 mg/kg caused significant ($p < 0.01$) reduction in cough reflexes as compared to the control. The standard or control antitussive drug (Hydryllin syrup) also significantly reduced (635.5 mg/kg, $p < 0.05$) the cough reflexes as compared to the control. In addition the test drug (Linkus) cough reflexes and blood profile displayed significant performance. Different herbs in Linkus have been combined so as to relieve different form of cough ailments. The selection of an herbal combination of Linkus is primarily based on the wide ethnomedical use as well as literature search. The mixing of individuals extracts of the given medicinal plants in the Linkus components causes significant difference in reducing cough in the animal model. From the experiment carried out and the data generated, Linkus syrup has shown good promise to control cough and has found greater acceptability in this respect and it was safe by observing acute and repeated dose toxicity. Linkus syrup did not show any mortality even at the doses of 1 to 5 gm/kg of body weight. Even by repeated dose toxicity, effects on urine, the blood profile and Liver Functions Test (LFT), the test drug has been found to be quite safe and there was no change in the highlighted signs in rats during 14 days *in vivo* study. There is an increasing use of herbal or traditional medicine in all over the developing countries due to their popularity and safety on long term use [28]-[30]. Even though these types of medicines are being used for centuries, in this modern world, there are safety concerns that these medicines may or may not produce affect on liver, brain or kidneys and thus cause abnormality [31] [32]. There are various herbal medicines available, but very few have been taken for clinical and preclinical trial studies to confirm their safety and efficacy [33]. Antitussive activity: aqueous and methonolic extract of Ocimum sanctum was studied for antitussive activity in guinea pigs at the doses of 1.55 gms and 0.875 gms/kg body wt respectively. Cough was induced by exposure to the aerosol of citric acid (7.5% w/v). The study showed that both the test extracts posses significant antitussive activity and aqueous extract showed a higher activity than the methonolic extract. The potential mechanism has not explored for this study. The body weight over the experimental time course before and during treatment did not change (see **Table 6**).

In the present *in vivo* study, it was observed that the test drug has not shown any acute and repeated dose toxicity even at higher doses.

Table 6. 14 days treatment (body weights means).

S. NO.	Dose (mg/kg)	Sex	Body Weight (g)		
			Day 1st	Day 7th	Day 14th
1	Control	Female	**266**	**268**	**268**
2	190.5	Female	**275**	**273**	**271**
3	635.3	Female	**238**	**237**	**235**
4	1270.0	Female	**373**	**371**	**368.8**
5	Control	Male	**300**	**302**	**302**
6	190.5	Male	**346**	**345**	**341.8**
7	635.3	Male	**289**	**288**	**286**
8	1270.0	Male	**374.8**	**373.6**	**370**

7. Conclusion

Acute toxicity test (LD_{50}) Wistar albino rats 10 in number weighing from 150 to 250 g received a single oral dose of 1000 mg/kg body weight of the test drug (Linkus). Animals were observed individually at least once during the first 30 min after dosing, periodically during the first 24 h, then first 4 h and finally for 7 days. Mortality and behavioral changes observed in skin and fur, eyes and mucus membrane (nasal), respiratory rate, circulatory signs (heart rate and blood pressure), autonomic effects (salivation, lacrimation, perspiration, piloerection, urinary incontinence and defecation) and central nervous system (ptosis, drowsiness, gait, tremors and convulsion) were noted. Dose toxicity was repeated in rats with doses of 20 mg/kg (whereas equivalent adult human dose = 1400 mg), 500 mg/kg (whereas equivalent adult human dose = 35,000 mg) and 1000 mg/kg (whereas equivalent adult human dose = 70,000 mg) of the test drug for 14 days. Usually cough is induced by citric acid but all coughs are not induced by it. It was concluded that test drug (Linkus) exhibited effectiveness as compared to the control drug (Hydryllin syrup) in alleviating the cough and has shown no toxicity or adverse reactions in experimental models.

Acknowledgements

This study was funded by Herbion Pakistan (Pvt) Limited, Karachi, Pakistan. The authors are thankful to Mr. Nadeem Khalid, CEO and Mr. Abid Mumtaz, COO as well as other colleagues for their support and contribution.

References

[1] Irwin, R.S. and Madison, J.M. (2000) The Diagnosis and Treatment of Cough. *New England Journal of Medicine*, **343**, 1715-1721. http://dx.doi.org/10.1056/NEJM200012073432308

[2] French, C.L., Irwin, R.S., Curley, F.J. and Krikorian, C.J. (1998) Impact of Chronic Cough on Quality of Life. *Archives of Internal Medicine*, **158**, 1657-1661. http://dx.doi.org/10.1001/archinte.158.15.1657

[3] Irwin, R.S., Boulet, L.P. and Cloutier, M.M. (1998) Managing Cough as a Defense Mechanism and as a Symptom. *Chest*, **114**, 133S-181S. http://dx.doi.org/10.1378/chest.114.2_Supplement.133S

[4] Salawu, O.A., Chindo, B.A., Tijani, A.Y., Obidike, I.C., Salawu, T.A. and Akingbasote, A.J. (2009) Acute and Sub-Acute Toxicological Evaluations of the Methanolic Stem Bark Extract of *Crossopteryx febrifuga* in Rats. *African Journal of Pharmacy and Pharmacology*, **3**, 621-626.

[5] Angell, M. and Kassierr, J.P. (1998) Alternative Medicine—The Risk of Untested and Unregulated Remedies. *New England Journal of Medicine*, **339**, 839-841. http://dx.doi.org/10.1056/NEJM199809173391210

[6] Nadig, P.D. and Laxmi, S. (2005) Study of Anti-Tussive Activity of Ocimum Sanctum Linn in Guinea Pigs. *Indian Journal of Physiology and Pharmacology*, **49**, 243-245.

[7] Dhawan, K. and Sharma, A. (2002) Antitussive Activity of the Methanol Extract of *Passiflora incarnate* Leaves. *Fitoterapia*, **73**, 397-399. http://dx.doi.org/10.1016/S0367-326X(02)00116-8

[8] Dhule, J.N. (1999) Antitussive Effect of Adhatoda Vasica Extract on Mechanical or Chemical Stimulation-Induced Coughing in Animals. *Journal of Ethnopharmacology*, **67**, 361-365. http://dx.doi.org/10.1016/S0378-8741(99)00074-4

[9] Chang, H.M. and Butt, P.P.H. (1986) Pharmacology and Applications of Chinese Materia Medica. Vol. 1, World Scientific, Singapore, 304. http://dx.doi.org/10.1142/0284

[10] Suekawa, M., Ishige, A., Yuasa, K., Sudo, K., Aburada, M. and Hosoya, E. (1984) Pharmacological Studies on Ginger. I. Pharmacological Actions of Pungent Constitutents, (6)-Gingerol and (6)-Shogaol. *Journal of Pharmacobio-Dynamics*, **7**, 836-848. http://dx.doi.org/10.1248/bpb1978.7.836

[11] Mandal, S.C., Kumar, C.K.A., Mohana Lakshmi, S., Sinha, S., Murugesan, T., Saha, B.P. and Pal, M. (2000) Antitussive Effect of *Asparagus racemosus* Root against Sulfur Dioxide-Induced Cough in Mice. *Fitoterapia*, **71**, 686-689.

[12] Srinath, K., Murugesan, T., Kumar, C.A., Suba, V., Das, A.K., Sinha, S., Arunachalam, G. and Manikandan, L. (2002) Effect of *Trichodesma indicum* Extract on Cough Reflex Induced by Sulphur Dioxide in Mice. *Phytomedicine*, **9**, 75-77. http://dx.doi.org/10.1078/0944-7113-00086

[13] Mandal, S.C., Ashok-Kumar, C.K., Lakshmi, S.M., Sanghamitra, S., Murugesan, T., Saha, B.P. and Pal, M. (2000) Antitussive Effect of *Asparagus racemosus* Root against Sulfur Dioxide-Induced Cough in Mice. *Fitoterapia*, **71**, 686-689. http://dx.doi.org/10.1016/S0367-326X(00)00151-9

[14] Nosál'ová, G., Mokrý, J. and Hassan, K.M. (2003) Antitussive Activity of the Fruit Extract of *Emblica officinalis* Gaertn. (Euphorbiaceae). *Phytomedicine*, **10**, 583-589. http://dx.doi.org/10.1078/094471103322331872

[15] Keter, L.K., Mwikwabe, N.M., Mbaabu, M.P., Sudhee, H.M., Tolo, F.M., Dhanani, P. and Orwa, J.A. (2013) Validation of Safety and Efficacy of Antitussive Herbal Formulations. *African Journal of Pharmacology and Therapeutics*, **2**, 26-31.

[16] Gupta, Y.K., Kaytyal, J., Kumar, G., Mehla, G., Katiyar, C.K., Sharma, N. and Yav, S. (2009) Evaluation of Antitussive Activity of Formulations with Herbal Extracts in Sulphur Dioxide (SO_2) Induced Cough Model in Mice. *Indian Journal of Physiology and Pharmacology*, **53**, 61-66.

[17] Calixto, J.B. (2000) Efficacy, Safety, Quality Control, Marketing and Regulatory Guidelines for Herbal Medicines (Phytotherapeutic Agents). *Brazilian Journal of Medical and Biological Research*, **33**, 179-189. http://dx.doi.org/10.1590/S0100-879X2000000200004

[18] Firenzuoli, F. and Gori, L. (2007) Herbal Medicine Today: Clinical and Research Issues. *Evidence-Based Complementary and Alternative Medicine*, **4**, 37-40. http://dx.doi.org/10.1093/ecam/nem096

[19] Greenblatt, D.J. and Shader, R.I. (1971) Uses and Toxicity of Belladonna Alkaloids and Synthetic Anticholinergics. *Seminars in Psychiatry*, **3**, 449-476.

[20] Red Book (2007) Guidance for Industry and Other Stakeholders Toxicological Principles for the Safety Assessment of Food Ingredients. Revised Edition, Chapter IV, 000045. http://www.cfan.fda.gov/guidance.html

[21] ICH Harmonized Tripartite Guideline (2002) Guidance for Good Clinical Practice. E6 (R1); PMP/ICH/135/95. European Agency, London.

[22] Yasmeen, I. and Siddiqui, H. (2012) Study of the Antitussive Potential of *Glycyrrhiza glabra* and *Adhatoda vasica* Using a Cough Model Induced by Sulphur Dioxide Gas in Mice. *International Journal of Pharmaceutical Sciences and Research*, **3**, 1668-1674.

[23] Nosal'ova, G., Saab, B.R., Pashayan, N. and El, C.S. (1992) Antitussive Efficacy of the Complex Extract and the Polysaccharide of Marshmallow (*Althaea officinalis* L. var. Robusta). *Pharmazie*, **47**, 224-226.

[24] Al-Snafi, A.I. (2013) The Pharmaceutical Importance of *Altahea officinalis* and *Althaea rosea*. *International Journal of PharmTech Research*, **5**, 1378-1385.

[25] Sutovska, M., Capek, P., Franova, S., Joskova, M., Sutovsky, J., Marcinek, J. and Kalman, M. (2011) Antitussive Activity of *Althaea officinalis* L. Polysaccharide Rhamnogalacturonan and Its Changes in Guinea Pigs with Ovalbumine-Induced Airways Inflammation. *Bratislavské lekárske listy*, **112**, 670-675.

[26] Clarke, M.L. and Clarke, E.G.C. (1967) Veterinary Toxicology. Bailliere Tindall, London.

[27] Zbinden, G. and Roversi, F. (1981) Significance of the LD_{50} Test for the Toxicological Evaluation of Chemical Substances. *Archives of Toxicology*, **47**, 77-99. http://dx.doi.org/10.1007/BF00332351

[28] Daswani, G.P., Brijesh, S. and Birdi, J.T. (2006) Preclinical Testing of Medicinal Plants: Advantages and Approaches. *Workshop Proceedings on Approaches towards Evaluation of Medicinal Plants Prior to Clinical Trial*, Foundation for Medical Research at Yashwantrao Chavan Academy of Development Administration (YASHADA), 60-77.

[29] Ogbonnia, S.O., Mbaka, G.O., Anyika, E.N., Osegbo, O.M. and Igbokwe, N.H. (2010) Evaluation of Acute Toxicity in Mice and Subchronic Toxicity of Hydro-Ethanolic Extract of *Chromolaena odorata* (L.) King and Robinson (Fam. Asteraceae) in Rats. *Agriculture and Biology Journal of North America*, **1**, 859-865. http://dx.doi.org/10.5251/abjna.2010.1.5.859.865

[30] Stewart, M.J., Moar, J.J., Steenkamp, P. and Kokot, M. (1999) Findings in Fatal Cases of Poisoning Attributed to Traditional Remedies in South Africa. *Forensic Science International*, **101**, 177-183. http://dx.doi.org/10.1016/S0379-0738(99)00025-0

[31] Saad, B., Azaizeh, H., Abu-Hijleh, G. and Said, O. (2006) Safety of Traditional Arab Herbal Medicine. *Evidence-Based Complementary and Alternative Medicine*, **3**, 433-439. http://dx.doi.org/10.1093/ecam/nel058

[32] Colson, C.R. and De Broe, M.E. (2005) Kidney Injury from Alternative Medicines. *Advances in Chronic Kidney Disease*, **12**, 261-275. http://dx.doi.org/10.1016/j.ackd.2005.03.006

[33] Cheng, C.W., Bian, Z.X. and Wu, T.X. (2009) Systematic Review of Chinese Herbal Medicine for Functional Constipation. *World Journal of Gastroenterology*, **15**, 4886-4895. http://dx.doi.org/10.3748/wjg.15.4886

25

Efficacy of Sea Buckthorn Therapy in Patients with Nonalcoholic Fatty Liver Disease

Zeli Gao[1*], Cheng Zhang[2], Liwen Jin[2], Wei Yao[2]

[1]Department of Gastroenterology, People's Hospital of Pudong New Area, Shanghai, China
[2]Department of Gastroenterology, Zhoupu Hospital, Pudong New Area, Shanghai, China
Email: [*]gzeli@163.com

Abstract

Aim: To evaluate the clinical efficacy of the traditional Chinese medicine sea buckthorn (SBT) in the treatment of patients with nonalcoholic fatty liver disease (NAFLD). Method: 94 patients with NAFLD were randomly divided into two groups: 48 cases of patients received oral sea buckthorn 1.5 g (3 times a day) for three months as the treated group, and 46 cases received only the vehicle for three months as the control group. Serum lipids, transaminase and serum liver fibrosis indices were assessed at baseline and after SBT treatment. All patients underwent liver CT and Fibroscan examination at baseline and after treatment. Results: SBT treatment resulted in a significant decrease in the serum levels of alanine aminotransferase (ALT), LDL-C, hyaluronic acid and collagen type IV. The liver stiffness measurement (LSM) of the treated patients was significantly lower than that in the control or baseline. The CT liver/spleen ratio of the treated patients was also significantly increased. Conclusion: The results of our study demonstrated the beneficial effects of SBT on serum lipids, transaminase, and liver/spleen ratio and liver stiffness in patients with NAFLD, which may be further developed as a promising therapy for the treatment of NAFLD.

Keywords

Sea Buckthorn (*Hippophae rhamnoides L*), Nonalcoholic Fatty Liver Disease, Blood Lipid, Traditional Chinese Medicine

1. Introduction

Nonalcoholic fatty liver disease (NAFLD) is a one of the most common causes of chronic liver injury in the

[*]Corresponding author.

world [1] [2]. Although NAFLD is usually benign in early stages in most cases; about 40% - 50% NAFLD cases progress to fibrosis, and 15% - 20% cases progress to cirrhosis or even end-stage liver disease. In NAFLD cirrhosis, 30% to 40% of patients will experience a liver-related death [3]. So, it is important to find ways or medicines to treat this disease.

Multiple factors have been reported to interact with the development of NAFLD. It has been shown that insulin resistance (IR), oxidative stress, genetic and immune factors, obesity, dyslipidemia, diabetes, and hypertension, are key risk factors for the development and progression of NAFLD [4]. It has been proved that insulin sensitizers, weight loss medications, lipid lowering medications (Statins), antioxidants all have some therapeutic effects in treatment of NAFLD; however, there is no definitive therapeutic strategy for effective treatment of NAFLD [5].

SBT (*Hippophae rhamnoides L*) is a thorny nitrogen-fixing deciduous shrub, native to Asia and Europe. The pharmacological effects of sea buckthorn were recorded in some medicinal classics. Recently, sea buckthorn was reported to have diverse pharmacological effects [6]. It was found that, in a high-fat diet fed mouse model, administration of flavonoids isolated from seed residues of *Hippophae rhamnoides L* (FSH) markedly reduced the levels of both serum total cholesterol and low-density lipoprotein-cholesterol, and significantly lowered total cholesterol and triglyceride concentrations in liver. Furthermore, the FSH treatment not only significantly suppressed the rise in serum glucose, but also improved the impaired glucose tolerance. The sea buckthorn leaf extract was found to have significant anti-inflammatory activity in adjuvant induced arthritis (AIA) rat model and in lipopolysaccharide-induced inflammatory response [7] [8]. Crude extracts containing carotenoids from the berries of various cultivars of SBT have been shown to have antioxidant capacity [9]. The SBT leaves and seed oil also have hepatoprotective activity evaluated using CCl_4-induced hepatic damage in animals [10] [11]. In consideration of these demonstrated effects of SBT, we presume that SBT may have a therapeutic effect in patients with NAFLD. Therefore, the aim of this study was to investigate the effects of SBT in the treatment of patients with NAFLD.

2. Patients and Methods

This randomized, prospective, clinical trial was carried out at the outpatient department of Gastroenterology of Shanghai Pudong New District ZhouPu Hospital and Shanghai Baoshan Central Hospital. The recruitment of patients started in March 2008 and was concluded in March 2011. Of the patients diagnosed with NAFLD by ultrasonographic evidence and elevated aminotransferase activity, 94 cases were consistent with the inclusion and exclusion criteria as follows.

2.1. Inclusion Criteria

2.1.1. Diagnostic Criteria of NAFLD

NAFLD was diagnosed according to the criteria in Guidelines for Management of Nonalcoholic Fatty Liver Disease set by Workshop on Fatty Liver and Alcoholic Liver Disease specified by the Chinese Society of Hepatology.

Inclusion criteria were as follows: 1) patients with no history of alcohol consuming or an alcohol-drinking history of less than 140 g (ethanol) weekly for man and less than 70 g for women; 2) patients with no histories of viral hepatitis, drug-induced liver disease, total parenteral nutrition, and hepatolenticular degeneration or autoimmune liver disease that could cause fatty liver; 3) patients whose histological changes in liver biopsy met the pathological diagnostic criteria of fatty liver disease; 4) patients whose liver imaging met the imaging diagnostic criteria of diffuse fatty liver, which could not be explained by other reasons; and 5) patients whose serum ALT and/or AST or GGT continued to rise in recent six months or longer.

2.1.2. Exclusion Criteria

Patients were excluded if they were in agreement with the following criteria: 1) patients whose fatty liver was due to chronic cardiac insufficiency or malnutrition; 2) patients whose fatty liver was associated with viral hepatitis, hepaticdecompensation, positive testing for hepatitis B virus or hepatitis C virus, any other suspected causes of liver disease by history; 3) patients who had received treatment for fatty liver by other Chinese or modern medicines; 4) patients with serious primary diseases, alcohol or drug abuse; 5) patients with encyesis; 6) patients with genetic diseases; and 7) patients who did not cooperate with the treatment or could not guarantee completion of the treatment.

2.2. Grouping and Treatment Method

The patients enrolled (n = 94) were randomly divided into two groups: the study group (n = 48, 25 male and 23 female) and the control group (n = 46, 27 male and 19 female). The age of the patients ranged from 18 to 67 years. The patients of the two groups were comparable in sex, age, duration of disease and severity of the pathological condition.

The study group was given SBT capsules (Hebei Shengxing Seabuckthorn Pharmaceuticals, Shijiazhuang City, China) at a dose of 1.5 g in capsules 3 times/day for 90 consecutive days. The control group was given starch 1.5 g in capsules 3 times a day (manufactured by the same company). Both groups were advised to follow a diet tailored on the individual requirement, a regimen of daily physical exercise of walking for 30 - 60 min/day for 3 months during the treatment. Patients with diabetes or hypertension were given the corresponding treatment at the same time.

Changes in symptoms and signs, blood pressure (BP), physical fitness index and adverse drug reactions were assessed during the 3-month treatment period.

Diabetes was considered present if patients took medications for diabetes (metformin or sulfamides) or if the fasting serum glucose level was 7 mmol/L or above in untreated patients. Arterial hypertension was considered present if patients took antihypertensive drugs.

2.3. Evaluation and Monitoring

2.3.1. Laboratory Tests

Laboratory tests were performed at the baseline and at the end of treatment. Fasting blood was collected from peripheral vein at observational points, using the automatic multi-parameter analyzer (Siemens, Germany). The following liver function associated laboratory parameters including serum aspartate aminotransferase (AST) and ALT levels, gamma glutamyl transferase (r-GT), blood glucose, serum lipid indices including triglycerides, (TG), total cholesterol (TC), high density lipoprotein cholesterol (HDL-C), low density lipoprotein cholesterol, (LDL-C), were evaluated. Liver fibrosis indices, including: laminin (LN), hyaluronic acid (HA, procollagen III), PC III and collagen Type IV (C IV), were measured by radioimmunoassay (RIA).

2.3.2. B-Ultrasound Examination and Quantitative Standard

Liver ultrasounds measurement were performed at baseline and post-treatment, by a single, blinded, radiologist in the two hospitals in order to avoid personal errors. The ultrasonographic diagnosis of fatty liver was confirmed in the presence of the following four findings: 1) a diffuse hyperechoic echotexture (bright liver); 2) increased liver echotexture compared with the kidneys; 3) vascular blurring; and 4) deep attenuation.

2.3.3. Transient Elastography

Liver stiffness measurement (LSM) was performed with a Fibroscan (EchoSens, Paris, France), based on elastometry or one dimensional transient elastography. Details of the technique and the examination procedure have been described in previous reports [12] [13].

2.3.4. CT Examination and Quantitative Standard

The patients with NAFLD of both groups underwent liver CT scan. The degree of NAFLD was determined by the liver/spleen ratio: 1) mild fatty liver: liver density decreased, the liver CT value was less than the spleen CT value, and the liver/spleen ratio was smaller than 1.0; 2) moderate fatty liver: the liver/spleen ratio was smaller than 0.7, and the intrahepatic vascular display was unclear; and 3) severe fatty liver: liver density decreased significantly and was even below zero, the liver/spleen ratio was ≤ 0.5, and the intrahepatic vascular display was clear.

2.4. Statistical Analysis

The obtained data were analyzed by SAS 6.12 software. The clinical and laboratory findings within groups were compared by analysis of variance (ANOVA). A confidence interval of 95% was used and a two-tailed, values of

$p < 0.05$, $p < 0.01$ and $p < 0.001$ were considered statistically significant. For non-parametric data were compared using chi-square test.

3. Results

3.1. Characteristics of the Study Population

94 patients were enrolled in the study and no patients in the two groups dropped out or were excluded from the study during the whole research period. During the treatment period no patient complained significant side-effects. Demographic characteristics of patients of both groups were well matched between groups with respect to age, gender and BMI (**Table 1**).

3.2. Change in Liver Function, Blood Glucose and Serum Lipid

The serum levels of ALT of the patients in the treated group decreased significantly from 69.6 ± 16.5 IU/L to 50.1 ± 13.7 IU/L ($p \leq 0.05$) after three months SBT treatment. By contrast, there was no significant difference in the control group (67.6 ± 15.8 vs. 65.4 ± 18.4 IU/L; $p > 0.05$) (**Table 1**). Furthermore, there were significant decreases in the levels of both blood TG (from 2.26 ± 0.73 to 1.74 ± 0.51 mmol/L, $p \leq 0.05$) and LDL-C (3.2 ± 0.5 vs. 2.6 ± 0.5 mmol/L) in the treated group. However, there were no significant differences in AST, r-GT, TC, glucose and HDL-C before and after treatment between two groups (**Table 2** and **Table 3**).

Table 1. Demographic characteristics of patients.

	Treatment group (n = 48)	Control group (n = 46)
Sex		
Male	28	24
Female	20	22
Age (years)		
Mean ± SD	37.42 ± 7.53	42.77 ± 9.36
BMI		
Mean ± SD	73.34 ± 11.3	69.58 ± 9.92

Table 2. Comparison of liver function indices between the treated and control groups (X ± SD).

Group	N	Time	ALT	AST	r-GT	TBA	BG (mmol/L)
Treated group	48	Before	69.6 ± 16.5	44.3 ± 6.9	79.8 ± 21.3	12.6 ± 1.4	5.24 ± 1.27
		After	50.1 ± 13.7*#	45.5 ± 8.9	76.7 ± 16.2	13.6 ± 1.2	4.68 ± 1.16
Control group	46	Before	67.6 ± 15.8	38.8 ± 8.3	78.5 ± 12.3	11.8 ± 3.2	5.52 ± 1.62
		After	65.4 ± 18.4	35.5 ± 6.4	75.6 ± 18.6	10.8 ± 2.4	5.36 ± 1.23

*Compared with the same group before treatment, $p < 0.05$; #Compared with the control group after treatment, $p < 0.05$.

Table 3. Comparison of blood lipids between the treated and control groups (X ± SD).

Group	N	Time	TC	TG	HDL-C	LDL-C
Treated group	48	Before	4.84 ± 1.10	2.26 ± 0.73	1.3 ± 0.2	3.2 ± 0.5
		After	4.76 ± 1.03	1.74 ± 0.51*#	1.4 ± 0.3	2.6 ± 0.5*#
Control group	46	Before	4.73 ± 0.7	2.43 ± 0.72	1.5 ± 0.3	3.3 ± 0.8
		After	4.5 ± 0.7	2.27 ± 0.64	1.4 ± 0.2	3.1 ± 0.7

*Compared with the same group before treatment, $p < 0.05$; #Compared with the control group after treatment, $p < 0.05$.

3.3. Liver Fibrosis Indices

After three months SBT treatment, the level of blood HA of the patients in treated group decreased significantly from 86.3 ± 22.3 to 73.5 ± 16.3 μg/L and collagen Type IV decreased from 37.3 ± 19.8 to 25.1 ± 3.5 ng/L ($P \leq 0.05$). By contrast, there was no significant difference in the control group (**Table 4**).

3.4. Findings of CT and Fibroscan

In consistency, significant decrease in LSM was observed as demonstrated by Fibrosca in the treatment group (7.2 ± 1.5 vs. 5.8 ± 1.2; $p \leq 0.05$), whereas the liver/spleen ratio as demonstrated by CT scan increased from 0.62 ± 0.12 to 0.86 ± 60.15, compared with the baseline parameters and that in the control group. There was significant differencc between the two groups ($p < 0.05$, **Table 5**).

4. Discussion

This seems to be the first report of a therapeutic benefit of SBT in humans with NAFLD. In this study, we found that SBT treatment of NAFLD patients could significantly decreased the liver/spleen ratio, which has been well documented closely correlated with the degree of steatosis on histopathology [14] [15]. It has been proved a good correlation between the liver fat content and the spleen-minus-liver attenuation difference elicited by CT in NAFLD patients, can accurately estimate the amount of hepatic fatty infiltration in NAFLD. Therefore, the results derived from this clinical study strongly indicated that SBT treatment can ameliorate hepatic fatty infiltration NAFLD, which was further supported by the result of lowered LSM as demonstrated by Fibroscan transient elastography as compared with that in the control group and baseline. Fibroscan is a novel non-invasive method to assess hepatic fibrosis in patients with chronic liver disease by measuring liver stiffness. The result by Yoneda *et al.* indicated that Fibroscan transient elastography liver KPa closely correlated with the degree of liver fibrosis in patients with NAFLD [16]. The accuracy of TE to detect ≥F3 and F4 fibrosis were 0.77 and 0.95 in patients with histologically proven [17]. Studies by Cast'era *et al.* have compared the METAVIR classification with stiffness values reported by the Fibroscan R system showing excellent correlation with fibrotic stages [18]. This was in agreement with serum liver fibrosis indices, as demonstrated in this study that hyaluronic acid and collagen type IV in the treatment group were significantly lower than in the control and baseline indicating the therapeutic effect of SBT on hepatic fibrosis.

Interestingly, after three months SBT treatment in this study, serum ALT levels of the patients in the treated group decreased significantly compared with pre-intake baseline levels from 69.6 ± 21.56 IU/L to 50.1 ± 18.5 IU/L ($p < 0.05$). Moreover, blood triglycerides and low density lipoprotein cholesterol were also significantly

Table 4. Comparison of liver fibrosis indices between the treated and control groups (X ± SD).

Group	N	Time	HA	Lamnin	III	IV
Treated group	48	Before	86.3 ± 22.3	56.5 ± 31.7	5.5 ± 0.8	37.3 ± 19.8
		After	73.5 ± 16.3*#	52.6 ± 18.5	5.5 ± 0.6	25.1 ± 3.5*#
Control group	46	Before	85.4 ± 19.7	55.5 ± 12.4	6.1 ± 2.2	34.5 ± 9.1
		After	78.3 ± 15.8	51.9 ± 14.2	6.8 ± 1.8	36.1 ± 8.8

*Compared with the same group before treatment, $p < 0.05$; #Compared with the control group after treatment, $p < 0.05$.

Table 5. Comparison of CT value and liver/spleen ratio between the treated and control groups (X ± SD).

Group	N	Time	L/S CT value	LSM
Ttreated group	48	Before	0.62 ± 0.12	7.2 ± 1.5
		After	0.86 ± 0.15*#	5.8 ± 1.2*#
Control group	46	Before	0.62 ± 0.11	7.1 ± 1.4
		After	0.64 ± 0.10	6.9 ± 1.1

*Compared with the same group before treatment, $p < 0.05$; #Compared with the control group after treatment, $p < 0.05$.

decreased after 3 month SBT treatment. This result derived from human study was consistent with the that reported by Wang *et al.* [19], in that a total SBT flavone could significantly reduce serum cholesterol and TG levels, and increase HDL-C level in mice with experimental hyperlipidemia. These results indicated that SBT may play important roles in hepatoprotection and improvement of lipid metabolism in NAFLD.

Until now, the exact pathogenesis of NAFLD remains unclear. The pathogenesis of NAFLD and NASH has classically been considered as a "two hit" theory: i) increased fat flux to the liver resulting in hepatic triglyceride accumulation, which predisposes a patient to the second hit; ii) increased oxidative stress, lipoperoxidation, and increased reactive oxygen species resulting in hepatocyte death and scar formation [20]. The major methods for the treatment of NAFLD at present include optimizing diet and increasing physical activity for the sake of curing obesity, diabetes and hyperlipidemia. The main aim of these treatments is to improve insulin resistance through using lipid-lowering and liver-protecting drugs such as fibrates and insulin sensitizers to maintain lipid metabolism, energy metabolism and antioxidant balance. However, these agents may also induce some adverse effects such as hepatic and muscular injuries, thus limiting their wider clinical applications [21] [22].

The present study was attempted to find effective drugs from the pool of traditional Chinese medicines that have no or significant less toxic effects, and known therapeutic effects in improving lipid metabolism and promoting NAFLD reversal.

SBT, also called *Hippophae rhamnoides L*, is an edibble plant and used as a traditional Chinese medicine, Tibetan medicine and Mongolian medicine. Various pharmacological activities of SBT, such as cytoprotective, anti-stress, immunomodulatory, radioprotective, anti-atherogenic, anti-tumor, anti-microbial and tissue regeneration, have been reported [7]. Moreover, it was also reported that SBT has antihypertensive effects at least in part through improving insulin sensitivity and blocking angiotensin signal pathway indicating its potential use in the management of hyperinsulinemia in non-diabetic state with cardiovascular diseases [23]. A recent study reported that SBT can significantly increase the activities of superoxide dismutase (SOD), glutathione peroxidase (GSH-Px), and GSH content in liver, and significantly reduced the elevated levels of alanine aminotransferase (ALT), aspartate aminotransferase (AST), alkaline phosphatase (ALP), triglyceride (TG), and cholesterol in carbon tetrachloride (CCl_4)-induced hepatic damage in ICR mice [11]. In agreement, other studies also demonstrated a protective effect of SBT against chronic hypoxic injury using primary rat hepatocytes through maintaining better levels/activities of GSH, GPx, and SOD [24].

Lipid accumulation in the liver is the major hallmark of NAFLD. In this study, we found that SBT has an effect of ameliorating lipid metabolism in NAFLD patients, although the mechanism is yet unknown. Alterations in immune response have been implicated in the pathogenesis of NAFLD. It has been proved that abnormalities in lipid and lipoprotein metabolism accompanied by chronic inflammation are considered to be the central pathway for the development of several obesity-related co-morbidities such as NAFLD and cardio-vascular disease (CVD) [25] [26]. NAFLD is associated with increased levels of the proinflammatory T helper 1-associated cytokines TNF-α and interleukin-12 (IL-12) [20]. Adipocytokines including TNF-α, IL-6, leptin and adiponectin, are important inflammatory proteins generated by visceral adipose. They all flow directly to the liver via the portal vein and have been implicated in the pathogenesis of NAFLD and NASH [27]. It was reported that intraperitoneal injection of SBT flavone could significantly increase the white blood cell and bone marrow nucleated cell counts, stimulate the production of interleukin-6 (IL-6) and tumor necrosis factor-alpha (TNF-α) in human blood mononuclear cells (PBMCs) [28] [29]. SBT leaf extract also has a significant anti-inflammatory activity in arthritis (AIA) rat mode

5. Conclusions

Our study demonstrated the beneficial effects of SBT treatment on serum lipids, transaminase; liver/spleen ratio and liver stiffness in patients with NAFLD; we thought that the SBT mediated effects of amelioration of lipid metabolism, manipulation of adipocytokine. SBT is especially suitable for complicating with hepatic dysfunction, obese patients with non-alcoholic fatty liver disease. SBT can improve insulin resistance, which has significantly reduced effect on TG accumulation in the liver, inhibit lipid peroxidation in liver cells, and improve liver microcirculation and liver fibrosis.

SBT provides a new medication for the treatment of NAFLD with traditional Chinese medicine. Clinical practice needs to be further implemented.

The limitation of this study is that the diagnosis of NAFLD was made mainly based on ultrasound, lacking pathological evidence. Pathological type and histological characteristic of the subjects enrolled in this study are quite unknown. Although ultrasound and CT studies demonstrated the significant improvement of the histological features of liver in NASH patients after SBT treatment, the supporting evidence of the liver pathology is desired. The second limitation of this study is that we cannot exclude the synergetic effect of other factors, such as the limited diet and physical exercise *et al.* Furthermore, in some patient with diabetes, hypoglycemic agents were used. It has been reported that diformin in itself can be used for the treatment of NAFLD. Furthermore, the observation period is too short for observation of the long-term effects of SBT treatment on NAFLD. Nonetheless, more extensive studies are needed for identification and isolation of the effective components or compound(s) in SBT and for elucidation of the underlying mechanism of SBT in the treatment of fatty liver. In conclusion, the promising results derived from this study will open up a new horizon for substantial treatment of fatty liver.

Acknowledgements

The authors are grateful to Professor Zhang Yusheng from the Department of Radiology for providing CT examination; Professor Tang Mingrong from the Department of Clinical Laboratory for the laboratory test; and Professor Ma Yuan from the Department of B-ultrasound for providing support for the present study.

Funding

Supported by the Laboratory of Liver and Kidney Disease (Shanghai University of Traditional Chinese Medicine) under the Ministry of Education of China (No. GS090501).

Authors Contribution

Gao Zeli designed the research strategy, performed the literature search and drafted the paper, analyzed the data and drafted the paper. Zhang Cheng, Jin Liwen and Yao Wei collected the clinical materials.

References

[1] Park, H., Shima, T., Yamaguchi, K., *et al.* (2011) Efficacy of Long-Term Ezetimibe Therapy in Patients with Nonalcoholic Fatty Liver Disease. *Journal of Gastroenterology*, **46**, 101-107. http://dx.doi.org/10.1007/s00535-010-0291-8

[2] Smith, B.W. and Adams, L.A. (2011) Non-Alcoholic Fatty Liver Disease. *Critical Reviews in Clinical Laboratory Sciences*, **48**, 97-113. http://dx.doi.org/10.3109/10408363.2011.596521

[3] Fon Tacer, K. and Rozman, D. (2011) Nonalcoholic Fatty Liver Disease: Focus on Lipoprotein and Lipid Deregulation. *Journal of Lipids*, **2011**, Article ID: 783976. http://dx.doi.org/10.1155/2011/783976

[4] Targher, G., Bertolini, L. and Poli, F. (2005) Nonalcoholic Fatty Liver Disease and Risk of Future Cardiovascular Events among Type 2 Diabetic Patients. *Diabetes*, **54**, 3541-3546. http://dx.doi.org/10.2337/diabetes.54.12.3541

[5] Chuthan Sourianarayanane, A., Pagadala, M.R. and Kirwan, J.P. (2013) Management of Non-Alcoholic Fatty Liver Disease. *Minerva Gastroenterologica e Dietologica*, **59**, 69-87.

[6] Kruczek, M., Swiderski, A., Mech-Nowak, A., *et al.* (2012) Antioxidant Capacity of Crude Extracts Containing Carotenoids from the Berries of Various Cultivars of Sea Buckthorn (*Hippophae rhamnoides L*). *Acta Biochimica Polonica*, **59**, 135-137.

[7] Ganju, L., Padwad, Y., Singh, R., Karan, D., Chanda, S., Chopra, M.K., Bhatnagar, P., Kashyap, R. and Sawhney, R.C. (2005) Anti-Inflammatory Activity of Seabuckthorn (*Hippophae rhamnoides*) Leaves. *International Immunopharmacology*, **5**, 1675-1684. http://dx.doi.org/10.1016/j.intimp.2005.03.017

[8] Padwad, Y., Ganju, L., Jain, M., Chanda, S., Karan, D., Kumar, R., Banerjee, P.K. and Sawhney, R.C. (2006) Effect of Leaf Extract of Sea Buckthorn on Lipopolysaccharide Induced Inflammatory Response in Murine Macrophages. *International Immunopharmacology*, **6**, 46-52. http://dx.doi.org/10.1016/j.intimp.2005.07.015

[9] Wang, J., Zhang, W., Zhu, D., *et al.* (2011) Hypolipidaemic and Hypoglycaemic Effects of Total Flavonoids from Seed Residues of *Hippophae rhamnoides L* in Mice Fed a High-Fat Diet. *Journal of the Science of Food and Agriculture*, **91**, 1446-1451. http://dx.doi.org/10.1002/jsfa.4331

[10] Geetha, S., Jayamurthy, P., Pal, K., Pandey, S. and Sawhney, R.C. (2008) Hepatoprotective Activity of Sea Buckthorn (*Hippophae rhamnoides L*) against Carbon Tetrachloride Induced Hepatic Damage in Rats. *Journal of Science of Food and Agriculture*, **88**, 1592-1597. http://dx.doi.org/10.1002/jsfa.3255

[11] Hsu, Y.W., Tsai, C., Chen, W.K. and Lu, F.J. (2009) Protective Effects of Seabuckthorn (*Hippophae rhamnoides L*)

Seed Oil against Carbon Tetrachloride-Induced Hepatotoxicity in Mice. *Food and Chemical Toxicology*, **47**, 2281-2288. http://dx.doi.org/10.1016/j.fct.2009.06.015

[12] Sandrin, L., Tanter, M., Gennisson, J.L., Catheline, S. and Fink, M. (2002) Shear Elasticity Probe for Soft Tissues with 1-D Transient Elastography. *IEEE Transactions on Ultrasonics, Ferroelectrics, and Frequency Control*, **49**, 436-446. http://dx.doi.org/10.1109/58.996561

[13] Sandrin, L., Fourquet, B., Hasquenoph, J.M., Yon, S., Fournier, C., Mal, F., *et al.* (2003) Transient Elastography: A New Noninvasive Method for Assessment of Hepatic Fibrosis. *Ultrasound in Medicine and Biology*, **29**, 1705-1713. http://dx.doi.org/10.1016/j.ultrasmedbio.2003.07.001

[14] Oliva, M.R., Mortele, K.J., Segatto, E., Glickman, J.N., Erturk, S.M., Ros, P.R. and Silverman, S.G. (2006) Computed Tomography Features of Nonalcoholic Steatohepatitis with Histopathologic Correlation. *Journal of Computer Assisted Tomography*, **30**, 37-43. http://dx.doi.org/10.1097/01.rct.0000193818.31749.84

[15] Tobari, M., Hashimoto, E., Yatsuji, S., Torii, N. and Shiratori, K. (2009) Imaging of Nonalcoholic Steatohepatitis: Advantages and Pitfalls of Ultrasonography and Computed Tomography. *Internal Medicine*, **48**, 739-746. http://dx.doi.org/10.2169/internalmedicine.48.1869

[16] Castera, L., Forns, X. and Alberti, A. (2008) Non-Invasive Evaluation of Liver Fibrosis Using Transient Elastography. *Journal of Hepatology*, **48**, 835-847. http://dx.doi.org/10.1016/j.jhep.2008.02.008

[17] Mahadeva, S., Mahfudz, A.S., Vijayanathan, A., Goh, K.L., Kulenthran, A. and Cheah, P.L. (2013) Performance of Transient Elastography (TE) and Factors Associated with Discordance in Nonalcoholic Fatty Liver Disease. *Journal of Digestive Diseases*, **14**, 604-610. http://dx.doi.org/10.1111/1751-2980.12088

[18] Yoneda, M., Yoneda, M., Mawatari, H., Fujita, K., Endo, H., Iida, H., *et al.* (2008) Noninvasive Assessment of Liver Fibrosis by Measurement of Stiffness in Patients with Nonalcoholic Fatty Liver Disease (NAFLD). *Digestive and Liver Disease*, **40**, 371-378. http://dx.doi.org/10.1016/j.dld.2007.10.019

[19] Wang, J., Zhang, W., Zhu, D., Zhu, X.L., Pang, X.F. and Qu, W.J. (2011) Hypolipidaemic and Hypoglycaemic Effects of Total Flavonoids from Seed Residues of *Hippophae rhamnoides L* in Mice Fed a High-Fat Diet. *Journal of the Science of Food and Agriculture*, **91**, 1446-1451. http://dx.doi.org/10.1002/jsfa.4331

[20] Smith, B.W. and Adams, L.A. (2011) Non-Alcoholic Fatty Liver Disease. *Critical Reviews in Clinical Laboratory Sciences*, **48**, 97-113. http://dx.doi.org/10.3109/10408363.2011.596521

[21] Rallidis, L.S., Drakoulis, C.K. and Parasi, A.S. (2004) Pravastatin in Patients with Nonalcoholic Steatohepatitis: Results of a Pilot Study. *Atherosclerosis*, **174**, 193-196. http://dx.doi.org/10.1016/j.atherosclerosis.2004.01.008

[22] Lewis, J.H. (2012) Clinical Perspective: Statins and the Liver—Harmful or Helpful? *Digestive Diseases and Sciences*, **57**, 1754-1763. http://dx.doi.org/10.1007/s10620-012-2207-3

[23] Tulsawani, R., Gupta, R. and Misra, K. (2013) Efficacy of Aqueous Extract of *Hippophae rhamnoides* and Its Bio-Active Flavonoids against Hypoxia-Induced Cell Death. *Indian Journal of Pharmacology*, **45**, 258-263. http://dx.doi.org/10.4103/0253-7613.111943

[24] Pang, X., Zhao, J., Zhang, W., Zhuang, X.Y., Wang, J.S., Xu, R.Q., Xu, Z.L. and Qu, W.J. (2008) Antihypertensive Effect of Total Flavones Extracted from Seed Residues of *Hippophae rhamnoides L* in Sucrose-Fed Rats. *Journal of Ethnopharmacology*, **117**, 325-331. http://dx.doi.org/10.1016/j.jep.2008.02.002

[25] Targher, G., Bertolini, L., Padovani, R., Rodella, S., Zoppini, G., Pichiri, I., *et al.* (2010) Prevalence of Non-Alcoholic Fatty Liver Disease and Its Association with Cardiovascular Disease in Patients with Type 1 Diabetes. *Journal of Hepatology*, **53**, 713-718. http://dx.doi.org/10.1016/j.jhep.2010.04.030

[26] Loria, P., Lonardo, A., Bellentani, S., Day, C.P., Marchesini, G. and Carulli, N. (2007) Non-Alcoholic Fatty Liver Disease (NAFLD) and Cardiovascular Disease: An Open Question. *Nutrition, Metabolism and Cardiovascular Diseases*, **17**, 684-698. http://dx.doi.org/10.1016/j.numecd.2007.01.007

[27] Kremer, M., Thomas, E., Milton, R.J., Perry, A.W., van Rooijen, N., Wheeler, M.D., *et al.* (2010) Kupffer Cell and Interleukin-12-Dependent Loss of Natural Killer T Cells in Hepatosteatosis. *Hepatology*, **51**, 130-141. http://dx.doi.org/10.1002/hep.23292

[28] Ganju, L., Padwad, Y., Singh, R., Karan, D., Chanda, S., Chopra, M.K., *et al.* (2005) Anti-Inflammatory Activity of Seabuckthorn (*Hippophae rhamnoides L*) Leaves. *International Immunopharmacology*, **5**, 1675-1684. http://dx.doi.org/10.1016/j.intimp.2005.03.017

[29] Mishra, K.P., Chanda, S., Karan, D., Ganju, L. and Sawhney, R.C. (2008) Effect of Seabuckthorn (*Hippophae rhamnoides*) Flavone on Immune System: An *in Vitro* Approach. *Phytotherapy Research*, **22**, 1490-1495. http://dx.doi.org/10.1002/ptr.2518

26

Primary Study of Novel Method for Determination of Saponin in Ziziphi Spinosae Semen (*Suan-Zao-Ren*) by Digitally Scanning the Photo of the HPTLC Image without Configuration of TLC Scanner Facility

Longgang Guo[1], Shuai Sun[2], He Li[1,3], Ruiyin Wang[1], Xinjun Xu[4*], Peishan Xie[1*]

[1]Guangdong UNION Biochemical Development Co. Ltd., Guangzhou, China
[2]Guangdong ImVin Pharmaceutical Co. Ltd., Guangzhou, China
[3]Livzon Group Pharmaceutical Factory, Zhuhai, China
[4]School of Pharmaceutical Sciences, Sun Yat-sen University, Guangzhou, China
Email: *xxj2702@sina.com, *psxie163@163.com, *xps340112@gmail.com

Abstract

Conventional quantity determination of Chinese herbal medicines by High-Performance Thin-Layer Chromatography (HPTLC) must be carried out on a TLC scanner for measuring the marker component on the HPTLC plate. Generally the HPTLC image of the herbal drug always takes the photograph as the permanent visual document. Considering the photo of the HPTLC image preserving all the visual quality-related parameters, there might be an alternative cost/effective approach worth studying. It would be presumably applicable to use the exclusively developed software as a virtual scanner instead of the TLC Scanner instrument to do digital scanning, integrating and calculating target components in the photo of the HPTLC image. It means digitally scanning the photo of the HPTLC image solely with software does the same thing as the instrumental scanner does. Based on this protocol, we primarily conducted the assay of the contents of the major saponins, jujuboside a and jujuboside b, in Ziziphi Spinosae Semen (*Suan-Zao-Ren*). Using home-developed software "*digiscan*" for acquiring the raw data and integrating the peaks area of the target components with "Origin Pro", the contents of jujuboside a and jujuboside b can then be calculated respectively. The primary investigated experiment results were well compatible with official HPLC-

*Corresponding authors.

ELSD method in Chinese Pharmacopoeia. The methodology validation and comparative analysis with HPLC confirmed that the unprecedented method is acceptable. The advantage of the recommended approach is far more simple, flexible and cost/effective than the conventional method, and it can be done at anytime and anywhere once only if the high quality HPTLC image photo is available. There would be a bright perspective for application to other herbal medicines. And the one-stop software for merging digital scanning, integration and calculation together is in progress.

Keywords

HPTLC Image Photo, Digital-Determination, Ziziphi Spinosae Semen (*Suan-Zao-Ren*), Jujuboside a and b

1. Introduction

One of the common-used Chinese herbal drugs, Spine Date Seed, Chinese name: *Suan-Zao-Ren* (abbr. *SZR*) is the dried ripe seed of *Ziziphus jujube* Mill. var. *spinosa* (Bunge) Hu et H.F. Chou (Family Rhamnaceae). Its acknowledged bioactive ingredients are saponins, flavonoids, polysaccharides, fatty acids [1]-[5]; amongst those, the major bioactive saponins—jujuboside a, jujuboside b and flavonoid spinosin are the chemical markers for identification and assay stipulated in Chinese Pharmacopoeia [6].

Generally determining the content of the selected marker component in the herbal drugs by means of chromatographic analysis such as HPLC, GC and HPTLC is the current basic requirement for herbal quality control. Amongst the chromatographic techniques, the off-line HPTLC technique is more convenient, economical, and flexible than others. In particular, the chromatogram pattern provided by HPTLC is a colorful picture-like image; all the images of the tested samples and the reference substances express on the same plate in parallel. The visual specific chemical composition functions effectively as either identification or quantitative analysis. That means multiple samples' qualitative (fingerprinting) and quantitative (marker quantification) testing in one-run on the same HPTLC plate is attractive for herbal medicines. The HPTLC quantitative analysis for herbal drugs' bioactive markers is conventionally carried out with expensive professional TLC scanner. The HPTLC image is considered as the permanent visual data bank, in which all of the parameters of relevant quality of the herbals are preserved. It can be presumed that the photo of the HPTLC image can play the role not only for fingerprinting identification as shown in the TLC Atlas [7] but also possibly for quantitative determination by digital scanning via software as a "virtual scanner" doing the same thing as the conventional determination of the HPTLC plate with the TLC scanner instrument. Based on such a protocol, we determined the jujuboside a and jujuboside b in Spine Date Seed (*Suan-Zao-Ren*, abbr. "*SZR*") on the HPTLC image photo with external standard method as pilot experiment in order to confirm the feasibility of the "*digiscan*" protocol.

2. Methods

2.1. Materials, Reagents

Ziziphi Spinosae Semen (*SZR*; Wild jujube seeds), purchased from the whole sale herbal drug markets in Hebei province and Guangzhou city in China; the defatted extractive of *SZR* (prepared in our lab; jujuboside a and jujuboside b, the purity: >98% via calibration by external standard method); n-butyl alcohol; methanol; ethanol; sulphuric acid; vanillin (analytical grades). HPTLC silica-gel plate (Merck, Germany).

2.2. Instrument and Software

Sample application device: Linomat 5; HPTLC development twin-trough chamber; HPTLC reagent dipping device; TLC visualizer (all from CAMAG, Mutenz, Switzerland) and/or digital single-lens reflex camera; "*digiscan*" software (home-developed by Franky Du) and Origin Pro 75 (**Figure 1**).

2.3. *SZR* Sample Solution

Add 100 mL of petroleum ether (b.p. 60˚C) to about 4.0 g of the powdered sample, sonicated at 30˚C for 60

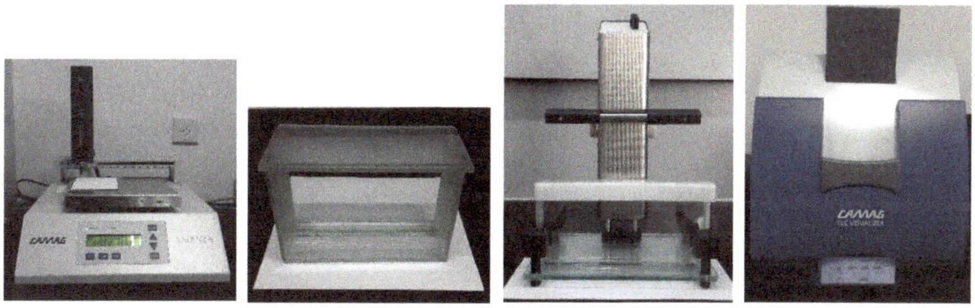

Figure 1. HPTLC facilities: Linomat 5, twin-trough chamber, reagent dipping device, CAMAG TLC Visualizer (CAMAG, Switzerland).

min, filter, discard the petroleum ether; evaporate the remnant solvent in the drug powder by flowing air, reflex extract the residue with methanol for 60 minutes, filter, evaporate the filtrate on water bath to dryness, dissolve the extract substance with 2.0 mL of methanol, the methanol solution ready for use.

2.4. Defatted *ESZR* (*ESZR*) Solution

Add 20 mL of methanol to 0.1 g defatted *ESZR*, sonicated for 15 min, filter, evaporate the methanol solution to dryness, re-dissolve the residue to 1 mL of methanol, and filter via 0.22 μL filter-membrane, the filtrate ready for use.

2.5. Chemical Reference Substance (CRS) Solution

Dissolve about 0.5 mg each of jujuboside a and jujuboside b in 0.5 mL of methanol respectively.

2.6. Sample Application

Apply appropriate amount (μL level, see **Table 1**) of the sample solution and CRS solution on HPTLC silica gel-60 plate (20 × 10 cm; Merck; Lot: OB678146) by means of Linomat 5 (CAMAG). Band width: 8 mm, interval between band to band: 4 mm. The sample-loaded plate was kept in a vacuum desiccator (P_2O_5 anhydrous) for 1 h before development.

2.7. Solvent System (Mobile Phase) and Development [6]

Aqueous-saturated n-butyl alcohol (cf. Chinese Pharmacopoeia [6]); ascending develop to 8 cm. T: 20˚C; RH: 40% - 50%.

2.8. Visualization

1) Dry the developed plate with flowing air to remove the remnant solvent and put it in a vacuum dessicator over P_2O_5 for 3 hours; 2) put the developed dry plate in the reagent dipping device in which 1% of vanillin/70% of sulphuric acid ethanol solution contained, the dipping time adjusted to 1 second; 3) take out the plate from the chamber, wipe out the residual reagent on the back of the plate as quickly as possible; the azure color of the two saponins are clearly visible. Caution: a crucial environment condition in lower relative humidity (RH < 50%) and lower temperature (T < 20˚C) during the visualization period must be kept.

2.9. The HPTLC Image Photograph Preparation

1) Take the visualized HPTLC plate in the TLC visualizer (CAMAG) as quickly as possible. The parameters in this case were: Exposure: Auto; Exposure time: 60.95 ms; Gain: 1.00; Digital level: 85%; Accentuation: 0.80; Color saturation: 1.30; Contrast: 1.0; Brightness: 0.00; White balance: Red gain: 1.39; Green gain: 1.00; Blue gain: 2.34. The alternative approach is by using a digital single-lens reflex camera to take the visible color image from the visualized plate and save the picture in jpg format; 2) the "modification" of the image photo was often necessary because some "noise" on the background caused by the remnant reagent and some unexpected contamination on the surface or the bright or the contrast too weak. The parameters adjusted by Photoshop® in this

Table 1. Recovery data.

Target	Jujuboside a/μg				Jujuboside b/μg			
amount	Before spiked ERS	After spiked (total)	Spiked amount	Recovery (%)	Before spiked ERS	After spiked (total)	Spiked amount	Recovery (%)
1st	0.882	1.594	0.696	102.43	0.647	1.140	0.441	111.88
2nd	0.886	1.589	0.696	101.17	0.653	1.1413	0.441	110.75
3rd	0.886	1.593	0.696	101.70	0.640	1.1297	0.441	111.03
Average		101.8				111.2		
RSD		**0.63**				**0.59**		

case were: surface blur (radius 4 pixel; threshold 100 gradation; luminance (luminance 45, contrast 18), smart sharpen (100%, radius 10 pixel); background replace color (luminance +33). The modification aimed at getting the clean and clear picture meanwhile keeping the image as what the naked-eye sighted as possible. The azure color of jujuboside a and jujuboside b bands on the greenish-yellow background of the HPTLC image photo observed (**Figure 2** and **Figure 3**).

2.10. Digital Scanning and Data Processing

1) Digital scanning the HPTLC image photo of *SZR* by self-developed software "*digiscan*", save the scanning raw data; 2) input the raw data to software "Origin Pro" for integration and getting the scanning profile; 3) output the integrated data into MS Excel for calculation. The facilities for HPTLC experiment refer to **Figure 1**.

3. Methodology Validation

3.1. Linearity

The equation of the linearity of jujuboside a: $y = 76820x - 14171$, $R^2 = 0.9993$; jujuboside b: $y = 87037x - 7949.4$, $R^2 = 0.9992$. The linearity range of the both compounds is within 0.25 - 1.5 μg.

3.2. Degree of Precision

Apply 7 bands of the CRS solution of jujuboside a and jujuboside b at 2 μL per band level and apply 9 bands of *ESZR*, 1.5 μL each on silica gel plate respectively. Developing, visualizing, photographing and digital scanning plus integration-calculation as described in 2.2. For ensuring the effective determination, the first step is to select the valid lanes and ignore the contaminated and the bands shape tortured lanes in the image. In this case 5 valid lanes of CRS and 6 valid lanes of Extractive of *Suan-Zao-Ren* (*ESZR*) (ignore the contaminated and tortured lanes) was carried out sequentially and integrated via Origin Pro. The RSD of integration peak area of the CRS were 1.61 for jujuboside a, 1.54 for jujuboside b (n = 5); in *ESZR*, jujuboside a 1.19; jujuboside b 1.31 (n = 6).

3.3. Recovery

Following the method in 2.3, spike jujuboside a 1.3 μL, jujuboside b 0.8 μL by means of Linomat 5 into band of the *ESZR* (0.7 μL per band), the measured data as **Table 1**.

4. Testing Results

4.1. The Contents of Jujuboside a and Jujuboside b in *SZR*

Determined by using the CRS as external standard (jujuboside a 1.049%, jujuboside b 0.619%) and by using *ESZRR* as external standard were carried out respectively. The results in crude drug *SZR* and extractive of *SZR* were shown in **Table 2** and **Table 3** (**Figures 2-4**).

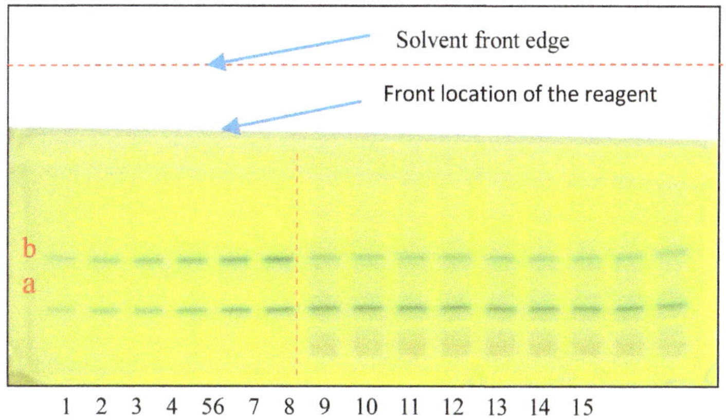

Figure 2. Calibration of jujuboside a and jujuboside b in *ESZR*. 1 - 6: CRS: jujuboside a and jujuboside b (1 μL, 1.5 μL, 2 μL, 2.5 μL, 3 μL, 3.5 μL); 7 - 15: *ESZR* samples, 1.5 μL each.

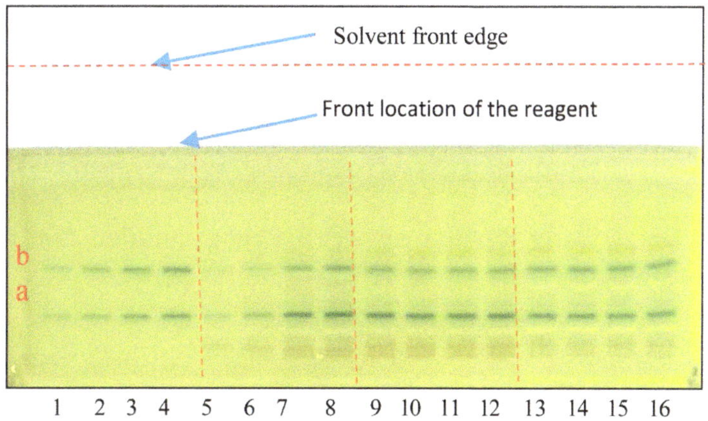

Figure 3. Assay of jujuboside a and jujuboside b in *SZR* by CRS and *ESZRR* respectively. 1 - 4: CRS: jujuboside a and jujuboside b (0.5 μL, 1 μL, 1.5 μL, 2 μL); 5 - 8: *ESZRR*, 0.3 μL, 0.6 μL, 1.2 μL, 1.5 μL; 9 - 12: crude drug *SZR* (**A**), 1.5 μL; 13 - 16: crude drug *SZR* (**B**), 1.5 μL.

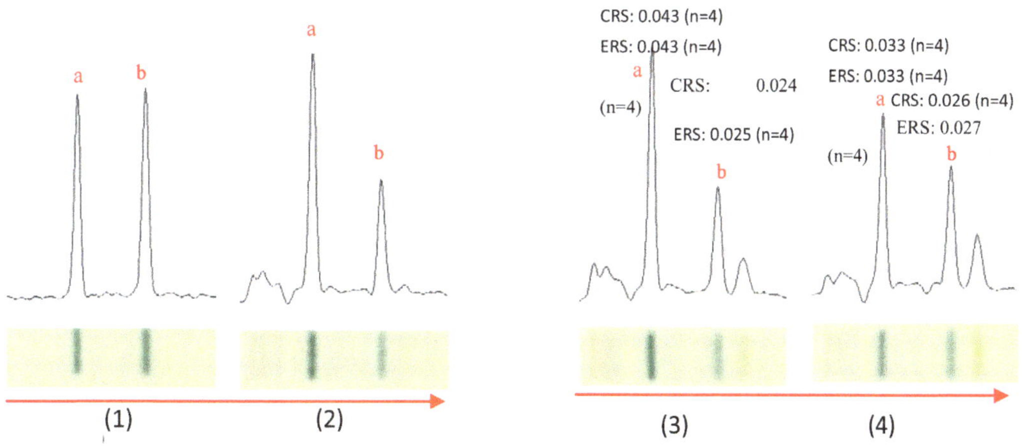

Figure 4. HPTLC photographic image of (1) CRS, (2) *ESZRR*, (3) Crude drug *SZR* (**A**), (4) *SZR* (**B**) and the corresponding digital scanning profiles. The contents (%) of jujuboside a and b determined with external standard method by CRS and ERS of *SZR* (=calibrated extractive *SZR*). CRS a = jujuboside a; b = jujuboside b.

Table 2. The contents of jujuboside a and jujuboside b in crude drug *SZR* (samples A and B).

Content	Crude drug *SZR* (**A**) (n = 4)		Crude drug *SZR* (**B**) (n = 4)	
	Jujubosidea	Jujuboside b	Jujuboside a	Jujuboside b
% (CRS)	0.0433	0.0244	0.0333	0.0259
% (*ESZRR*)	0.0431	0.0250	0.0332	0.0267
RSD	0.33	1.72	0.21	2.15

CRS (Chemical Reference Substance): jujuboside a, jujuboside b; *ESZRR* (Extractive Reference Substance) = Extractive Reference Substance of *Suan-Zao-Ren*.

Table 3. The contents of jujuboside a and jujuboside b in extractive of *SZR*.

content	*ESZR* (**A**) (n = 4)	
	Jujuboside a	Jujuboside b
% (CRS)	1.049	0.619
% (*ESZRR*)	1.047	0.621
RSD	0.135	0.228

4.2. The HPTLC Photographic Image and the Digital Scanning Profile

The HPTLC photographic image and the digital scanning profile were shown in **Figures 2-4**.

4.3. Comparison of the Testing Results between Recommended Method Here with the Official HPLC Method

For evaluating the feasibility of the HPTLC image photo *digiscan* method, a comparison between HPTLC image *digiscan* method and official HPLC method was also carried out [6]. It is shown that the recommended method is compatible with the official HPLC method (**Table 4**).

5. Discussion

1) The pilot experimental results showed that quantitative determination through digital scanning the photo of the HPTLC image via software reaches the expected effect which was validated by methodology (Linearity, precision, Recovery) (2.3.1) and the comparison with official HPLC-ELSD method in Chinese Pharmacopoeia.

2) Jujuboside a and jujuboside b reacted with vanillin/sulphuric acid reagent appeared characteristic azure color bands on the light greenish-yellow background of the silica gel plate (**Figure 2** and **Figure 3**). The chromatographic procedure must be carried out in lower relative humidity (<50%) and temperature (<25°C) environment of the lab to keep the air dry and cool. Otherwise no azure color produced. The color of the bands are not stable, it will be faded quickly. So taking the image's photo for quantitation (as well as identification) by digital scanning and measuring the data can be done at anywhere and anytime in convenience and functionality. The qualified HPTLC image is absolutely the prerequisite for conducting this method.

3) As external standard, in spite of the Chemical Reference Substance (CRS), we used the Extractive Reference Substance (ERS) calibrated with CRS (jujuboside a and jujuboside b reference substances) as alternative

Table 4. The contents of jujuboside a and jujuboside b incrude drug *SZR* by HPLC (ChP 2010) and by HPTLC image photo *digiscan* (cf. 5.2).

Content	Digiscan n = 4	HPLC-ELSD n = 4	RSD
Jujuboside a (%)	0.043	0.045	3.50
Jujuboside b (%)	0.025	0.024	2.32

S1: jujuboside a; S2: jujuboside b.

approach to determining the target marker compounds, the acceptable result showed using the calibrated ERS as standard substance to carry out quantitative analysis would be more simple and low cost [8].

4) The software package ("*digiscan*" for scanning the photo, "Origin Pro" for integration and "MS Excel" for calculation) were used at the pilot stage, the one-stop integrating software is in progress.

6. Conclusion

The photograph of the HPTLC image of herbal medicine as the permanent archive contains the visual quality-related data; it can be used as the substitute of HPTLC image plate for quantitative analysis, *i.e.*, digitally scanning the image photo by using software as the virtual scanner replaced the instrumental TLC scanner. The primary results of determination of saponin (jujuboside a and b) in *Suan-Zao-Ren* (Ziziphi Spinosae Semen) brought out the optimistic foreground. Such a rapid, inexpensive, flexible and feasible method will be expectedly welcomed by the herbal drug industry and sales markets for in-process quality control and market supervising.

Acknowledgements

The Author appreciates Franky Du who developed the software "*digiscan*".

References

[1] Xiao, P.-G. (2002) Chinese Meteria Medica (Upgraded Version) Vol. II. Beijing Chemical Industry Publishing Co., Beijing, 648.

[2] Ma, J.-J., Liu, P. and Ma, B.P. (2011) The Chemical Constituents of Semen Ziziphi Spinosae and Pharmacological Mechanism of Its Sedative and Hypnotic Effects: Research Advances. *International Research Journal of Pharmacy*, **38**, 206-211.

[3] Zeng, L., Zhang, R.Y. and Wang, X. (1986) Studies on the Constituents of Chinese Traditional Drug Suan Zao Ren. *Acta Botanica Sinica*, **28**, 517-522. (In Chinese with English Abstract)

[4] Zeng, L., Zhang, R.Y. and Wang, X. (1987) Studies on the Constituents of *Ziziphus spinosus* Hu. *Acta Pharmacologica Sinica*, **22**, 114-120. (In Chinese with English Abstract)

[5] Li, L.-M., Liao, X., Peng, S.L. and Ding, L.-S. (2005) Chemical Constituents from the Seeds of *Ziziphus jujube* var. *spinosa* (Bunge) Hu. *Journal of Integrative Plant Biology*, **47**, 494-498. http://dx.doi.org/10.1111/j.1744-7909.2005.00060.x

[6] Chinese Pharmacopoeia Commission (2010) Pharmacopoeia of People's Republic of China, Volume I. 343-344.

[7] Chinese Pharmacopoeia Commission (2009) TLC Atlas of Chinese Crude Drugs in Pharmacopoeia of the People's Republic of China Volume I. People's Medical Publishing House, Beijing.

[8] Xie, P.-S., Ma, S.-C., Tu, P.-F., Wang, Z.-T., Stoeger, E. and Bensky, D. (2013) The Prospect of Application of Extractive Reference Substance of Chinese Herbal Medicines. *Chinese Medicine*, **4**, 4125-4136. http://dx.doi.org/10.4236/cm.2013.44016

27

Quantitative Estimation of Gallic Acid as Biomarker in Lipitame Tablets by HPTLC Densitometry for Diabetic Dyslipidemia

Sheeraz Siddiqui[1], Khan Usmanghani[1,2], Aqib Zahoor[2], Zeeshan Ahmed Sheikh[2], Saleha Suleman Khan[2]

[1]Faculty of Eastern Medicine, Hamdard University, Karachi, Pakistan
[2]Research and Development Department, Herbion Pakistan (Pvt.) Limited, Karachi, Pakistan
Email: ugk_2005@yahoo.com

Abstract

Lipitame is a poly herbal formulation comprised of *Terminalia arjuna*, *Terminalia belerica*, *Commiphora mukul* and *Phyllanthus emblica*. The formulation is investigated for its analysis evaluation. Biomarkers of three herbs such as *Terminalia arjuna*, *Terminalia belerica*, and *Phyllanthus emblica* have been already cited to contain gallic acid, which was qualitatively and quantitatively estimated. In the present study rapid and inexpensive qualification methods for the quality control of *Terminalia arjuna*, *Terminalia belerica*, *Commiphora mukul* and *Phyllanthus emblica* on thin layer chromatography (TLC) were developed and validated. The solvent system used was toluene:ethyl acetate:formic acid:methanol (12:9:4:0.5). The scanning of plate was performed linearly at 273 nm (absorption) by use of a TLC Scanner III CAMAG with a deuterium source, and the area of spots corresponding to Gallic acid standard was integrated. It was found that gallic acid has been found in the Lipitame tablets on HPTLC densitometry assessment compared with authentic gallic acid reference standard.

Keywords

Lipitame, Tablets, Quantitative Estimation, Densitometry, Diabetic Dyslipidemia

1. Introduction

Inadequately controlled hyperglycemia has been cited as a primary cause of diabetic complications. Increased serum levels of lipids in diabetics (as observed by high levels of triglycerides, total cholesterol and LDL-cholesterol) are partially responsible for and further exacerbate the damaging effects of diabetic hyperglycemia. Because there has been no effective and inexpensive therapeutic option to control glycemic or lipidemic levels in diabetic patients; these patients often suffer severe complications, including nephropathy, retinopathy, neuropathy and atherosclerosis. Although improved glycemic control can reduce the incidence and progression of diabetic complications, implementation and monitoring of glycemic control are arduous and expensive. Many diabetic complications are believed to occur through the oxidative action of glucose. In particular, the high oxidant activity in diabetics coupled with dyslipidemia can lead to the formation of advanced glycation endproducts (AGEs). The presence of AGEs is associated with the formation of arterial atheromas and ultimately, to the development of atherosclerosis. These complications can be mitigated in part by certain antioxidants, including superoxide dismutase, catalase and gluathione. Blocking the oxidative action of glucose responsible for diabetic vascular dysfunction has been validated as one approach to reduce the occurrence of diabetic complications. For example, aldose reductase inhibitors have been shown to prevent or reduce different components of vascular dysfunction, cataract formation, neuropathy and nephropathy in animal model. Furthermore, antioxidants (such as vitamin E, vitamin C and alpha lipoic acid) and antiplatelet agents (such as aspirin and ticlopidine) are being tested to determine their efficacy against the progression of certain diabetic complications, such as non-proliferative diabetic retinopathy.

Although some strides have been made to control glycemic levels and the associated oxidant activity in diabetics, little progress has been made to address the underlying problem of diabetic dyslipidemia. By lowering levels of triglycerides, total cholesterol and LDL-cholesterol in diabetics, development or progression of atherosclerosis and other diabetic complications could be slowed or eradicated. Advantageously, such therapy could be combined with hypoglycemic medications to synergistically treat diabetic patients. Therefore, it is of great importance for the long-term quality of life for diabetic patients that therapeutic options can be made available to treat diabetic dyslipidemia.

The present study is directed to a polyherbal formulation Lipitame comprised of *Terminalia arjuna*, *Terminalia belerica*, *Commiphora mukul* and *Phyllanthus emblica* or a mixture of the active ingredients that have been extracted from such herbs. The herbal compositions of the present invention are effective for the treatment of conditions involving atherosclerosis, stress and anxiety, for use in cardioprotection, cardio-toning, and hyperlipidemia. The medicinal herbal composition such as *Terminalia arjuna* (Roxb.) Wight & Arn., *Terminalia belerica* (Gaertn.) Roxb., *Commiphora mukul* (*Hook ex Stock*) Linn. and *Phyllanthus emblica* Linn. have been used in 10% - 15% by weight of selection of herbal drugs for hyperlipidemia to formulate the dosage which is in tablet form. The Unani herbal drugs have been cited for ethnobotanaical and scientific evidences and are selected for hyperlipidemia after thorough Qarabadini and published literature from electronic journals.

2. Material and Methods

2.1. Formula of Tablet Lipitame (Unani Medicine)

The Unani medicine based tablets "Lipitame" has the following ingredients: *Terminalia arjuna* Bark (Arjun) powder, 1000 gm; *Commiphora mukul* gum resin (muqil), 1300 gm; *Terminalia chebula* (epicarp, harh) powder, 500 gm; *Phyllanthus emblica* fruit (amla) powder, 500 gm.

2.2. Manufacturing Process

All herbs are purchased from the local market then cleaned and examined for their impurities and adulteration. The herbs are weighted according to the formulation and three drugs respectively; ***Terminalia chebula***, ***Phyllanthus emblica*** and ***Terminalia arjuna*** are powdered through grinding machine and passed through the sieve no 50. The powder is further checked for its homogenous consistency. ***Commiphora mukul*** is soaked in water for a night and then boiled along with continuous stirring. After boiling and cooling the solution of *Commiphora mukul* is filtered and the impurities are separated. This cooled filter solution of ***Commiphora mukul*** is mixed with the powdered drug to develop the granules for tablet making by passing through the sieve no 80. The granules are mixed with binder gum acacia for half hour thoroughly in a mixer.

The granules are dried at 35˚C for a day in oven and then these granules were used to make the compressed tablets weighing each 1 gm on average and they were stored in air tight plastic jars. After the above testing the tablets are then send for blister allo-allo foil. Each blister contains ten tablets. Three blisters are put in a box for

30 days dosage (recommended dose 1 tablet at bedtime with plane water).

2.3. Testing Specification

The tablets are checked for disintegration time which is 15 minutes for Lipitame. Hardness of tablets are checked which is 6 kg. Friability test under limit *i.e.* 0.5%. Moisture test is 3%.

2.4. Indications

Primary hyperlipidemia and mixed dyslipidemia, hypertriglyceridemia.

2.5. Dosage and Administration

Recommended dose for Lipitame is one tablet (1 gm) at bedtime with plane water.

2.6. Dosage Form and Packaging

Tablet: 1 gm, 30 tablets (10 × 3 unit dose).

2.7. Contraindication

Active liver and renal diseases, pregnancy, nursing mothers.

2.8. Adverse Effects

Mostly tolerated but in certain cases mild constipation, dry mouth and mild hypotension with headache.

3. Quantitative Estimation of Gallic Acid in Lipitame Tablet by HPTLC Densitometry

Lipitame tablets consist of *Phyllanthus emblica*, *Terminalia chebula*, *Commiphora mukul* and *Terminalia arjuna.* On literature citation it has been found that all the three drugs contains gallic acids where as *Commiphora mukul* elaborate no gallic acid.

Equipment: CAMAG Scanner III, CAMAG Linomat 5 or Equivalent
TLC Plates: HPTLC silica gel $G60F_{254}$
Solvent system:Toluene:Ethyl acetate:Formic acid:Methanol
12:9:4:0.5
Wave length: 273 nm

3.1. Standard Preparation

Prepare standard solution containing known concentration (0.4 mg/ml) by dissolving 4 mg standard of gallic acid monohydrate in 10 ml of methanol.

3.2. Sample Preparation

Weigh about 2.5 g of tablet powder (note exact weight) in to 100 ml of conical flask. Add 30 ml of methanol heat to boil on water bath for 15 minute filter the solution in 250 ml round bottomed flask. Repeat extraction of the remaining residue of tablet powder four times more using 30 × 4 ml portions (5 times in total) as mention above. Collect methanol soluble fraction into the same round-bottomed flask. Evaporate the methanol under vacuum. Dissolve the dry residue in 5 ml of methanol and transfer quantitatively into a 10 ml volumetric flask. Bring the solution's volume to the mark with methanol.

3.3. Procedure

3.3.1. TLC Preparation

a) Perform analysis on 10 × 10 cm HPTLC silica gel $G60F_{254}$ plates with fluorescent indicator.
b) Before start the analysis, HPTLC plate cleans by predevelopment with methanol by ascending method. (Note:

immerse HPTLC Plate in a CAMAG glass chamber (20 × 20 cm), contains 30 ml methanol as solvent system cover the chamber with glass lid and wait to develop the plate to the top with methanol. After complete development, remove the plate from TLC glass chamber and dry it in an oven at 105˚C for 5 min.)

3.3.2. Application Procedure

a) Apply three spots of 10 µl (in the form of band) of standard preparation along with three spots of 10 µl of sample preparation as the bands on the same plate by means of a CAMAG Linomat 5 (automated spray-on applicator equipped with a 100 µl syringe and operated with the settings band length 6 mm, distance between bands 14 mm, distance from the plate side edge 15 mm, and distance from the bottom of the plate 15 mm).
b) After sample application, dry the plate in hot air oven at 105˚C for 5 min.

3.3.3. TLC Development

a) Develop the plate by immersing sample HPTLC Plate in a CAMAG glass chamber (20 × 20 cm) contained the solvent system (Toluene:Ethyl acetate:Formic acid:Methanol (12:9:4:0.5)), wait to develop the plate to the distance of 8 to 9 cm (see **Figure 1**).
b) After complete development, allow the plate to dry by keeping in fume cupboard for 10 minutes and then keep in hot air oven for 5 min at 105˚C.

3.3.4. TLC Scanning

a) Scan the plate in the densitometer by linear scanning at 273 nm (absorption) by use of a TLC Scanner III CAMAG with a deuterium source, and integrate the area of the spots of the sample (see **Figure 2**) and corresponding to gallic acid standard (see **Figure 3**).

Calculate the amount of gallic acid in mg per 10 ml in Lipitame tablet by following formula.

3.4. Content of Gallic Acid

$$\frac{A_{SMP} \times W_{STD} \times f \times \text{ Dilution of Smp} \times \text{Application vol. of Smp} \times P \times 0.5}{A_{STD} \times \text{ Dilution of Std} \times W_{SMP} \times \text{Application of vol. Std} \times 100}$$

A_{SMP} = Avg. Area of Sample;
A_{STD} = Avg. Area of Standard;
W_{STD} = Weight of Standard, mg;
W_{SMP} = Weight of Sample, g;
Dilution of Smp = Dilution of Sample, ml;
Dilution of Std = Dilution of Standard, ml;
P = Percent Purity of Standard;
$f(0.904)$ = conversion factor of gallic acid monohydrate in gallic acid.
Note: quantity of gallic acid in Lipitame tablet should be NLT 2.72 mg/tablet.

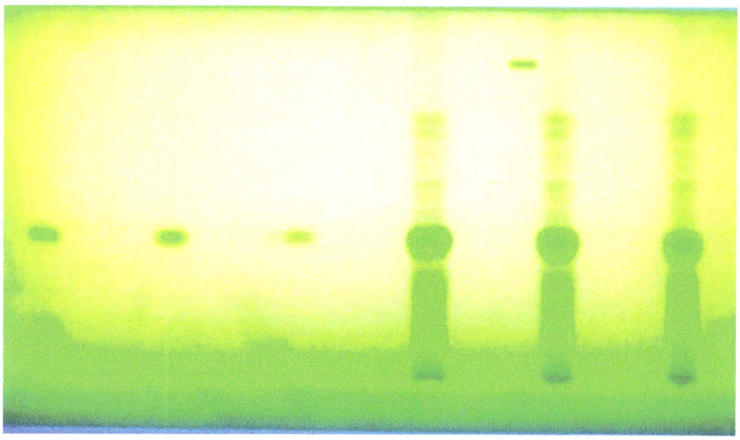

Figure 1. TLC image of gallic acid analysis in Lipitame tablet.

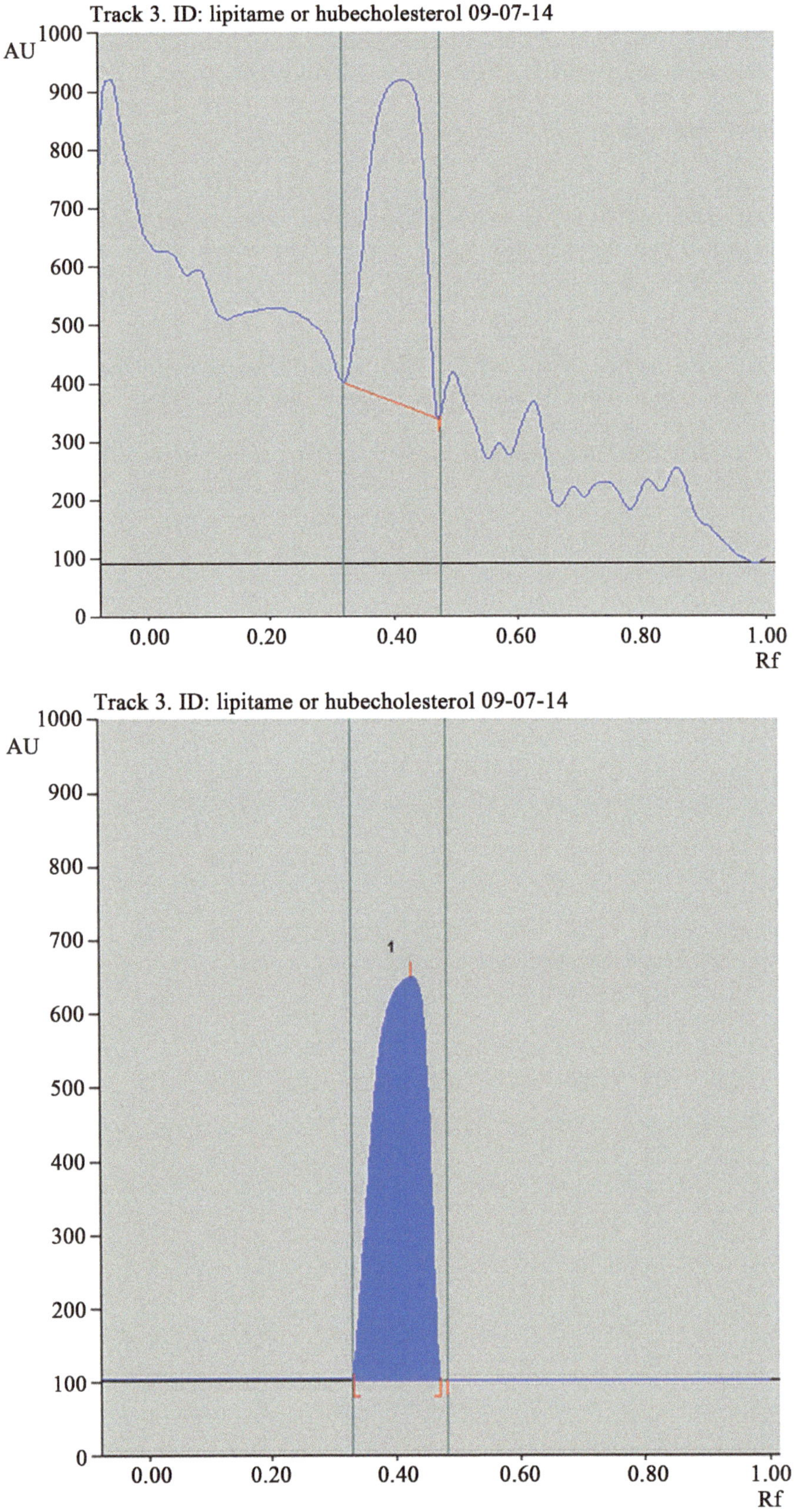

Figure 2. Peak response of gallic acid in Lipitame tablet.

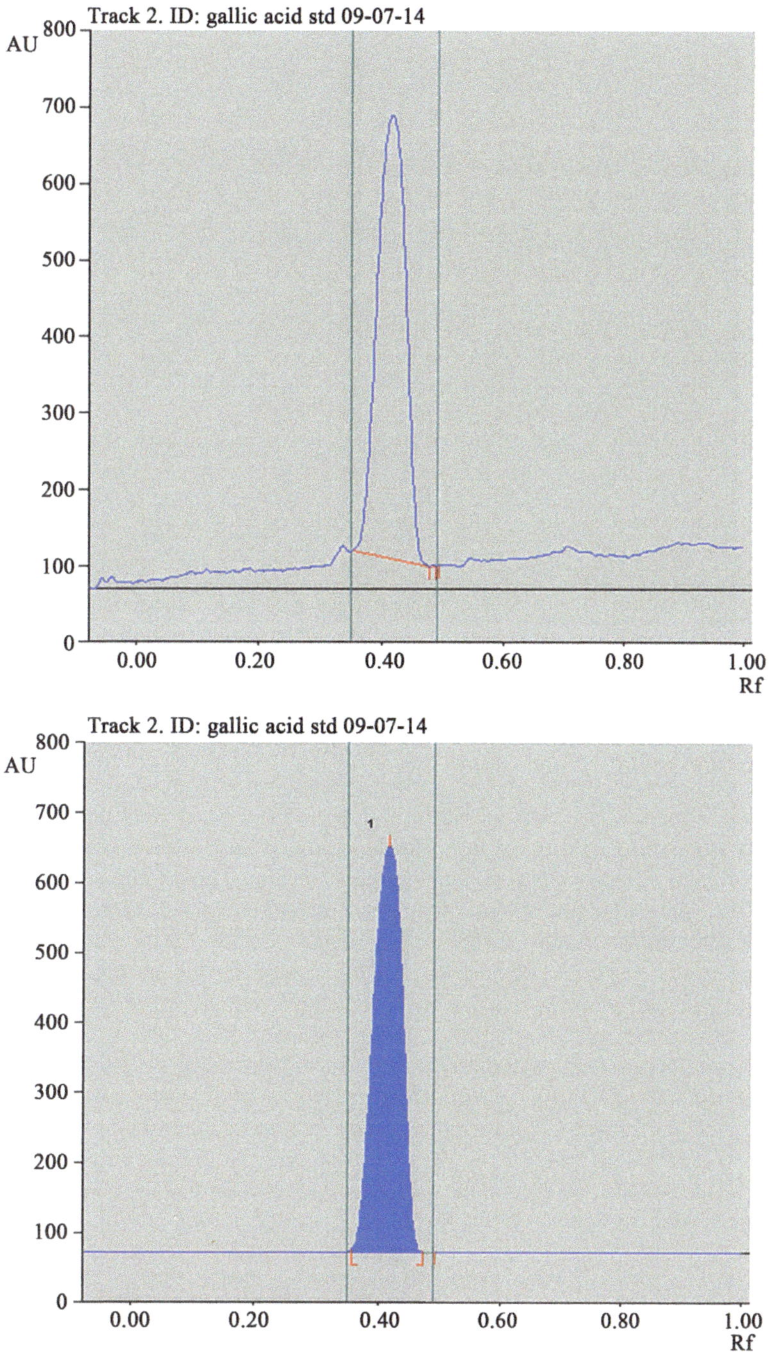

Figure 3. Peak response of gallic acid STD.

4. Results and Discussion

The quantity of gallic acid in Lipitame tablets is as follows:

$$X = \frac{34847.966 \times 4.0 \times 0.904 \times 10 \times 5 \times 99 \times 0.986}{17727.866 \times 2.5454 \times 10 \times 5 \times 100} = 2.72587\ \text{mg/tablet}$$

The gallic acid content was also tested in a tablet containing high gallic acid (positive controls) and a tablet which did not contain gallic acid (negative controls) with the same method and comparable results were observed, confirming the quantification of gallic acid in the formulation (see **Figure 4**).

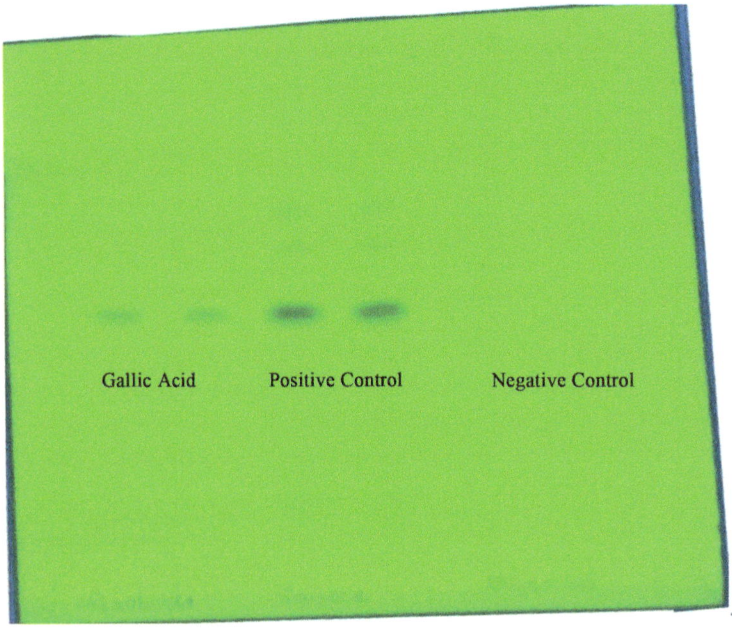

Figure 4. TLC image of Gallic acid, positive and negative control.

Standardization of specific biologically active gallic acid component was identified as material in the poly herbal formulation and quantitative analysis cover identification of chemical components where as quantitative assay measure the identification and level of bio marker in the extract establish the standard of that particular compound for validation. Lipitame is a poly herbal formulation designed by the candidate for clinical trials delineated here with in this research based study. So as to standardized the procedure of the finished tablet product and there in the four different herbal drugs such as *Terminalia arjuna*, *Terminalia belerica*, *Commiphora mukul* and *Phyllanthus emblica.* The formulation organoleptic and physic-chemical characteristics such as identification by TLC, foreign matter, total ash, acid insoluble ash, alcohol; soluble extraction and water soluble extraction are adequately presented herewith. Physico-chemical evaluation such as appearance, pH determination plays a significant role in the quality assessment. The identification with quantitative reaction and preparation of 0.1% alcohol solution exhibit the indication polarity concern of plant materials. TLC was done to augment the determination of gallic acid components and there in the identification was located. All these values show that the physic-chemical parameters adopted the values were within the limits and repeated experiments confirmed the verification. HPLC was performed to confirm the quantitative and qualitative presence of gallic acid for validation. The present standardization under taken reveal compliance with all the physic-chemical and analytical procedures, therefore it is concluded that Lipitame tablets is well standardized product at the base line parameters. As Lipitame consists of *Terminalia arjuna*, *Terminalia belerica*, *Commiphora mukul* and *Phyllanthus emblica* and where as all the three *Terminalia arjuna*, *Terminalia belerica* and *Phyllanthus emblica* contains gallic acid, therefore in the quantitative estimation gallic acid is well represented in different chromatogram. The gallic acid also inhibit the different forms of microbiological organisms so it is useful as well in diabetic dyslipidemia.

If these analytical profiles compared with the work of Modi *et al.* where Zeal cough syrup employing physico-chemical test and bioassay marker compounds agree with quality and potency [1]. In another study Desai and coworker validated the, manufacturing procedure of Vasu cough syrup with the poly herbal formulation for compliance for their reproducibility [2]. The work done by Khadair and associates validation analysis of hederacoside C, the marker of Ivy plant and percentage recovery was given as 99.6% [3]. In a patent of cough syrup the extract of *Adhatoda vasica* along with *Hedychium* spp. and *Curcuma* spp. cough syrup has been validated in greater details [4]. Therefore, Lipitame tablets standardization fall under the specific guide lines of quality herbal medicine and in line with different as mentioned earlier follow the prerequisite for global harmonization.

The bark of *Terminalia arjuna* is known for its heart-health benefits in ayurvedic literature. This has been further supported by *in vivo* studies on animal and human volunteers. But there is no detailed study on identification of the active ingredients such as polyphenols. Polyphenols possesses antioxidant properties and are well-known health actives, it is important to characterise polyphenols in *Terminalia arjuna.* Aqueous extract of *Ter-*

minalia arjuna bark was analysed for its composition and molecular weight distribution by dialysis. Compositional analysis revealed that it has 44% polyphenols and dialysis study showed that 70% of the polyphenols have molecular weight greater than 3.5 kDa. High performance liquid chromatography and liquid chromatography-mass spectrometry analysis of *Terminalia arjuna*, confirmed that it contains flavon-3-ols such as (+)-catechin, (+)-gallocatechin and (−)-epigallocatechin. Phenolic acids such as gallic acid, ellagic acid and its derivatives were also found in *Terminalia arjuna* extract. Ellagic acid derivatives were isolated and their spectral studies indicated that isolated compounds were 3-O-methyl-ellagic acid 4-O-aD-xylopyranoside, ellagic acid and 3-O-methyl ellagic acid 3-O-rhamnoside. Hydrolysis and thiolysis studies of high molecular weight polyphenols indicated that they are proanthocyanidins. Given these results, it may be possible to attribute the heart-health effects of *Terminalia arjuna* to these polyphenols which may be responsible for the endothelial benefit functions like tea [5].

Phyllanthus emblica A tannin containing gallic acid, ellagic acid and glucose in its molecule and naturally present in the fruit, prevents or retard oxidation of vitamin and renders the fruit a valuable antiscorbutic activity in the fresh as well as in the dry condition. The distribution of tannin percentage in the plant is as follows: fruit 28 percentage, twig bark 21 percentage, stem bark 8 - 9 percentage, and leaves 22 percentage respectively. The fruit contains two tannins, one giving on hydrolysis gallic acid, ellagic acid and glucose and the other giving ellagic acid and glucose only [6].

The anticholesterolaemic and antiatherogenic effects of the fruits of *Phyllanthus emblica* have been studied. The Department of Food and Nutrition, Lady Irwin College, University of Delhi did the research over the supplementation of diet with *Phyllanthus emblica* in normal and hypercholesterolaemic men aged 35 - 55 years and found to be effective hypocholesterolemic [7]. *Phyllanthus emblica* fruit juice has been proved to be hypolipidemic at the Department of Home Science (Food and Nutrition), University of Rajasthan, Jaipur, India. The fruit juice was administered at a dose of 5 ml/kg body weight per rabbit per day for 60 days reduced serum cholesterol, triglycerides, phospholipids and LDL levels by 82%, 66%, 77% and 90% respectively [8]. Similarly, the ethanol extract of *Phyllanthus emblica* at a dose of 10 or 20 mg/kg body weight/day for 20 days to rats fed 1% cholesterol diet significantly reduced total, free and LDL-Cholesterol levels in a dose-dependent manner [9]. Flavonoid extracts from the fruits of *Phyllanthus emblica* inhibited synthesis and enhanced degradation of cholesterol via increased hepatic HMG-CoA reductase [10]. In another study, the fruit juice of *Phyllanthus emblica* shown to reduce the oxidative stress induced by ischemic-reperfusion injury (IRI) in rat heart in three different doses 250, 500, 750 mg/kg for 30 days. These changes were due to increased production of myocardial endogenous antioxidants like superoxide dismutase (SOD), catalase and glutathione peroxidase (GPx) in rat [11]. Another study shown the dried fruit powder to be hypolipidemic in rabbits by reducing 42%, 29% and 31% of total cholesterol, triglycerides and LDL-Cholesterol and by increasing 33% of HDL-Cholesterol and reducing 38% of plaque areas in vascular system [12]. *Phyllanthus emblica* aqueous extract also reduces cholesterol in alloxan-induced diabetic rats along with glucose levels [13]. In another study in rabbits for 12 weeks showed increased lipid mobilization and catabolism and retarded deposition of lipids in the extrahepatic tissue [14].

Terminalia chebula fruit contains about 30% of an astringent substance called chebulinic acid, tannic acid about 20% to 40%, gallic acid, resin and some purgative principle of the nature of anthraquinone [15].

Terminalia chebula has been analyzed for its antioxidant activity at different magnitudes of potency [16]. Chebulanin of *Terminalia chebula* has its inhibitory effects on the lipid peroxidation and the production of superoxide radicals in the body [17]. It also possessed hypocholesterolemic activity against cholesterol-induced hypercholesterolemia and atherosclerosis in rabbits [18].

In conclusion, a HPTLC method has been developed and it can be used for the quantitative determination of gallic acid in lipitame tablet. Its mean advantages are its simplicity accuracy and selectivity. This method can also be used conveniently for the estimation of gallic acid in other herbal preparations and may be utilized for standardization purpose.

5. Conclusion

In this study for medicinal plants component, *Terminalia arjuna*, *Terminalia belerica*, *Commiphora mukul* and *Phyllanthus emblica* were formulated for the indication of diabetic dyslipidemia activity. TLC of extract and gallic acid reference standard were carried out. The R_f value (0.4) of gallic acid spot in both extract and reference standard was found comparable under UV light at 254 nm. Quantitative and spectrophotometric estimation of gallic acid was found between the range of 0.035% and 0.07%. HPLC in Liptame tablets was determined as 0.3 mg per 10 ml. The analytical profile of Lipitame tablets and that in gallic acid have been validated to prove that Lipitame tablets in different batches confirmed the verification.

References

[1] Modi, J., Soni, H., Pandya, K., Patel, G. and Patel, N. (2014) A Detail Phyto-Chemical Evaluation of Herbo-Mineral Formulation Used in Respiratory Diseases. *Journal of Pharmacognosy and Phytochemistry*, **2**, 36-42.

[2] Desai, L., Oza, J. and Khatri, K. (2012) Prospective Process Validation of Polyherbal Cough Syrup Formulation. *Journal of Advanced Pharmaceutical Technology & Research*, **2**, 225-231.

[3] Khdair, A., Mohammad, M.K., Tawaha, K., Al-Hamarsheh, E., AlKhatib, H.S., Al-khalidi, B., Bustanji, Y., Najjar, S. and Hudaib, M. (2010) A Validated RP HPLC-PAD Method for the Determination of Hederacoside C in Ivy-Thyme Cough Syrup. *International Journal of Analytical Chemistry*, **2010**, Article ID: 478143, 5 p.

[4] Herbal Formulation Comprising Extracts of Adhatoda, Hedychium and Curcuma as Cough Syrup, WIPO Patent Application (2005) WO/2005/077393 Kind Code: A1.

[5] Saha, A., Pawar, V.M. and Jayaraman, S. (2012) Characterisation of Polyphenols in *Terminalia arjuna* Bark Extract. *Indian Journal of Pharmaceutical Sciences*, **74**, 339-347.

[6] Said, H.M. (1970) Emblica Officinalis. In: *Hamdard Pharmacopoeia of Eastern Medicine*, The Times Press, Karachi, 383.

[7] Jacob, A., Pandey, M., Kapoor, S. and Saroja, R. (1988) Effect of the Indian Gooseberry (Amla) on Serum Cholesterol Levels in Men Aged 35 - 55 Years. *European Journal of Clinical Nutrition*, **42**, 939-944.

[8] Mathur, R., Sharma, A., Dixit, V.P. and Varma, M. (1996) Hypolipidaemic Effect of Fruit Juice of *Emblica officinalis* in Cholesterol-Fed Rabbits. *Journal of Ethnopharmacology*, **50**, 61-68. http://dx.doi.org/10.1016/0378-8741(95)01308-3

[9] Kim, H.J., Yokozawa, T., Kim, H.Y., Tohda, C., Rao, T.P. and Juneja, L.R. (2005) Influence of Amla (*Emblica officinalis* Gaertn.) on Hypercholesterolemia and Lipid Peroxidation in Cholesterol-Fed Rats. *Journal of Nutritional Science and Vitaminology*, **51**, 413-418.

[10] Anila, L. and Vijayalakshmi, N.R. (2002) Flavonoids from *Emblica officinalis* and *Mangifera indica*—Effectiveness for Dyslipidemia. *Journal of Ethnopharmacology*, **79**, 81-87. http://dx.doi.org/10.1016/S0378-8741(01)00361-0

[11] Rajak, S., Banerjee, S.K., Sood, S., Dinda, A.K., Gupta, Y.K., Gupta, S.K. and Maulik, S.K. (2004) *Emblica officinalis* Causes Myocardial Adaptation and Protects against Oxidative Stress in Ischemic-Reperfusion Injury in Rats. *Phytotherapy Research*, **18**, 54-60. http://dx.doi.org/10.1002/ptr.1367

[12] Liu, L., Li, B. and Wang, L. (2005) Effect of *Emblica officinalis* on Formation of Atherosclerotic Plaque in Hypercholesterolemia Rabbits. *Applied Journal of General Practice*, **2**, 97-98.

[13] Qureshi, S.A., Asad, W. and Sultana, V. (2009) The Effect of Phyllanthus Emblica Linn on Type-II Diabetes, Triglycerides and Liver-Specific Enzyme. *Pakistan Journal of Nutrition*, **8**, 125-128. http://dx.doi.org/10.3923/pjn.2009.125.128

[14] Mand, J.K., Soni, J.L., Gupta, P.P. and Singh, R. (1991) Effect of Amla (*Ebmlica officinalis*) on the Development of Artherosclerosis in Hypocholesterolemic Rabbits. *Journal of Research and Education in Indian Medicine*, **10**, 1-7.

[15] Pharmacopoeia Committee (2003) Monographs on Herbal Drugs of Unani Medicine. Drugs Control and Traditional Medicine Division, National Institute of Health, Islamabad, Vol. 1, 530.

[16] Kapoor, L.D. (1990) Ayurvedic Medicinal Plants. In: *CRC Handbook of Ayurvedic Medicinal Plants*, CRC Press, India, 322.

[17] Cheng, H.Y., Lin, T.C., Yu, K.H., Yang, C.M. and Lin, C.C. (2003) Antioxidant and Free Radical Scavenging Activities of *Terminalia chebula. Biological & Pharmaceutical Bulletin*, **26**, 1331-1335.

[18] Chattopadhyay, R.R. and Bhattacharyya, S.K. (2007) Plant Review *Terminalia chebula*: An Update. *Pharmacognosy Reviews*, **26**, 1331-1335.

28

Effects of Exogenous Growth Hormone on Growth Hormone-Insulin-Like Growth Factor Axis of Human Gastric Cancer Cell

Daoming Liang*, Yi Zhang, Jiayong Chen, Hua Wang, Tao Huang, Xin Xue

Gastrointestinal Surgery Department, Second Affiliated Hospital of Kunming Medical University, Kunming, China
Email: *daomingliang@sina.cn

Abstract

Aim: To study effects of recombinant human growth hormone (rhGH) on growth hormone-insulin-like growth factor axis (GH-IGFs) of human gastric cancer cell *in vivo* in order to reveal part mechanism of growth effects of rhGH on gastric cancer. Methods: Nude mice were randomly divided into control group, cisplatin (DDP) group, rhGH group and DDP + rhGH group after human gastric cancer xenograft model of node mice was successfully founded and drugs were used for 6 days. We investigated volume of tumor, inhibitory rate of tumor and cell cycle by slide gauge and flow cytometry. In addition, We also respectively investigated insulin-like growth factor-I (IGF-I) and insulin-like growth factor binding protein-3 (IGFBP-3) of blood serum of nude mice, IGF-ImRNA, insulin-like growth factor-I receptor (IGF-IR) mRNA and IGFBP-3 mRNA of xenograft of nude mice by enzyme linked immunosorbent assay (ELISA) and semiquantitative reverse transcriptase-polymerase chain reaction (RT-PCR) on the first day of completing use of drugs later. Results: Tumor grew obviously slowly and tumor inhibitory rate obviously rose in DDP group and DDP + rhGH group compared with control group and rhGH group ($p < 0.05$), but they were not remarkably different between DDP group and DDP + rhGH group or between control group and rhGH group. Cells of gastric cancer xenograft in S phase distinctly diminished in DDP group and DDP + rhGH group compared with control group and rhGH group ($p < 0.05$), but they were not statistically significant between DDP group and DDP + rhGH group or between control group and rhGH group. IGF-I and IGFBP-3 of blood serum of nude mice obviously rose, but ratio of IGF-I and IGFBP-3 obviously lowered in rhGH group and DDP + rhGH group compared with control group and DDP group ($p < 0.05$). Expressions of IGF-I mRNA and IGF-IR mRNA were not obviously different in all groups. But expression of IGFBP-3 mRNA obviously increased in rhGH group, DDP group and DDP + rhGH group compared with control group; meanwhile, expression of IGFBP-3 mRNA also obviously increased in DDP + rhGH group compared with control group, DDP group and rhGH group. Conclu-

*Corresponding author.

sion: Our results indicated rhGH in short-time use did not improve proliferation of human gastric cancer cells and its mechanism was possible that rhGH in short-time use raised simultaneously IGF-I and IGFBP-3 of blood serum and increased IGFBP-3 mRNA, but degraded ratio of IGF-I and IGFBP-3 of blood serum in human gastric cancer cells.

Keywords

Human Growth Hormone, Stomach Neoplasm, Insulin-Like Growth Factor, Insulin-Like Growth Factor Binding Protein-3, RT-Polymerase Chain Reaction

1. Introduction

The effect of growth hormone/insulin-like growth factor (GH/IGF) axis on normal cells was very clear; meanwhile, many evidences manifested that GH/IGF axis promoted growth of tumor tissue [1] [2]. Furthermore, epidemiologic survey hinted that GH/IGF axis and long-term use of growth hormone (GH) were tumorigenic possible factors. But other data showed that long-term use of GH could not promote tumorigenesis [3]-[6]. Since 1996, we have always undertaken the clinical research that recombinant human growth hormone (rhGH) was applied in postoperative patients with gastrointestinal malignant tumor for metabolic intervention. We found that rhGH improved patients' rehabilitation, raised patients living quality and did not raise relapse rate and transfer rate of cancer compared with control group [7] [8]. Lots of overseas clinical data showed that hGH did not improve cancer growth and could decrease peroperative complications incidence and death rate in postoperative patients with gastrointestinal malignant tumor [9]-[13]. Our previous empirical study has also demonstrated that rhGH did not accelerate the proliferation of human gastric cancer cell line BGC823 *in vitro* and *in vivo* [14] [15]. But mechanism that rhGH did not accelerate the proliferation of human gastric cancer cell was unknown. GH should upgrade the blood level of IGF-I by promoting the transcription and expression of IGF gene. The major effects of IGF were induced by IGF-1R. 1% of IGF was free and effective *in vivo*, while 99% was combined with insulin-like growth factor binding protein (IGFBP). It showed that IGFBP was important to the regulation of IGF effects *in vivo*. We analyzed contents of insulin-like growth factor-I (IGF-I), insulin-like growth factor binding protein-3 (IGFBP-3) of blood serum and expression IGF-ImRNA, insulin-like growth factor-I receptor (IGF-IR) mRNA, and IGFBP-3 mRNA of transplantation tumor of nude mice with gastric cancer after rhGH was used in nude mice for short term. Our experiment results would reveal part mechanism of growth effects of rhGH on gastric cancer.

2. Materials and Methods

2.1. Materials

Nu/Nu nude mice were obtained from Beijing Wei Tong Li Hua experimental animal technology limited company and animal certificate number was SCXK (Jing) 2002-003. The mice were 6 wk old, with weights ranging between 15 - 21 g and they were allowed free access to the normal diets and water in specific-pathogen free laboratory in the emphasis natural drugs and pharmacology laboratory of Yunnan province China. The animal experiments were performed according to the European Community guidelines for the care and use of animals, and approved by the Animal Research Ethics Committee, Kunming Medical University. Human gastric cancer cell line MKN45 was supplied by the Cell Bank of Shanghai Cell Biology Institute of Chinese Academy of Sciences. rhGH (Saizen) was supplied by Serono (Switzerland), cisplatin (DDP) by Gejiu Biotechnology and Pharmacology Limited Company. Immunoreagent kit of insulin-like growth factor-I (IGF-I) and insulin-like growth factor binding protein-3 (IGFBP-3) was supplied by Immunodiagnostic Systems Limited, USA and 5× Reverse Transcriptase Buffer, dNTP Mixture, RNase Inhibitor, Oligo (dT) 18 Primer and AMV Reverse Primer all by Takara Biotechnology (Dalian) Limited Company. In addition, enzyme linked immunosorbent assay implement was M262154, USA. PCR implement was supplied by Biometra Company, Germany and its type was UNO-Thermoblock.

2.2. Methods

The cells of human gastric cancer cell line MKN45 were cultured in laboratory and the density of single cell suspension was adjusted to 1 × 10^7/L for further use. Later, cell suspension (0.2 mL) was inoculated subcutaneously into right gluteal of nude mice.

After long diameter of gastric cancer xenograft was observed to be 1.0 centimeter by measuring its long diameter and short diameter, nude mice were executed and xenograft was divided into lots of mass-their volume were 2 × 2 × 2 mm^3. Then, the mass were respectively inoculated subcutaneously into right gluteal of 30 nude mice and gastric cancer xenograft models of nude mice were founded.

On the fourteenth day of inoculation, nude mice whose xenograft grew well were randomly divided into 4 groups: control group, rhGH group, DDP group and rhGH + DDP group, and 6 in each group. Later, the following drugs were administrated for 6 consecutive days: normal saline (NS) was subcutaneously injected in control group, 0.1 mL/d; rhGH group with rhGH, 2 IU/kg per day; L-OUP group with L-OHP by celiac injection, 1.3 mg/kg per day; and rhGH + L-OHP group with both rhGH and L-OHP of the same dosage as rhGH group and L-OHP group, respectively. The nude rice was killed on the first day of completing administration.

After length and breadth of tumor were measured by slide gauge, volume of tumor was computed before use of drug. On the first day of drugs completing administration, tumor was measured by slide gauge also and volume of tumor and tumor inhibitory rate was computed. In addition, the xenograft was confirmed in pathological observation by HE dyeing. Then, 1 - 1.5 mL eyeballs blood of nude mice was obtained and was centrifuged 3000 rpm/second centrifugal separation of serum 10 min, drawing the upper serum, placed in −20˚C refrigerator for enzyme-linked immunosorbent assay (ELISA) detection of IGF-I and IGFBP-3. ELISA detection methods include: coating, dispensing, plus HRP, substrate Yexian add color, to terminate the reaction; results found: on a white background can be a direct observation with the naked eye: the deeper the color reaction hole, the positive degree stronger negative reaction is a colorless or very light, measured by ELISA detector optical density (OD) of each hole.

Calculation formula:

$$\text{Volume of tumor } V = ab^2/2$$

(V: volume of tumor, a: length of tumor, b: breadth of tumor) [16]

$$\text{Tumor growth inhibitory rate } (\%) = \frac{\text{volume in control group} - \text{volume in experiment group}}{\text{volume in control group}} \times 100\%$$

Tissue of tumor was taken and was detected by flow cytometry and by reverse transcriptase-polymerase chain reaction (RT-PCR) after nude mice were killed on the first day of drugs completing administration respectively.

Flow cytometry procedures:

Part of tumor was made into a single-cell suspension for flow cytometry by grinding, centrifugating and washing. After fixed with 70% alcohol, the cells were kept at 4˚C overnight, then, dyed with fluorescence. Finally the cell cycle was examined at 488 nm wavelength. Barlogie cell cycle assay was used.

RT-PCR procedures:

1) Extraction of total tissue RNA

1 μg RNA was taken and the first chain of cDNA was synthesized by reverse transcription. Then, according to the instruction of AMV reverse transcriptase, the liquid was shifted in 42˚C thermostatic bath and incubated one hour and cooling 2 minutes in ice water in turn after it was lightly stirred and was placed for 10 minutes in room temperature. The last, the reaction product was used for PCR reaction.

2) Primer sequence and reaction condition were shown in **Table 1** and PCR carried out in the volume of 25 μl:

PCR reaction included 94˚C denaturing for 3 minutes and lots of cycles which were 94˚C denaturing for 30 seconds, annealing for 30 seconds, extending 72˚C for 30 seconds and the last extending 72˚C for 3 minutes.

3) Electrophoresis after agarose gel electrophoresis, 5 μg/mL ethidium bromide dyeing for 10 minutes and pure water flush, gel was analyzed by Quantity-One software (BIO-RAD, Hercules, CA) and was image analyzed.

2.3. Statistical Analysis

Statistics were computed using the statistics program SPSS 13.0 software (SPSS Inc., Chicago, Ill., USA) for

Table 1. Primer sequence and reaction conditions of RT-PCR.

	Primer sequence	Annealing temperature (˚C)	Product (bp)
IGF-1	ATTTCAACAAGCCCACAG TCCCTCTACTTGCGTTCT	56	219
IGF-1R	CCTACAACATCACCGACCCG CCACGACCCATTCCCAGA	58	464
IGFBP-3	CCCTCTACTTGCTCGATTC ACGTGCCTACCCACCTTC	54	240
GAPDH	GGAGCCAAACGGGTCATCATCTC GAGGGGCCATCCACAGTCTTCT	62	233

Windows. Data are presented as mean ± SEM and differences among experimental groups were analyzed by one-way analysis of variance or rank test. Statistical significance was set at $p < 0.05$.

3. Results

3.1. Pathomorphology of Xenograft by HE Dyeing

We observed pathomorphology of xenograft in optical microscope by HE dyeing and we found that the tumor cells of xenograft were round, amount, big nucleus, more pathological division, multiple nucleoli, tumor cells arranging in disorder, plentiful blood sinusoid (**Figure 1**). So we thought that gastric cancer xenograft models of nude mice were successfully founded.

3.2. Volume of Tumor and Tumor Inhibitory Rate

Tumor grew obviously slowly and tumor inhibitory rate obviously rose in DDP group and DDP + rhGH group compared with control group and rhGH group ($p < 0.05$); but they were not remarkably different between DDP group and DDP + rhGH group or between control group and rhGH group (**Table 2**).

3.3. ELISA Detection

As shown in **Table 3**, IGF-I and IGFBP-3 of blood serum of nude mice obviously stepped up in rhGH group or DDP + rhGH group compared with Control group or DDP group but ratio of IGF-I and IGFBP-3 obviously lowered and there was significant difference among them.

3.4. Cell Cycle

Cells of gastric cancer xenograft in S phase distinctly diminished in DDP group and DDP + rhGH group compared with control group and rhGH group ($p < 0.05$); but there was not statistically significant between DDP group and DDP + rhGH group or between control group and rhGH group (**Table 4**, **Figure 2**).

3.5. RT-PCR Detection

Relative abundance of mRNA was accounted in accordance with glyceraldehyde phosphate dehydrogenase (GAPDH) strap which optical density value was set for 1.000. Expression of IGF-ImRNA IGF-IR and mRNA has no statistical difference among all groups, but expression of IGFBP-3 mRNA obviously raised in DDP group, rhGH group and DDP + rhGH group compared with control group and it also obviously raised in DDP + rhGH group compared with other groups ($p < 0.05$) (**Table 5**, **Figure 3**).

4. Discussions

In our experiment, we successfully founded gastric cancer xenograft models of nude mice and cancer models were confirmed by HE dying. Then, after we detected volume of tumor, tumor growth inhibitory rate and cell cycle, we thought that the short term usage of rhGH would not accelerate the growth of human gastric cancer cells and it was in accord with our earlier studies and other data [14] [15] [17]. The results lay the foundation for next study.

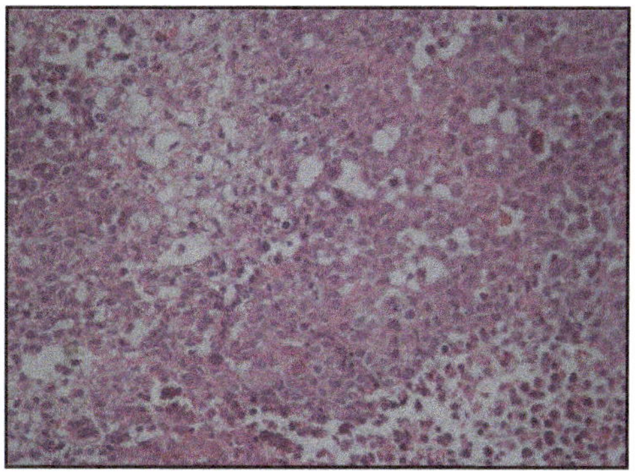

Figure 1. Pathomorphology of xenograft in control group by HE dyeing (×40). There were big nucleus, more pathological division, multiple nucleoli, tumor cells arranging in disorder.

Table 2. Volume of tumor and tumor inhibitory rate of gastric cancer before and after use of drug.

Groups	Volume of tumor before use of drug (cm^3)	Volume of tumor after use of drug (cm^3)	Tumor inhibitory rate (%)
Control Group	0.56 ± 0.35	1.54 ± 0.96	0
DDP Group	0.55 ± 0.27	0.60 ± 0.22*	60.75*
rhGH Group	0.58 ± 0.36	1.57 ± 0.93	−0.21
DDP + rhGH Group	0.40 ± 0.22	0.45 ± 0.24*	70.76*

*$p < 0.05$, control group or rhGH group vs DDP group or DDP + rhGH group.

Table 3. IGF-I, IGFBP-3 and IGF-I/IGFBP-3 of blood serum of nude mice by ELISA ($\bar{x} \pm s$).

Groups	IGF-I (ng/mL)	IGFBP-3 (ng/mL)	IGF-I/IGFBP-3
Control Group	1727.3 ± 69.2	565.0 ± 106.3	3.20 ± 0.94
DDP Group	1735.3 ± 80.2	627.5 ± 176.4	2.84 ± 0.84
rhGH Group	1916.1 ± 93.7*	1194.2 ± 245.9*	1.65 ± 0.28*
DDP + rhGH Group	1909.5 ± 118.7*	1181.7 ± 342.8*	1.71 ± 0.42*

*$p < 0.05$, rhGH group or DDP + rhGH group vs control group or DDP group.

Table 4. Cell cycle of gastric cancer after use of drug.

Groups	G0-G1 phase	S phase	G2-M phase
Control Group	66.80 ± 4.95	11.13 ± 5.33	20.03 ± 2.72
DDP Group	71.33 ± 6.23	5.27 ± 3.21*	23.37 ± 3.65
rhGH Group	66.03 ± 5.59	12.68 ± 4.41	21.28 ± 4.11
DDP + rhGH Group	69.87 ± 8.51	5.72 ± 2.41*	24.42 ± 10.65

*$p < 0.05$, control group or rhGH group vs DDP group or DDP + rhGH group.

Table 5. Expression of IGF-I, IGF-IR and IGFBP-3mRNA in tumor by RT-PCR.

Groups	IGF-ImRNA	IGF-IR mRNA	IGFBP-3 mRNA
Control Group	0.675 ± 0.221	0.646 ± 0.282	0.021 ± 0.001#
DDP Group	0.724 ± 0.224	0.681 ± 0.203	0.283 ± 0.103*#
rhGH Group	0.566 ± 0.184	0.495 ± 0.212	0.215 ± 0.087*#
DDP + rhGH Group	0.618 ± 0.243	0.652 ± 0.193	0.534 ± 0.189*

*$p < 0.05$, DDP group, rhGH group or DDP + rhGH group vs control group; #$p < 0.05$, control group, DDP group or rhGH group vs DDP + rhGH group.

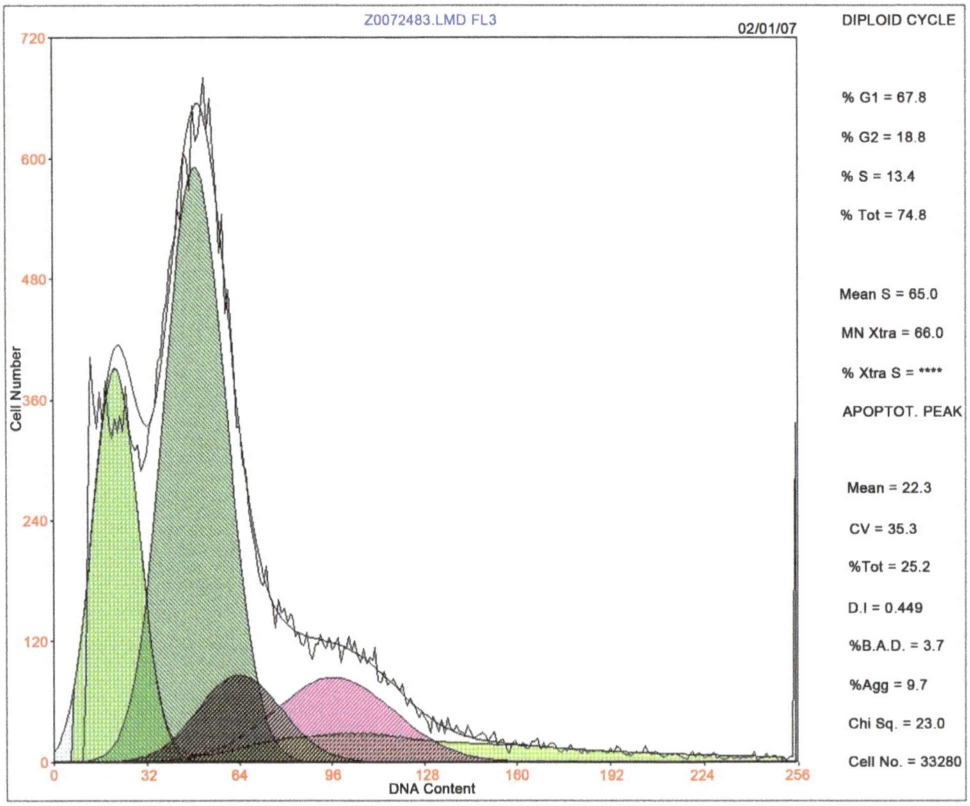
Z0072483.LMD FL3
02/01/07
DIPLOID CYCLE
% G1 = 67.8
% G2 = 18.8
% S = 13.4
% Tot = 74.8
Mean S = 65.0
MN Xtra = 66.0
% Xtra S = ****
APOPTOT. PEAK
Mean = 22.3
CV = 35.3
%Tot = 25.2
D.I = 0.449
%B.A.D. = 3.7
%Agg = 9.7
Chi Sq. = 23.0
Cell No. = 33280
Cell Number
DNA Content
0
120
240
360
480
600
720
32
64
96
128
160
192
224
256

(a)

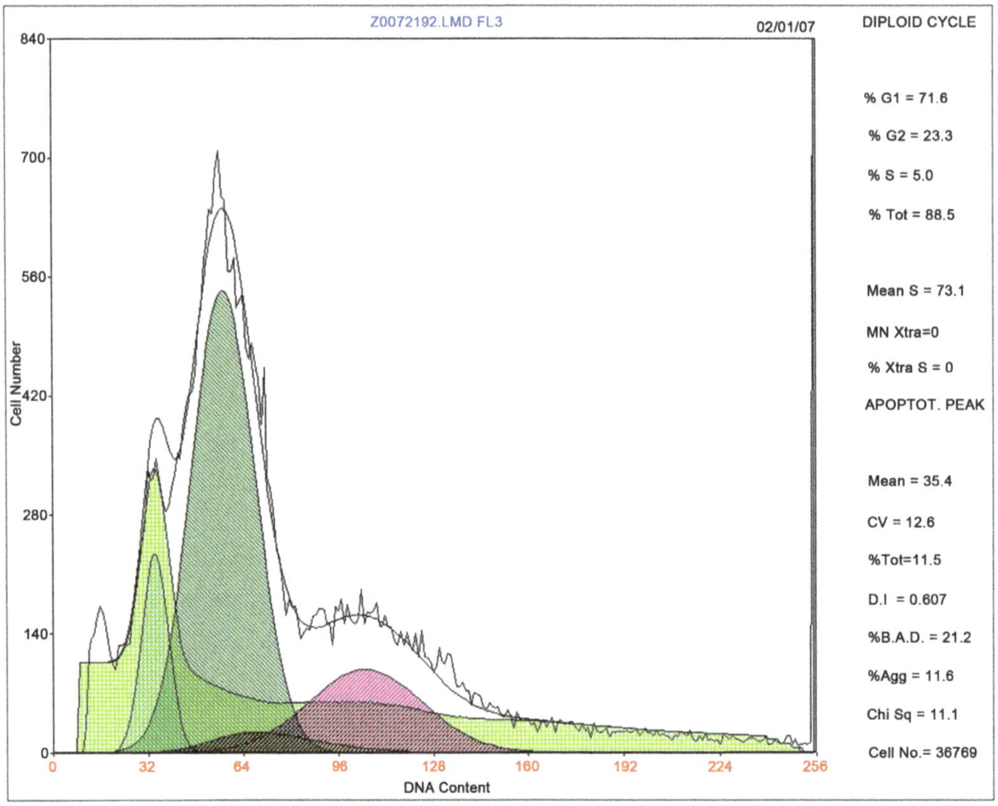
Z0072192.LMD FL3
02/01/07
DIPLOID CYCLE
% G1 = 71.6
% G2 = 23.3
% S = 5.0
% Tot = 88.5
Mean S = 73.1
MN Xtra=0
% Xtra S = 0
APOPTOT. PEAK
Mean = 35.4
CV = 12.6
%Tot=11.5
D.I = 0.607
%B.A.D. = 21.2
%Agg = 11.6
Chi Sq = 11.1
Cell No.= 36769
Cell Number
DNA Content
0
140
280
420
560
700
840
32
64
96
128
160
192
224
256

(b)

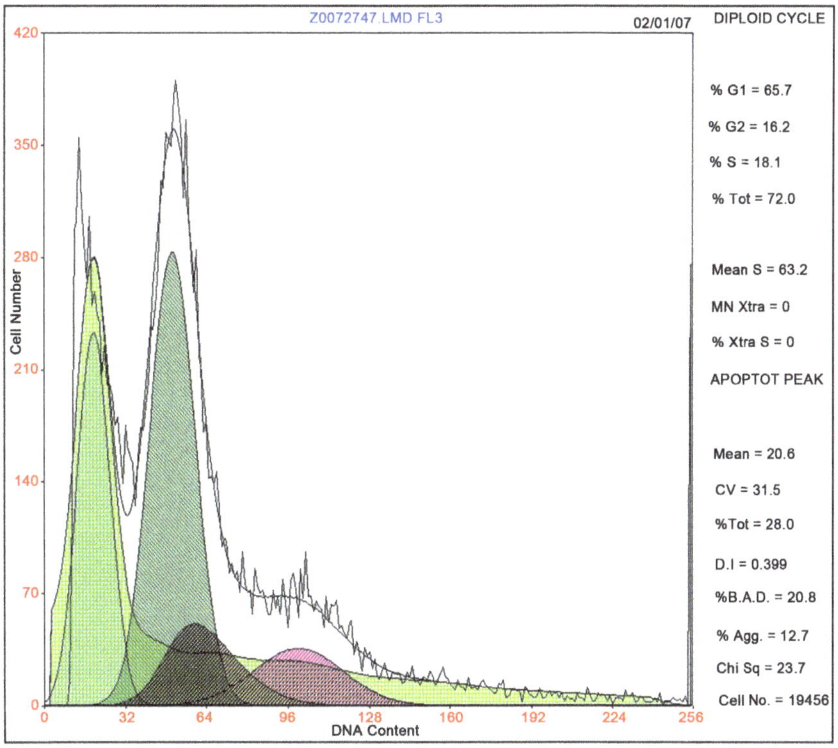

(c)

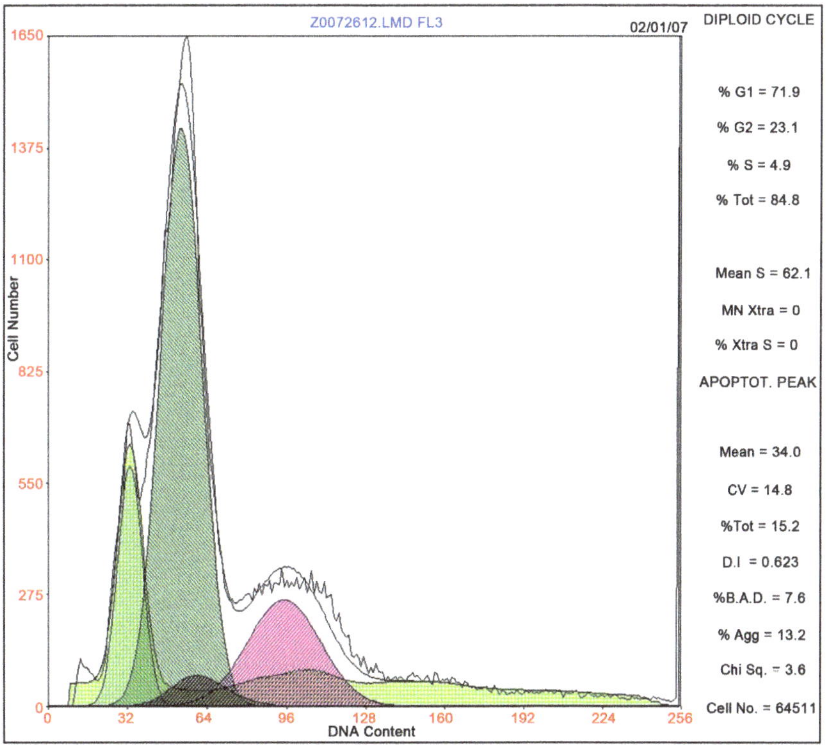

(d)

Figure 2. Scanogram of cell cycle of gastric cancer cells after use of drug by flow cytometry: (a) control group; (b) DDP group; (c) rhGH group; (d) DDP + rhGH group green stands for G0-G1 phase gray stands for S phase; pink stands for G2-M cells in S phase distinctly diminished in DDP group and DDP + rhGH group compared with control group and rhGH group ($p < 0.05$).

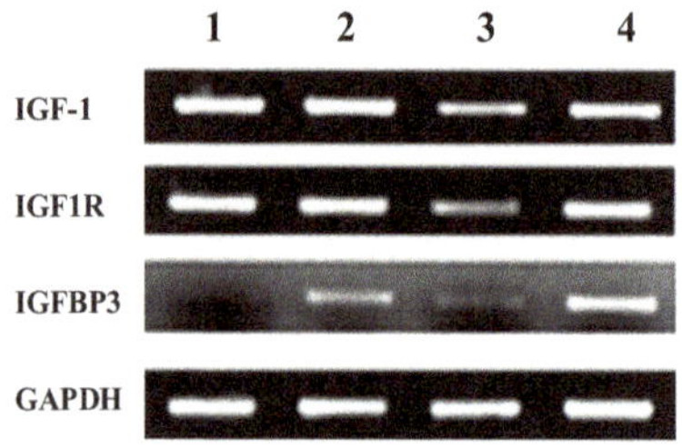

Figure 3. Expression of IGF-I, IGF-IR and IGFBP-3mRNA in tumor by RT-PCR. 1: control group, 2: DDP group, 3: rhGH group, 4: DDP + rhGH group. Expression of IGFBP-3 mRNA obviously raised in DDP group, rhGH group and DDP + rhGH group compared with control group and it obviously raised in DDP + rhGH group compared with other groups ($p < 0.05$).

The growth hormone-insulin-like growth factor axis (GH-IGFs) contains GH, IGFs, IGFR, IGFBP, and IGFBP protease. IGF-1, one of the IGFs, was effective on cell caryocinesia and metabolism. GH could stimulate liver to produce and release IGF, and there was positive correlation between the GH level and the released IGF level. Growth hormone played on its metabolic effects in directly or indirectly by IGF-I [18] [19]. Simultaneously, IGF-I mediated multiple roles of growth hormone promoting growth and synthesis [20]. Furthermore, both growth hormone and IGF-I have roles of saving lean body tissue and maintaining anabolic effect of protein synthesis [21]-[24].

The GH-IGFs acted as a strong promoter not only on cell proliferation in normal tissue but also on tumor formation, development and transference. In many prospective researches, the investigated people were distributed into different 4 groups by their IGF-I levels, and the tumor such as prostatic carcinoma, lung cancer, rectal cancer and breast cancer occurred double or triple times in the highest IGF-I level group than in the lowest IGF-I level group [25] [26]. IGF-I was detected in almost every normal tissue type, it was positive on cell proliferation and differenciation. IGF-1 was also a strong motigen in tumor tissues, and it was regarded as a messenger of GH which was related with several tumor occurrence [27]. Research has shown IGF-I to stimulate the proliferation of pancreatic [28], colon [29], and breast [30] adenocarcinoma cell lines, with blockade of the IGF-1R leading to a downregulation in growth [28] [31] [32]. Studies about breast [33] and colon cancer [34] have demonstrated higher IGF-I levels to be associated with increased risk of adenocarcinoma development. But in recent researches, it was suggested that GH should act differently in tumor tissues according to the IGF-I gene polymorphism and the tumor tissue type [35]-[37]. In addition, Shitara *et al.* found that genetic polymorphisms of IGF-I may have a substantial effect on recurrence for gastric cancer patients who have undergone curative gastrectomy [38]. Felice *et al.* thought GH action in the T47D cells was independent of changes in IGF-I and IGF-I receptor (IGF-IR) expression and IGF-IR signaling, suggesting that GH can exert direct effects on breast cancer cells [39].

IGFBP included IGFBP-1, 2, 3, 4, 5, 6 and them were separated and were identified, and IGFBP-3 was regarded as the major binding protein. In some special cases, IGFBP-3 could increase the activities of IGF-I by its self-degradation. The dual regulating mechanisms were controlled by IGFBP protease and GH *et al.* Because IGFBP was more effective than IGF-1R on binding with IGF-I, it should decrease the activity of IGF-I by the way of competitive inhibition. Besides, IGFBP should suppress cell growth directly. In tumor tissue, the level of IGF-I and IGFBP was effective on tumor occurrence, development, and prognosis, as well as the ratio between IGF-I and IGFBP. It was reported in a research of tumor-bearing mice that the tumor grew little when the mice had ingested the compound protein of IGF-I and IGFBP-3 while the protein production and nutritional status of the mice were improved apparently [40]. It was believed in part of researchers that the proper usage of GH should be related to the treatment periods and the doses of GH as well as the blood level of IGF-1 and IGFBP-3 [41]. It was reported that IGF-1 and IGF-1/IGFBP-3 molar ratio might increase the risk of cancer by increasing mammographic density [42]. In our experiment, the short term treatment of exogenous human growth hormone had increased not only the blood level of IGF-I and IGFBP-3 but also the mRNA expression of IGFBP-3 gene in tumor tissue, but had decreased the rate of IGF-I/IGFBP-3 in the mean time. The increased blood level of IGF-I and IGFBP-3 was also reported in the research of applying rhGH to the dystrophic patients who had been treated with total parenteral nutrition [43].

In the experiment, the short term treatment of exogenous human growth hormone had increased not only the blood level of IGF-I and IGFBP-3 but also the mRNA expression of IGFBP-3 gene in tumor tissue. In the mean time, the short term treatment of which rhGH had decreased the rate of IGF-I/IGFBP-3, especially when the treatment was associated with chemical therapy. In our earlier and before researches, it showed that the short term usage of rhGH would not accelerate the growth of human gastric cancer cells [13] [14]. Considering the results of both research, it should be suggested that the short term usage of rhGH would decrease the rate of IGF-I/IGFBP-3 in blood and would increase the protein level of IGFBP-3 in blood and gastric cancer tissue both, and the increased IGFBP-3 would bind with IGF-I as well as competitively inhibited the combination between IGF-I and its receptors, so it was one of mechanism of that the short term usage of rhGH would not accelerate the growth of human gastric cancer cells.

5. Conclusions

RhGH in short-time use did not improve proliferation of human gastric cancer cells and its mechanism was possible that rhGH in short-time use raised simultaneously IGF-I and IGFBP-3 of blood serum and increased IGFBP-3 mRNA, but degraded ratio of IGF-I and IGFBP-3 of blood serum in human gastric cancer cells.

Finally, we didn't do some long-term experiments about the research for death of nude mice in DDP group, and this also is the defect of our experiment.

Acknowledgements

We are grateful to anonymous reviewers for their valuable suggestions and comments. This work was supported by research grants from Natural Science Foundation of China (No. 81060114).

Conflict of Interest

The authors state no conflict of interest.

Foundation

Supported by the Natural Science Foundation of China, No. 81060114.

References

[1] Smith, G.D., Gunnell, D. and Holly, J. (2000) Cancer and Insulin-Like Growth Factor-I. A Potential Mechanism Linking the Environment with Cancer Risk. *BMJ*, **321**, 847-848. http://dx.doi.org/10.1136/bmj.321.7265.847

[2] Samani, A.A., Yakar, S., LeRoith, D. and Brodt, P. (2007) The Role of the IGF System in Cancer Growth and Metastasis: Overview and Recent Insights. *Endocrine Reviews*, **28**, 20-47. http://dx.doi.org/10.1210/er.2006-0001

[3] Bogarin, R. and Steinbok, P. (2009) Growth Hormone Treatment and Risk of Recurrence or Progression of Brain Tumors in Children: A Review. *Child's Nervous System*, **25**, 273-279. http://dx.doi.org/10.1007/s00381-008-0790-6

[4] Losa, M., Gatti, E., Rossini, A. and Lanzi, R. (2008) Replacement Therapy with Growth Hormone and Pituitary Tumor Recurrence: The Relevance of the Problem. *Journal of Endocrinological Investigation*, **31**, 75-78.

[5] Arnold, J.R., Arnold, D.F., Marland, A., Karavitaki, N. and Wass, J.A. (2009) GH Replacement in Patients with Non-Functioning Pituitary Adenoma (NFA) Treated Solely by Surgery Is Not Associated with Increased Risk of Tumor Recurrence. *Clinical Endocrinology*, **70**, 435-438. http://dx.doi.org/10.1111/j.1365-2265.2008.03391.x

[6] Rohrer, T.R., Langer, T., Grabenbauer, G.G., Buchfelder, M., Glowatzki, M. and Dörr, H.G. (2010) Growth Hormone Therapy and the Risk of Tumor Recurrence after Brain Tumor Treatment in Children. *Journal of Pediatric Endocrinology and Metabolism*, **23**, 935-942. http://dx.doi.org/10.1515/jpem.2010.150

[7] Chen, J.Y., Zhang, J., Tan, J., Gan, P., Sun, M. and Chen, X.Z. (1999) Evaluation of Human Growth Hormone on Gastric and Gastric Cancer Patients after Surgery. *Chinese Journal of Base and Clinics in General Surgery*, **6**, 365-367.

[8] Chen, J.Y., Gan, P., Xu, P.Y., Zhang, J., Tan, J. and Sun, M. (2000) Effects of Growth Hormone on Protein Catabolism and Immunologic Function of Postoperative Old Age Patients with Digestive Tract Tumor. *Chinese Journal of Gerontology*, **20**, 162-163.

[9] Harrison, L.E., Blumberg, D., Berman, R., Ng, B., Hochwald, S., Brennan, M.F. and Burt, M. (1996) Effect of Human Growth Hormone on Human Pancreatic Carcinoma Growth, Protein and Cell Cycle Kinetic. *Journal of Surgical Research*, **61**, 317-322. http://dx.doi.org/10.1006/jsre.1996.0123

[10] Tacke, J., Bolder, U., Herrmann, A., Berger, G. and Jauch, K.W. (2000) Long-Term Risk of Gastrointestinal Tumor Recurrence after Postoperative Treatment with Recombinant Human Growth Hormone. *JPEN*, **24**, 140-144.

http://dx.doi.org/10.1177/0148607100024003140

[11] Bartlett, D.L.T., Stein, P., Torosian, M.H., Philadelphia, P.A. and Camden, N.J. (1995) Effect of Growth Hormone and Protein Intake on Tumor Growth and Host Cachexia. *Surgery*, **117**, 260-267. http://dx.doi.org/10.1016/S0039-6060(05)80199-0

[12] Beentjes, J.A., van Gorkom, B.A., Sluiter, W.J., de Vries, E.G., Kleibeuker, J.H. and Dullaart, R.P. (2000) One Year Growth Hormone Replacement Therapy Does Not Alter Colonic Epithelial Cell Proliferation in Growth Hormone Deficient Adults. *Clinical Endocrinology*, **52**, 457-462. http://dx.doi.org/10.1046/j.1365-2265.2000.00993.x

[13] Blethen, S.L., Allen, D.B., Graves, D., August, G., Moshang, T. and Rosenfeld, R. (1996) Safety of Recombinant Deoxyribonucleic Acid-Derived Growth Hormone: The National Cooperative Growth Study Experience. *Journal of Clinical Endocrinology and Metabolism*, **81**, 1704-1710.

[14] Chen, J.Y., Liang, D.M., Gan, P., Zhang, Y. and Lin, J. (2004) *In Vitro* Effects of Recombinant Human Growth Hormone on Growth of Human Gastric Cancer Cell Line BGC823 Cells. *World Journal of Gastroenterology*, **10**, 1132-1136.

[15] Liang, D.M., Chen, J.Y., Zhang, Y., Gan, P., Lin, J. and Chen, A.B. (2006) Effects of Recombinant Human Growth Hormone on Growth of a Human Gastric Carcinoma Xenograft Model in Nude Mice. *World Journal of Gastroenterology*, **12**, 3810-3813.

[16] Osieka, R., Houchens, D.P., Goldin, A. and Johnson, R.K. (1977) Chemotherapy of Human Colon Cancer Xenografts in Athymic Nude Mice. *Cancer*, **40**, 2640-2650.

[17] Lin, Y., Li, S., Cao, P., Cheng, L., Quan, M. and Jiang, S. (2011) The Effects of Recombinant Human GH on Promoting Tumor Growth Depend on the Expression of GH Receptor *in Vivo*. *Journal of Endocrinology*, **211**, 249-256. http://dx.doi.org/10.1530/JOE-11-0100

[18] Heemskerk, V.H., Daemen, M.A. and Buurman, W.A. (1999) Insulin-Like Growth Factor-I (IGF-1) and Growth Hormone (GH) in Immunity and Inflammation. *Cytokine & Growth Factor Reviews*, **10**, 5-14.

[19] Berneis, K. and Keller, U. (1996) Metabolic Actions of Growth Hormone: Direct and Indirect. *Baillière's Clinical Endocrinology and Metabolism*, **10**, 337-352. http://dx.doi.org/10.1016/S0950-351X(96)80470-8

[20] LeRoith, D. and Yakar, S. (2007) Mechanisms of Disease: Metabolic Effects of Growth Hormone and Insulin-Like Growth Factor I. *Nature Clinical Practice. Endocrinology & Metabolism*, **3**, 302-310.

[21] Hayes, V.Y., Urban, R.J., Jiang, J., Marcell, T.J., Helgeson, K. and Mauras, N. (2001) Recombinant Human Growth Hormone and Recombinant Human Insulin-Like Growth Factor I Diminish the Catabolic Effects of Hypogonadism in Man: Metabolic and Molecular Effects. *Journal of Clinical Endocrinology & Metabolism*, **86**, 2211-2219.

[22] Mauras, N. and Haymond, M.W. (2005) Are the Metabolic Effects of GH and IGF-I Separable? *Growth Hormone & IGF Research*, **15**, 19-27.

[23] Mauras, N., Martinez, V., Rini, A. and Guevara-Aguirre, J. (2000) Recombinant Human Insulin-Like Growth Factor Has Significant Anabolic Effects in Adults with Growth Hormone Receptor Deficiency: Studies on Protein, Glucose, and Lipid Metabolism. *Journal of Clinical Endocrinology & Metabolism*, **85**, 3036-3042.

[24] Shimoda, N., Tashiro, T., Yamamori, H., Takagi, K., Nakajima, N. and Ito, I. (1997) Effects of Growth Hormone and Insulin-Like Growth Factor I on Protein Metabolism, Gut Morphology, and Cell-Mediated Immunity in Burned Rats. *Nutrition*, **13**, 540-516.

[25] Shaneyfelt, T., Husein, R., Bubley, G. and Mantzoros, C.S. (2000) Hormonal Predictors of Prostate Cancer: A Meta-Analysis. *Journal of Clinical Oncology*, **18**, 847-853.

[26] Toniolo, P., Bruning, P.F., Akhmedkhanov, A., Bonfrer, J.M., Koenig, K.L., Lukanova, A., Shore, R.E. and Zeleniuch-Jacquotte, A. (2000) Serum Insulin-Like Growth Factor-I and Breast Cancer. *International Journal of Cancer*, **88**, 828-832. http://dx.doi.org/10.1002/1097-0215(20001201)88:5<828::AID-IJC22>3.0.CO;2-8

[27] Ibrahim, Y.H. and Yee, D. (2004) Insulin-Like Growth Factor-I and Cancer Risk. *Growth Hormone & IGF Research*, **14**, 261-269. http://dx.doi.org/10.1016/j.ghir.2004.01.005

[28] Tomizawa, M., Shinozaki, F., Sugiyama, T., Yamamoto, S., Sueishi, M. and Yoshida, T. (2010) Insulin-Like Growth Factor-I Receptor in Proliferation and Motility of Pancreatic Cancer. *World Journal of Gastroenterology*, **16**, 1854-1858. http://dx.doi.org/10.3748/wjg.v16.i15.1854

[29] Koenuma, M., Yamori, T. and Tsuruo, T. (1989) Insulin and Insulin-Like Growth Factor I Stimulate Proliferation of Metastatic Variants of Colon Carcinoma 26. *Cancer Science*, **80**, 51-58. http://dx.doi.org/10.1111/j.1349-7006.1989.tb02244.x

[30] Lippman, M.E. (1985) Growth Regulation of Human Breast Cancer. *Clinical Research*, **33**, 375-382.

[31] Li, S.L., Liang, S.J., Guo, N., Wu, A.M. and Fujita-Yamaguchi, Y. (2000) Single-Chain Antibodies against Human Insulin-Like Growth Factor I Receptor: Expression, Purification, and Effect on Tumor Growth. *Cancer Immunology*,

Immunotherapy, **49**, 243-252. http://dx.doi.org/10.1007/s002620000115

[32] Reinmuth, N., Liu, W., Fan, F., Jung, Y.D., Ahmad, S.A., Stoeltzing, O., Bucana, C.D., Radinsky, R. and Ellis, L.M. (2002) Blockade of Insulin-Like Growth Factor I Receptor Function Inhibits Growth and Angiogenesis of Colon Cancer. *Clinical Cancer Research*, **8**, 3259-3569.

[33] Key, T.J., Appleby, G.N., Reeves, G.K. and Roddam, A.W. (2010) Insulin-Like Growth Factor I (IGF1), IGF Binding Protein 3 (IGFBP3), and Breast Cancer Risk: Pooled Individual Data Analysis of 17 Prospective Studies. *Lancet Oncology*, **11**, 530-542. http://dx.doi.org/10.1016/S1470-2045(10)70095-4

[34] Ma, J., Pollak, M.N., Giovannucci, E., Chan, J.M., Tao, Y., Hennekens, C.H. and Stampfer, M.J. (1999) Prospective Study of Colorectal Cancer Risk in Men and Plasma Levels of Insulin-Like Growth Factor (IGF)-I and IGF-Binding Protein-3. *Journal of the National Cancer Institute*, **91**, 620-625. http://dx.doi.org/10.1093/jnci/91.7.620

[35] Cleveland, R.J., Gammon, M.D., Edmiston, S.N., Teitelbaum, S.L., Britton, J.A., Terry, M.B., Eng, S.M., Neugut, A.I., Santella, R.M. and Conway, K. (2006) IGF1 CA Repeat Polymorphisms, Lifestyle Factors and Breast Cancer Risk in the Long Island Breast Cancer Study Project. *Carcinogenesis*, **27**, 758-765. http://dx.doi.org/10.1093/carcin/bgi294

[36] Zecevic, M., Amos, C.I., Gu, X., Campos, I.M., Jones, J.S., Lynch, P.M., Rodriguez-Bigas, M.A. and Frazier, M.L. (2006) IGF1 Gene Polymorphism and Risk for Hereditary Nonpolyposis Colorectal Cancer. *Journal of the National Cancer Institute*, **98**, 139-143. http://dx.doi.org/10.1093/jnci/djj016

[37] McGrath, M., Lee, I.M., Buring, J. and De Vivo, I. (2011) Common Genetic Variation within IGFI, IGFII, IGFBP-1, and IGFBP-3 and Endometrial Cancer Risk. *Gynecologic Oncology*, **120**, 174-178. http://dx.doi.org/10.1016/j.ygyno.2010.10.012

[38] Shitara, K., Ito, S., Misawa, K., Ito, Y., Ito, H., Hosono, S., Watanabe, M., Tajima, K., Tanaka, H., Muro, K. and Matsuo, K. (2012) Genetic Polymorphism of IGF-I Predicts Recurrence in Patients with Gastric Cancer Who Have Undergone Curative Gastrectomy. *Annals of Oncology*, **23**, 659-664. http://dx.doi.org/10.1093/annonc/mdr293

[39] Felice, D.L., El-Shennawy, L., Zhao, S., Lantvit, D.L., Shen, Q., Unterman, T.G., Swanson, S.M. and Frasor, J. (2013) Growth Hormone Potentiates 17β-Estradiol-Dependent Breast Cancer Cell Proliferation Independently of IGF-I Receptor Signaling. *Endocrinology*, **154**, 3219-3227. http://dx.doi.org/10.1210/en.2012-2208

[40] Wang, W., Iresjö, B.M., Karlsson, L. and Svanberg, E. (2000) Provision of rhIGF-I/IGFBP-3 Complex Attenuated Development of Cancer Cachexia in an Experimental Tumor Model. *Clinical Nutrition*, **19**, 127-132. http://dx.doi.org/10.1054/clnu.1999.0090

[41] Cohen, P., Clemmons, D.R. and Rosenfeld, R.G. (2000) Does the GH-IGF Axis Play a Role in Cancer Pathogenesis? *Growth Hormone & IGF Research*, **10**, 297-305. http://dx.doi.org/10.1054/ghir.2000.0171

[42] Izzo, L., Meggiorini, M.L., Nofroni, I., Pala, A., De Felice, C., Meloni, P., Simari, T., Izzo, S., Pugliese, F., Impara, L., Merlini, G., Di Cello, P., Cipolla, V., Forcione, A.R., Paliotta, A., Domenici, L. and Bolognese, A. (2012) Insulin-Like Growth Factor-I (IGF-1), IGF-Binding Protein-3 (IGFBP-3) and Mammographic Features. *Il Giornale di Chirurgia*, **33**, 153-162.

[43] Justová, V., Lacinová, Z., Melenovský, V., Marek, J., Holly, J.M. and Hass, T. (2001) The Changes of IGF Binding Proteins after rhGH Administration to Patients Totally Dependent on Parenteral Nutrition. *Growth Hormone & IGF Research*, **11**, 407-415. http://dx.doi.org/10.1054/ghir.2001.0257

29

Effects of mRNA, Protein Expression and Activity for Myocardial SOD2 by a Single Bout of or Long-Term Strenuous Endurance Exercise in Rats

Simao Xu*, Weichun Liu, Minhua Li

Department of Physical Education, Guangxi Normal University, Guilin, China
Email: *xusimao666@163.com

Abstract

Objective: To explore the effects of myocardial SOD2 by strenuous endurance exercise. Methods: 27 grown male SD rats were randomly divided into control group (C), a single bout of strenuous endurance exercise group (E1) and seventh-week strenuous endurance exercise group (E2). Real-time PCR was used to observe the changes of mRNA expression for myocardial SOD2. Western bolt was used to observe the changes of SOD2 protein expression. In addition, SOD2, T-SOD and SOD1 activity changes were observed. Results: Myocardial SOD2 expression level at mRNA and protein of Group E1, E2 was significantly higher than that in group C, and SOD2 and T-SOD activity in group E2 were significantly higher than those in group C. Those changes were more obvious in group E2. Conclusions: Strenuous endurance exercise can improve level of myocardial SOD2 expression at mRNA and protein, and enhance the activity for SOD2, thus increasing the activity for T-SOD. Effect of long-term strenuous endurance exercise was better than a single bout of one.

Keywords

SOD2, Strenuous Endurance Exercise, Myocardia

1. Introduction

In recent years, with the development of economy and society, people's diet and lifestyle change, and heart

*Corresponding author.

health is also seriously threatened, *i.e.*, the incidence of ischemic heart disease was on the rise "year by year". Therefore, heart health maintenance has always been an important issue. According to the researches, the damage of Reactive Oxygen Species (ROS) plays a considerable role in the process of myocardial pathological changes. It is of great significance to maintain the heart health, such as the prevention of ischemic cardiomyopathy, to increase the ability of heart's antioxidant as well as to effectively remove ROS. Numerous studies have indicated that appropriate exercises can promote heart health and resist to myocardial ischemia-reperfusion injury [1]-[4]. What's more, according to powers and other researchers, the effect of exercise on heart health is closely related to the improved myocardial antioxidant capacity [5]. However, it has yet to explore the improved myocardial antioxidant capacity caused by exercise and cardioprotective effects.

As it's known to all, enzymatic defensive system acts as a considerable part in body issue's antioxidant and ROS removal, among which Superoxide Dismutase (SOD) is regarded as the first protective barrier to defense ROS. Therefore, the improvement of SOD activity marks the myocardial antioxidant capacity enhancement. A great number of researches have shown that exercise can improve the activity of myocardial Total Superoxide Dismutase (T-SOD). However it is not difficult to find that exercise models in studies concerned focus on the high-intensity intermittent exercise or moderate-intensity endurance exercise model; other possibly existed and targeted suitable exercise models needed further exploration. On the other hand, SOD has two types in higher animal vivo, one being Cu, Zn Superoxide Dismutase (SOD1) existed in cytoplasm, another Manganese Superoxide Dismutase (SOD2) in mitochondria; therefore, strengthening in-depth study of SOD types will contribute a further understanding of protective effects of exercise on the heart and its possible mechanisms. Since mitochondria play a crucial role in the maintenance of cardiomyocytes normal function and structural integrity. In addition, they are main sites of ROS production. Theoretically, the increase of SOD2 function has a significant effect on ROS removal as well as myocardial protection. Taking the above reasons into consideration, this study is to observe whether strenuous endurance exercise can accelerate the improvement of myocardial SOD2 expression at mRNA and protein as well as their activity level or not, trying to prove that this effect can be enhanced by long-term endurance exercise. It's also expected to rich the theory of exercise's protective effect on the heart, and to improve practical applications of sports and fitness on cardioprotective effects.

2. Materials and Methods

2.1. Research Objects

27 grown male Sprague Dawley (SD) rats (SPF grade), weighting 146 ± 15 g, are bought from Guangxi Medical University Laboratory Animal Center. They are raised in standard rodent cages, feeding freely. Favorable ventilated conditions, controlling room temperature at about 27˚C and natural light are provided.

2.2. Experiment Methods

2.2.1. Groups and Exercise Modes

After one week adaptive feeding, 27 grown male SD rats were randomly divided into control group (group C, n = 9), a single bout of strenuous endurance exercise group (group E1, n = 9) and seventh-week strenuous endurance exercise group (group E2, n = 9). Group E1 and E2 trained endurance running on treadmills (Type DSPT 202 made by Hangzhou Litai S & T Co. Ltd.). Before formal training, the both groups firstly conducted three-day adaptive treadmill exercise (0˚, 15 m/min), and then strenuous endurance running at a speed of 22 m/min and gradient of +10˚ (85% $VO2_{max}$) for 30 min daily referred to Bedford and other researchers standards [6]. Group E1 only exercised one day while group E2 exercised 6 days/week (Sunday off) for continuous 7 weeks.

2.2.2. Drawing Materials

Intraperitoneal anesthesia with urethane (1.2 g/kg) were performed when group E1 after exercise within 24 h - 48 h, group E2 after the last exercise within 24 h - 48 h together with group C, and then hearts were quickly taken and ventricular myocardia were cut, washing with PBS. Ventricular myocardia were cut into small pieces during an ice-bath. Most ventricular myocardial pieces, placed immediately into the −80˚C ultra-low temperature refrigerator after liquid nitrogen flash freeze, were used for determining SOD2 expression at mRNA and protein; that remaining small portion was used for the observation of SOD activity after weighing (about 100 mg) and recording.

2.2.3. Real-Time Fluorescent Quantitative PCR

SYBR Green I method was adopted, with necessary reagent provided by American Life Technologies Co. Ltd. Real-time PCR primers were synthesized by Invitrogen Corporation Shanghai Representative Office.

Upstream of SOD2: AAGGAGAGTTGCTGGAGGCTATC

Downstream: CTCCTTATTGAAGCCAAGCCAG

Upstream of β-actin: CATTGTCACCAACTGGGACGATA

Downstream: GGATGGCTACGTACATGGCTG

1) RNA extraction

A portion of frozen myocardial tissue was taken, weighted (100 mg) and recorded. Grind into powder after adding liquid nitrogen, and then the total myocardial RNA were immediately extracted under the guidance of Trizol kit instructions after the liquid nitrogen were evaporated.

2) Synthesize cDNA by Reverse Transcription (RT)

5 μl (5 μg) of extracted myocardial RNA samples, together with 0.5 μl of Oligo (dt) primer (50 uM), 0.5 μl of random primer, 1 μl of dNTP Mix (10 mM), and 5 μl of DEPC-treated water added one after another, gets a Mix I of 12 μl, 5 min warm bath at 65˚C and then 1 min ice bath at once. Afterwards, 20 μl of Mix II, received by adding 4 μl of 5× First-Strand buffer, 2 μl of 0.1 M dTT, 1 μl of RNaseout (40 U/μl), and 1 μl of SuperScrip III RT (200 U/μl) into Mix I, was treated with 5 min bath at 25˚C, 60 min bath at 50˚C and 15 min bath at 70˚C. The resulting cDNA was placed on ice immediately.

3) Real-time PCR

PCR solution was carried out PCR amplification reaction in real-time PCR instrument (Type 7500 Fast, Life technologies' product). The real-time PCR reaction system is: 14 μl of ultrapure water, 2 μl of 10× PCR buffer solution, 1 μl of magnesian ion (50 mM), 0.5 μl of upstream primer (10 uM), 0.3 μl of SYBR (20×) fluorescent dye, 0.5 μl of downstream primer (10 uM), 0.2 μl of Taq DNA Polymerase, 1 μl of template, accounting for 20 μl. Reaction parameters are: initial denaturation for 2 min at 95˚C; 40 PCR cycles (95˚C, 10 S; 60˚C, 30 S; 70˚C, 45 S). During this course, Ct values (cycled threshold values) of tested products were recorded when fluorescence signal intensity was significantly enhanced; three wells were made in each test sample, calculating the average of each sample's Ct value. Continue to slowly heat from 70˚C to 95˚C after completion, and then melting curves of PCR products were established in order to observe the specificity of amplified products.

After that, the Relative Expression (RE) of target gene SOD2 mRNA was calculated by the $2^{-\Delta\Delta Ct}$ Method [7], using housekeeping gene β-actin as reference gene. Average value of each sample was taken as Ct, $\Delta Ct = (Ct_{\text{target gene}} - Ct_{\text{reference gene}})$, $\Delta\Delta Ct = (Ct_{\text{experimental group}} - Ct_{\text{control group}})$, $2^{-\Delta\Delta Ct}$ was RE of mRNA for SOD2.

2.2.4. Western Bolt for Myocardia SOD2

The remaining frozen myocardial tissues, weighted and recorded, were speedily ground into powder with liquid nitrogen. They were immediately placed in EP tube after evaporation, and then RIPA lysate (a concentration of 1 mM) formulated from PMSF buffer was added to fully lyse in the proportion of 20 mg of myocardial tissues to 200 μl of lysate (protein extraction reagent); supernatant was collected by hypothermic centrifugal machine (centrifugal force 10,000 - 14,000 ×g, 3 - 5 min). BSA (Bicinchoninic acid) Method was adopted to determine the total protein concentration.

50 μg of myocardial total protein, using prestained maker as protein molecular weight marker, were carried out 12% SDS-PAGE protein electrophoresis (constant pressure electrophoresis with separating gel at 80 V and stacking gel at 100 V) until the front edge of color marker-bromophenol blue stopped electrophoresis when went down to the end of gel. The separated protein bands (0.20 μm of SOD2 and 0.45 μm of i-actin) were transferred to a PVDF membrane by wet cell transmembrane method (250 mA constant current for 1 h). 5% BSA buffer was closed at room temperature for 2 h. After that, SOD2 primary antibodies (diluted rabbit anti-human polyclonal antibody at the ratio of 1 to 1000) and β-actin primary antibodies (diluted mouse anti-human monoclonal antibody at the ratio of 1 to 1000) were added into these two membranes correspondingly. Incubate them overnight at 4˚C, and then wash the membrane with TBST three times (10 min/time). Secondary antibodies marked by rabbit anti-horseradish peroxidase (dilute at the ratio of 1 to 2000) and by mouse anti-horseradish peroxidase (dilute at the ratio of 1 to 2000) were mixed in correspondingly. The two mixtures were incubated on the shaking table at room temperature for 1 h, and then washed with TBST three times (10 min/time) as well as developed with chemiluminescence. Electrophoretic bands were treated by Gel-pro analyzer software to analyze the gray value of each band area, the ratio of target band (SOD2)'s grey value to reference band (β-actin)'s grey

value representing the expression level at target protein.

For the main reagents used in experiments, RIRA lysate, BCA kit as well as ECL kit were bought from Shanghai Beyotime Biotechnology Co., Ltd., PMSF buffer is provided by Amresco Company, BSA by Sigma-Aldrich Co. LLC; *β*-actin primary antibodies, secondary antibodies labeled rabbit anti-horseradish peroxidase as well as secondary antibodies labeled mouse anti-horseradish peroxidase were bought from Beijing Zhongshan Golden Bridge Biotechnology Co., Ltd. while SOD2 primary antibodies from Epitomics Biotechnology Co., Ltd.; TBST from Beijing Solarbio Science & Technology Co., Ltd. Electrophoresis was Powerpac Basic Electrophoresis bought from American Bio-Rad Laboratories, Inc.

2.2.5. Determination of Myocardial SOD2 Activity

10% homogenates were made and then supernatant was collected by centrifuge (4000 rpm, 30 min). SOD1 and T-SOD activity were detected with hydroxylamine method, and finally SOD2 activity was obtained by T-SOD activity minus SOD1 activity. SOD kits were bought from Nanjing Jiancheng Biotechnology Co., Ltd.

2.2.6. Statistical Analysis

Experimental data were presented as "mean ± standard deviation" ($\overline{X} \pm S$). Statistical analysis was completed by SPSS for windows version 17.0 software. The experimental results were all analyzed with One-Way Analysis of Variance (ANOVA). After-effect test was conducted by Least-Significant Difference (LSD) Method in the case of homogeneity of variance, otherwise by Tamhane's T2 Method. $P < 0.05$ was regarded as the standard of significant differences.

3. Results

3.1. Comparisons of RE of mRNA for Myocardia SOD2 in Rats

Melting curve of amplification products in SYBR Green I real-time PCR reflects that solubility changes with temperature, with temperatures as ordinate against solubility as abscissa. In this study, melting curve of both myocardia SOD2 gene and myocardia *β*-actin gene in rats only appeared a single peak; besides, the melting temperature (Tm) were about 85.35˚C and 88.43˚C respectively, approximately nearing to the annealing temperature of the corresponding products: amplification products were in preferable specificity.

Real-time PCR amplification curve was used cycles as ordinate against real-time fluorescence intensity as abscissa during PCR. According to statistics, RE of mRNA for myocardia SOD2 in group E1 and E2 was obviously higher than that in group C (control group), marking significant differences; RE in group E2 were more distinct than those in group E1, marking significant differences (**Table 1**; **Figure 1**).

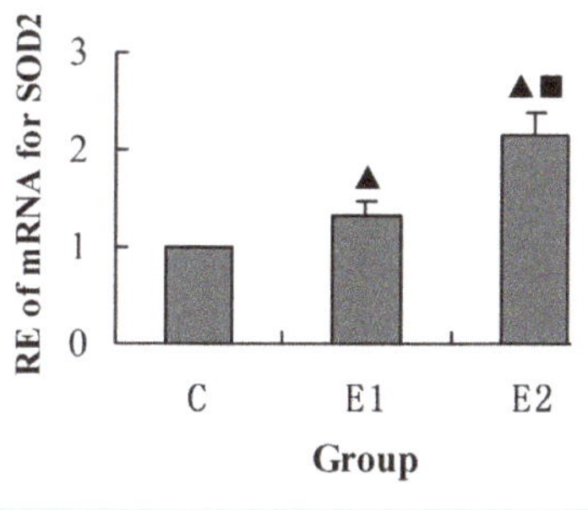

Figure 1. Diagram of changes in RE of mRNA for myocardia SOD2 in rats. ▲Compared with group C, $p < 0.05$; ■Compared with group E1, $p < 0.05$.

Table 1. Changes in RE of mRNA for myocardia SOD2 in rats.

Group	N	SOD2 mRNA
C	9	1.00 ± 0.00
E1	9	1.32 ± 0.16[a]
E2	9	2.16 ± 0.23[ab]

[a]Compared with group C, $p < 0.05$; [b]Compared with group E1, $p < 0.05$.

3.2. Changes in RE of Protein for Myocardia SOD2 in Rats

Group E1 and E2 myocardia SOD2 expression level at protein was clearly improved compared with group C, marking meaningful differences; levels in group E2 were more distinct than those in group E1, marking meaningful differences (**Figure 2**; **Table 2**; **Figure 3**).

3.3. Changes of Activity Level for Myocardia SOD2 in Rats

SOD2 activity was gotten by T-SOD activity subtracting the SOD1. The activity of myocardia SOD2 and T-SOD in group E1 and E2 was clearly improved compared with group C, marking significant differences; improvements in group E2 were more distinct than those in group E1, marking significant differences (**Table 3**; **Figure 4**).

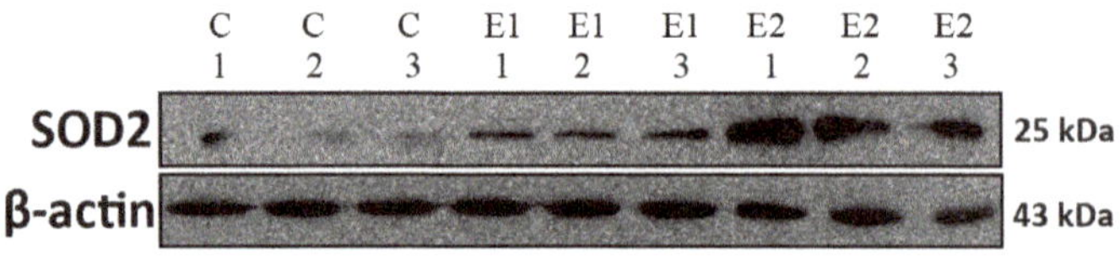

Figure 2. Diagram of western blotting for myocardia SOD2 in rats. 1, 2, 3, three different individual samples in each group rats for C, E1, E2.

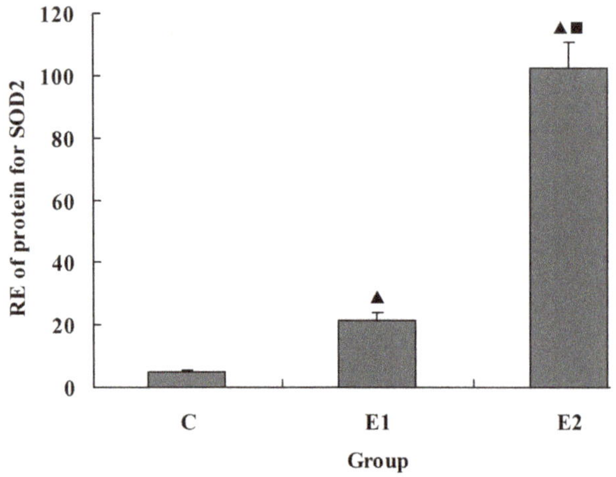

Figure 3. Diagram of changes in RE of protein for myocardia SOD2 in rats. ▲Compared with group C, $p < 0.05$; ■Compared with group E1, $p < 0.05$.

Table 2. Changes in RE of protein for myocardia SOD2 in rats.

Group	n	SOD2
C	9	4.743 ± 0.652
E1	9	21.367 ± 2.787[a]
E2	9	102.424 ± 8.336[ab]

[a]Compared with group C, $p < 0.05$; [b]Compared with group E1, $p < 0.05$.

Table 3. Changes in activity of myocardia SOD2, T-SOD in rats (U/mg·prot).

Group	n	SOD1	SOD2	T-SOD
C	9	77.820 ± 8.955	39.653 ± 6.032	117.473 ± 13.852
E1	9	76.674 ± 9.743	54.274 ± 7.257[a]	131.948 ± 14.285[a]
E2	9	77.221 ± 9.724	79.314 ± 8.456[ab]	156.535 ± 15.755[ab]

[a]Compared with group C, $p < 0.05$; [b]Compared with group E1, $p < 0.05$.

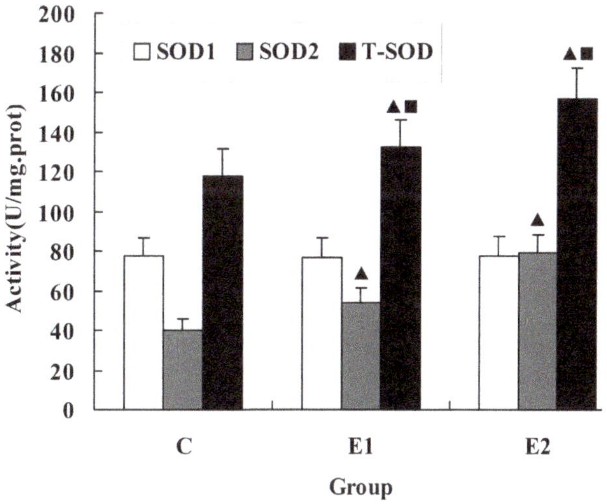

Figure 4. Diagram of changes in activity of myocardia SOD2, T-SOD in rats. ▲Compared with group C, $p < 0.05$; ■Compared with group E1, $p < 0.05$.

4. Discussion

Studies on the impact of exercise on the heart earliest started in an anatomy find, Robinson, an Englishman, pointed out that relative weight of heart in high-intensity physical activity animal was heavier than that in low-intensity physical activity animal in 1748. As humans, Henschen, a Swedish scholar, first discovered the enlargement of skier's heart by percussion in 1899, and then put forward the term of "Athlete's Heart". Afterwards, the field of sports medicine had committed to the study of "effect of exercises on cardiac structure and function", and gradually penetrated into the field of molecular biology. Up to now, it's generally viewed that the exercise is a "double-edged sword" for excessive exercises may be harmful to heart health while moderate exercises are beneficial to it, being able to pre-treat various cardiovascular diseases. In the past reports about "exercise and heart health", most intervention models were moderate-intensity endurance exercise. In recent years, some researches had been conducted by using high-intensity intermittent exercise as intervention model at home, e.g. some references pointed out that intermittent high-intensity exercise can protect the heart and improve myocardial tolerance of ischemia [8] [9]. However, it still needed to build more sports models for reference how to enhance heart health by rationally using physical exercise with targets, such as the improvement of myocardial antioxidant capacity. What's more, this study suggested that excessive exercise, such as intermittent high-intensity exercise, may not be practical for the old and infirm as well as for the crowd urgently needing for sports and fitness, and was somewhat difficult to popularize. That is why endurance exercise was more widespread in physical exercise at present. Taking these conditions into consideration, this study chose the model of "a single bout of or seven-week strenuous endurance exercise" to investigate the effects of myocardial antioxidase SOD by strenuous endurance exercise. It's clear that there were two kinds of SOD in myocardial tissue, namely SOD1 and SOD2.

According to this study, a single bout of or seven-week strenuous endurance exercise can outstandingly improve the level of myocardial SOD2 expression at mRNA and protein. SOD's main function was to remove ROS in vivo, which was mainly produced in mitochondria, where also lay SOD2, a type of SOD. In this study, the increase of myocardial SOD2 expression level may be adaptive changes of ROS increase and oxidative stress stimulate made by mitochondrial. It was found that a single bout of long-term high-intensity endurance exercise can give rise to the increase of myocardial malondialdehyde (MDA) content [10], suggesting the increase of myocardial oxidative stress level. The author considered that the improving myocardial oxidative stress level after exercise resulted from exercise-induced myocardial ischemia and hypoxia. In one recent study, rats were carried out a single bout of strenuous endurance exercise at a speed of 19 - 21 m/min and gradient of +10° (80% $VO2_{max}$) to "exhaustion" [11]. And then they found that rats' ECG presented characteristic changes of myocardial ischemia and myocardial stunning, and myocardia had ischemic necrosis, both of which showing that exercise can induce myocardial ischemia [11]. In addition, other similar studies showed that a single bout of exhaustive strenuous endurance exercise can induce myocardial ischemia in rats [12]. The model of a single bout of "exhaustive" strenuous endurance exercise in the above references, differing from that of a single bout of or long-term strenuous endurance exercise with quantitative loads in the present study, still suggested the existence of myocardial ischemia phenomenon by strenuous endurance exercise. Great amount of studies had proved that effects of exercise-induced myocardial ischemia and hypoxia on myocardial structure and function were bitterly similar to the clinical pathological myocardial ischemia; Large quantity of ROS were generated and oxidative stress levels were significantly increased in myocardium in the process of exercise-induced myocardial ischemia (hypoxia) and reperfusion. Distinguished from clinical pathological myocardial ischemia, exercise-induced myocardial ischemia was relative myocardial ischemia and hypoxia due to the high level of myocardial metabolic as well as initiative ischemia and hypoxia occurred under the protective monitoring system [13]. When cannot tolerate hypoxia, the body will reduce the degree of ischemia and hypoxia by reducing exercise intensity or stopping exercise, thus avoiding myocardial irreversible damage resulted from excessive ischemia and hypoxia [13]. Therefore, combined this study's results and analyses, the author held that relative myocardial ischemia and hypoxia of reasonable duration caused by strenuous endurance exercise gave impetus to a certain amount of ROS and some degree of oxidative stress in mitochondria, which were extremely sensitive to ischemia, as long as exercise will not be too durative. Adaptive changes, occurring after mitochondria were stimulated by oxidative stress, manifested as increased expression at SOD2 mRNA as well as at protein. Their heighten guarantees the increase of activity with the consequences of enhanced mitochondrial elimination ability of ROS. Furthermore, from the comparisons of changes in a single bout of strenuous endurance exercise group (group E1) and seven-week strenuous endurance exercise group (group E2), those changes were more obvious in group E2, which demonstrated that the improving amount of SOD2 mRNA and protein expression of long-term endurance exercise was clearly more than that of a single bout of exercise.

Yamashita and other researchers certified that long-term moderate-intensity endurance exercise increased the activity of myocardial SOD2 by antisense oligonucleotides technology [14]. Hou and other scholars detected that myocardial SOD2 activity in rats can be improved by swimming without load, 1 h per day for three days while SOD1 activity was unchanged [15]. In this study, a single bout of or seven-week strenuous endurance exercise gave rise to distinguished improvement of SOD2 and T-SOD activity; meanwhile, SOD1 activity showed no significant change. Some references discovered that endurance exercise stepped up muscle SOD2 protein expression and activity [16] [17]. Moreover, in this study, myocardial SOD2 activity trends were consistent with those of SOD2 mRNA and protein expression. Therefore, exercise can increase myocardial SOD2 protein expression, enhance its activity as well as improve T-SOD activity by stimulating SOD2 mRNA expression in this study. Moreover, it was found that both the increasing level of myocardial mRNA and protein expression and improvement level of SOD2 and T-SOD activity after seven-week strenuous endurance exercise were much better than those after a single bout of strenuous endurance exercise, which revealed that long-term endurance exercise can improve exercise effects.

5. Conclusions

Strenuous endurance exercise can stimulate myocardial SOD2 expression at mRNA and protein and enhance the activity for SOD2, thus increasing the activity for T-SOD.

The improvements of myocardial mRNA and protein expression as well as the activity for SOD2 by seven-week strenuous endurance exercise were all more obvious than those by a single bout of strenuous endurance exercise, demonstrating that long-term endurance exercise can improve exercise effects.

Research Support

Guangxi Natural Science Foundation of China (Project Number: 2013GXNSFBA019146).

References

[1] Ascensao, A., Ferrira, R. and Magalhaes, J. (2007) Exercise-Induced Cardioprotection-Biochemical, Morpho-Logical and Functional Evidence in Whole Tissue and Isolated Mitochondria. *International Journal of Cardiology*, **117**, 16-30. http://dx.doi.org/10.1016/j.ijcard.2006.04.076

[2] Brown, D.A., Chicco, A.J., Jew, K.N., Johnson, M.S., Lynch, J.M., Watson, P.A. and Moore, R.L. (2005) Cardioprotection Afforded by Chronic Exercise Is Mediated by the Sarcolemmal, and Not the Mitochondrial, Isoform of the KATP Channel in the Rat. *The Journal of Physiology*, **569**, 913-924. http://dx.doi.org/10.1113/jphysiol.2005.095729

[3] Budiono, B.P., Hoe, L.E.S., Peart, J.N., Sabapathy, S., Ashton, K.J., Haseler, L.J. and Headrick, J.P. (2012) Voluntary Running in Mice Beneficially Modulates Myocardial Ischemic Tolerance, Signaling Kinases, and Gene Expression Patterns. *American Journal of Physiology-Regulatory Integrative and Comparative Physiology*, **302**, R1091-R1100. http://dx.doi.org/10.1152/ajpregu.00406.2011

[4] French, J.P., Quindry, J.C., Falk, D.J., Staib, J.L., Lee, Y., Wang, K.K.W. and Powers, S.K. (2006) Ischemia-Reperfusion-Induced Calpain Activation and SERCA2a Degradation Are Attenuated by Exercise Training and Calpain Inhibition. *American Journal of Physiology. Heart and Circulatory Physiology*, **290**, H128-H136. http://dx.doi.org/10.1152/ajpheart.00739.2005

[5] Powers, S.K., Sollanek, K.J., Wiggs, M.P., Demirel, H.A. and Smuder, A.J. (2014) Exercise-Induced Improvements in Myocardial Antioxidant Capacity: The Antioxidant Players and Cardioprotection. *Free Radical Research*, **48**, 43-51. http://dx.doi.org/10.3109/10715762.2013.825371

[6] Bedford, T.G., Tipton, C.M., Wilson, N.C., Oppliger, R.A. and Gisolfi, C.V. (1979) Maximum Oxygen Consumption of Rats and Its Changes with Various Experimental Procedures. *Journal of Applied Physiology: Respiratory, Environmental and Exercise Physiology*, **47**, 1278-1283.

[7] Pfaffl, M.W. (2001) A New Mathematical Model for Relative Quantification in Real-Time PT-PCR. *Nucleic Acids Research*, **29**, e45. http://dx.doi.org/10.1093/nar/29.9.e45

[8] Peng, F.L., Lu, Y.L., Zhang, L., Chen, D.Q. and Deng, S.X. (2009) The Cardioprotective Effect of Intermittent Exercises on Ischemia-Reperfusion Rats' Myocardium. *Chinese Journal of Rehabilitation Medicine*, **24**, 910-913.

[9] Peng, F.L., Guo, Y.J. and Zhang, L. (2010) The Effects of Interval Training and Acute Interval Exercise on Ischemia-Reperfusion Rats' ECG and Serum Myocardial Enzymes. *China Sport Science and Technology*, **46**, 102-105.

[10] Xu, S.M., Liu, T.B. and Su, Q.S. (2011) Study on Heavy Load Training-Induced Cardiac Contractility Changes of Rats, and the Relationship between This Changes and the Levels of Cardiac Free Radical, Calcium Ions. *China Sport Science*, **31**, 73-78.

[11] Li, S.C., Duan, Y.M. and Su, Q.S. (2012) The Establishment of Exercise-Induced Myocardial Stunning Model of Rat with Repeated Exhaustive Exercise on Treadmills. *China Sport Science*, **32**, 49-54.

[12] Xu, S.M, Zhou, Y. and Wang, J. (2014) Abnormal ECG Changes and Energy Metabolic Disturbance after an Exhaustive Exercises in Rats. *Journal of Tianjin University of Sport*, **29**, 132-135.

[13] Su, Q.S. (2004) Effect on the Structure of Heart during Re-Oxygen Process. *Journal of Chengdu Physical Education Institute*, **30**, 61-64.

[14] Yamashita, N., Hoshida, S., Otsu, K., Asahi, M., Kuzuya, T. and Hori, M. (1999) Exercise Provides Direct Biphasic Cardioprotection via Manganese Superoxide Dismutase Activation. *The Journal of Experimental Medicine*, **189**, 1699-1706. http://dx.doi.org/10.1084/jem.189.11.1699

[15] Hou, Y.Y, Ma, Z.Y. and Fan, X.Z. (2010) Protective Effect of Short-Term Exercise on Rat Ischemic/Reperfused Myocardium and Its Mechanism. *Suzhou University Journal of Medical Science*, **30**, 50-53.

[16] Wenz, T., Diaz, F., Hernandez, D. and Moraes, C.T. (2009) Endurance Exercise Is Protective for Mice with Mitochondrial Myopathy. *Journal of Applied Physiology*, **106**, 1712-1719. http://dx.doi.org/10.1152/japplphysiol.91571.2008

[17] Smuder, A.J., Min, K., Hudson, M.B., Kavazis, A.N., Kwon, O., Nelson, W.B. and Powers, S.K. (2012) Endurance Exercise Attenuates Ventilator-Induced Diaphragm Dysfunction. *Journal of Applied Physiology*, **112**, 501-510. http://dx.doi.org/10.1152/japplphysiol.01086.2011

List of Abbreviations

Reactive Oxygen Species (ROS); Superoxide Dismutase (SOD); Total Superoxide Dismutase (T-SOD); Cu, Zn Superoxide Dismutase (SOD1); Manganese Superoxide Dismutase (SOD2); Sprague Dawley (SD); Reverse Transcription (RT); Relative Expression (RE); Analysis of Variance (ANOVA); Least-Significant Difference (LSD); Temperature (Tm); Malondialdehyde (MDA).

30

Cosmological Origins of the Obverse-Reverse Zang Fu Pairing in Chinese Medicine

Electra Peluffo

Faculty of Medicine, Universidad de Valencia, Valencia, Spain
Email: electra.peluffo@gmail.com

Abstract

Most of the rich philosophical and scientific concepts which nurtured the Chinese thought we know today, were developed during the troubled final end of the era before ours, from V to II centuries. After reading reputed sinologists' work on the cosmological origin and subsequent evolution of the Chinese concept of parallelism-pairing in poetry, literature, mathematic and other disciplines and since it is a tradition that all branches of knowledge in China are based on the development of those initiatory thoughts, the author asked herself if such knowing on the cosmological genesis of the parallelism concept could also be applied to Chinese medicine, science that describes its coupled structures and functions in pairs, simply based on yinyang, matrix of all pairings. Therefore, this paper proposes to apply those foundations, to explain the pairing of dynamisms in medicine. This work starts out from the oracular inscriptions in ancient times, cosmological basis of these ideas and their applications to Chinese literature and from there translates this approach to the study of the pairings described by Chinese medicine, and thanks to which (qi xue) blood-energy circulation occurs in human beings. Organic and functional pairs described by Chinese medicine are the basic element to understand the concept of health and disease, and this paper is about the cosmological roots of those pairings, the cosmic resonance influence and the numerology influence in them, and the whole is illustrated both through the description of the (obverse-reverse) biao li pair, different from (inside-outside) nei wai, and the functional relationship between these two couples.

Keywords

Chinese Medicine, Cosmology, Oracles, Parallelism, Pairing, Yin Yang, Biao Li, Nei Wai, Zang Fu

1. Introduction

"one **Yin**, one **Yang**, that's the **Dao**"
Yi Jing Xi Ci

Between the subtle celestial **yang** and the dense earthy **yin**, ten thousand combinations impregnated by all movements of life move, explain *Su Wen* 5 [1] because everything that exists is a particular composition of **yin yang**. And thus, the Chinese civilization tells us once and again that the process of pairing is *natural*; that is to say under the laws of universe from the origin to the end of times and according to expert voices, this immanence is an effective way to ensure the perdurability of all aspects of the authoritarian imperial regime and its consequences [2].

Whichever the reason, from the **yinyang** dynamisms, Chinese medicine pairs up, energetically couples and pairs up organs with bowels (**zangfu**) and the corresponding meridians establish the **biao li** relationship, obverse and reverse each couple, building basis for an important guide theory for clinical practice.

There are classic treatises where parallelism is analyzed as an important rhetoric way of Chinese literature [3] and contemporary studies describing the notion of parallelism in Chinese mathematics too [4]. Thus, knowing about the existence of energetic-organic pairings in Chinese medicine, we hereby shall inquire about the reasoning which led from the cosmological parallelism to the medical organ-function pairs and the coupling of meridians in acupuncture.

2. Chinese Vision of the World

Chinese thought gives us a vision of the world based on the *pairing* among other concepts. And by using this word we want to describe becomingness or a *process* which starts from a duality in permanent interaction: opposition and complementariness as a result of a *parallelism* that in ancient times was already shown by oracular inscriptions from the second BC millennium. These inscriptions, considered the origin of Chinese writing, essentially constitute the embryonic written expression of Eastern thought.

Parallelism (*para* = near, close to, *allos* = other, alien) is not just a simple formal operation to distribute and align without modifying the paired members, procedure which, being concepts threaded in a two-to-two basis without any possibility of change, would reflect a symmetry solely geometrical and therefore static [5].

To the Chinese tradition, the pairing is a basic dynamism, conceptually opposite and complementary which allows existence, subject the author has already considered in one of her previous books [6]. This is not to say that Western culture had not elaborate concepts on antinomic contrapositions, but to point out that it had and has always been done in the West on an excluding basis of rigid and limiting antithesis: either it exists or it does not exist.

Chinese intuition perceives the real as a dynamic process starting from a binomial of phenomena in constant interaction, because opposition and complementarity are presented as a generalized bipolarity and "parallelism" is both initial and dynamic: ever since the originator **yinyang**, Heaven and Earth have been coupled cosmological realities which encourage and regulate each other. As **Wang Fuzhi** says the initial harmony [5] (**Dao**) already contains the opposition-complementarity relationship which is the quintessential pairing of **yinyang** for which the rest-movement alternation within constitutes its own conception and it is not a consequence of the pairing because which would the factor (external) initiating that dynamism be if it were not originated by the original interaction of the pair? The Chinese thinker did not conceive "creation" as a development of *succession*: first the sky, then the earth and after that man or as a *progression* according to which **Tai Yi** as an originator would gradually separate itself and progressively heaven and earth would be born from the original chaos [7]. Instead of that, Chinese philosophy gives us the notion of **Dao**, a word that among other terms, some Western sinologists translate as "process" (immanent laws) in opposition to "creation".

Then, what was the reflection? Heaven and earth represent the oppositional archetype, and they could not exist as two isolated halves. This interdependency is not only territorial but it is at the basis of all experiences, either because one element conditioned the other (high-low, back-forward) or because both mutually substitute each other: move-be still; be born-die... Each term in the pair depends on the other one and communicates with it, which means that one does not exist except through its relationship with the other.

Consequences arising from this correlation are used to elaborate all knowledge or knowing: no reality can be unilaterally and individually considered because everything that is real is perceived through the understanding of the relationships which bind and make the couples. Nothing exists isolated but by mutual implication; talking about one is talking simultaneously about the other and thus the parallelism or pairing relationship is neither exterior nor subaltern but rather what intrinsically makes existence. There is nothing existing outside this couple relationship which expresses a duality in unity mode. **Tai Yi**, the unity, is named by two characters.

The omnipresent expressions of parallelism in Chinese culture show a way of reflecting, of reasoning, a way of conceiving the universe according to the intuitive Chinese grasping of reality, a way of nature observation, a way of the real perceived as a becoming which elapses from a duality of elements in constant interaction.

Not surprisingly, physicians, scholars trained in this conception of cosmos and nature reasoned to applying it to the energetic dynamisms they described for the organic functionality in the human being.

3. Divinational Oracles

To show evidence of this, we go back to those oracular inscriptions where a "literary" parallelism of writing can be found in what sinologists call now *symmetrical divinations* in plastromancy (on turtle shells) and scapulomancy (bovine scapula) practiced by the **yin** people and later by the **Shang** centuries BC. As there are no other ancient divination treaties it is not possible to trace the original features of the archaic method.

It is clear that the tortoise shells drawings provided a picture of the cosmos which conditioned the writing on both sides of the midline: parallelism and symmetry **Figure 1**.

I hope this brief historical introduction serves to facilitate the understanding of both the origin and the development of the parallelism-symmetry notion (antinomy-complementarity) in the attempt to explain the origin of the concept of energetic pairing of viscera and their meridians in Chinese medicine.

Parallelism is "literary" in the broadest sense of the adjective, *i.e.* textual, and it is also included in the most disparate extra-literary subjects, in mathematics or medicine because these are texts in which the physician, the mathematician, or... the scholars in general, registered their theoretical and/or practical reasoning. Certainly, the conception of parallelism is primarily manifested in literary creation because the first texts already gave testimony of elementary impressions of parallelism which are considered spontaneous, natural as expressed by **Liu Xie** (465-522) in his presentation of this subject [3].

Moreover, parallelism in China is the representation of a principle derived from its conception of the world, *i.e.* it is a cosmological figure and its production was greatly contributed to by *Yi Jing*, divinatory practice with a specific cosmological basis of its culture which does not constitute a simple technique to just predict but a procedure to decipher the course of things because it seeks to clarify the hidden meaning of the events where the subject of the consultation lies [8].

From the initial parallelism comes the pairing of things which, as F. Jullien says, constitutes the basis which allows the understanding of the chance to exist [5], because nothing takes place in isolation, everything has access to existence through pairs. The turtle shell, rounded on top (heaven) and square at the bottom (earth) resembles the universe, not that it just represents the universe, it is the universe; a reduced model of the universe thanks to its identity in shape and longevity to the animal which embodies a fundamental virtue of cosmos: its duration. That is, making a query to the turtle was making it to the very universe itself, even when it was pre-

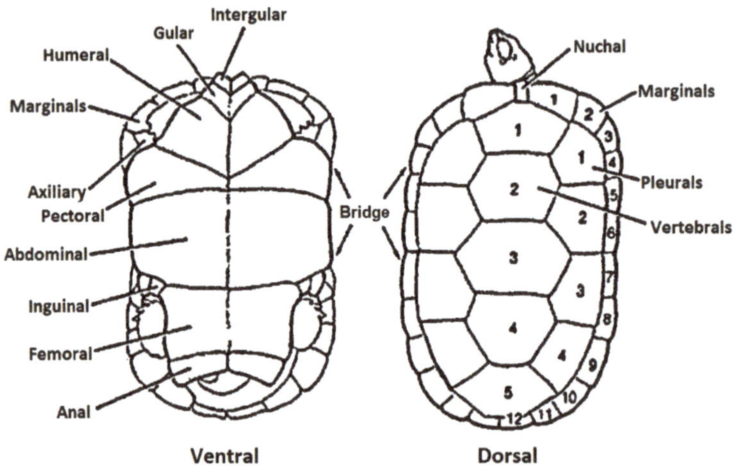

Figure 1. Turtle shell.

ferred to use the plastron (consultation was on earthly matters) rather than the dorsal portion. Both parts have a fixed number of geometrical patterns that favours a parallel evaluation of them. One first consequence seems to have been that both sides of the plastron, external and internal, naturally led to the **yinyang** notion: one turtle, two possibilities, the millenary uniduality of Chinese reflection. The shell drawings allowed the symmetrical distribution of the inscriptions marked by the red-hot awl on the ink smeared shell. It is said without hesitation, that this technique conditioned the ulterior written expression, specially poetry, and canonical literature as well, among the latter *Nei Jing Su Wen Ling Shu*, the great classical medical text.

In Chinese language the interrogative form does not exist, nor does the inversion of subject and verb which specifies an interrogative form: "Are you here?" and the modern question mark does not exist either, nor do the words "yes" and "no" natural consequence of this Chinese form of asking. Simplifying, in Chinese language questions are made by an affirmative double sentence-question: "we do this/we don't do this" and the answer is made by using the already used verb preceded, or not, by negation according to the chosen option: "we do this/ we don't do this" (**Figure 2**).

We can see that ever from interrogation there is symmetry, a parallelism which reveals a way of thinking with no absolute rules. And this double, dualistic way of questioning was scrupulously applied from the early divination spellings. The bilateral symmetry of the turtle shell led to consider that a hypothetical event always has two sides and that it is very important to consider them both, there is no **yin** without **yang** or **yang** without **yin**. And the matchable elements are the ten thousand things, everything that exists because everything exists in the very simple one of uniduality.

We said that, etymologically, parallelism comes from the idea of getting closer to the other and in the medical subject at hand, parallelism becomes *pairing*, *i.e.* approaching, and staying together in a complementary and opposite interchange, a bipolarity where the dynamic effect of parallelism is manifested from the very beginning.

Chinese medicine describes the parallel path of the main meridians on the surface, symmetrically mirror-like duplicated on both sides of the two mid lines of the body. Acupuncture maps only show the "visible" obverse which, according to Chinese thought is necessarily paired up with the hidden reverse, that of the nexus between organs and coupled meridians and the **zang fu** between themselves, as well as the relationship between internal and external **nei wai**.

Ling Shu 11 show us the broad meaning of **jingluo**

*...through the **jingmai** and the five **zang** and six **fu** the body armonizes itself with the **Dao** in heaven...*

which also defines the anatomical three-dimensionality of human being.

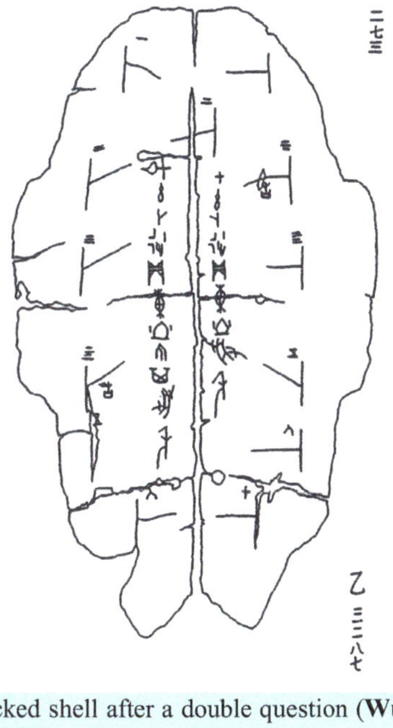

Figure 2. Cracked shell after a double question (**Wu Ding** period, XV century BC [9]).

Illustrations with meridians do not reveal the total fullness of the network of relationships woven among meridians and with the internal side of the body thus not favouring the understanding of the anatomical and functional vision of the **qi xue** flow (energy blood) basic concept in health and in sickness. So, how are the body components related? How do energy and blood circulate? How does the therapeutic function of Acupuncture take place? The **biao li** pair gives us answers.

As our interest is to look for the conceptual roots of the **biao li** pairing of **zang fu** inside the cosmological notions, we highlight the information provided by the oracle studies on the origins of this way of reflection in China since the mantic practices have influenced the evolution of the Chinese reasoning.

Concepts arisen from the observation of cosmos-nature slowly impose themselves as intellectual movement in IV-III centuries BC and culminate their maturation during the early part of **Han** dynasty in II century BC with the formalization of the basis of what would be the subsequent "nature philosophy". It is in this time when the **yinyang** school (parallelism paradigm) which specially deals with the relationship Heaven-Man, arises.

In *Zuozhuan*, first year of Duke **Zhao**, the physician **He** lists the six breaths of heaven: **yinyang** (shade-sun) *wind*, *rain*, *darkness*, *lights* which also inhabit the human body and whose harmonious interrelationship the doctor has to keep [8].

It is precisely at this time (IV-III centuries) when **yinyang** transform themselves, cleaved themselves from the initial group and turn to represent the two primary energies which constitute the uniduality, matrix to all binomials.

Chinese medicine as a discipline emerged during the Warring States (**Zhou** dynasty), period called "*Different Teachers*, *One Hundred Schools*", intense and very fertile philosophical and scientific movement in which the "Academy of **Jixia** Gate" that typified the naturalist thought stood out; teachers from all over China went there to teach under imperial patronage. Its most prominent member due to his cosmologic naturalism, **Zou Yan** (305 - 240) was counselor to sovereigns eager to increase their political prestige [10].

And these teachings had a strong influence on the theoretical development of *Neijing Su Wen Ling Shu.*

4. Biao Li Binding

Numerous are the ways of pairing described in Chinese medicine based on the variety of dynamic **yinyang**. In this case we are going to focus on the **biao li** pair.

As *Su Wen* 6 explains in "*Separations and Reunions of **Yin** and* **Yang**", it is through the **biao li** binding that are specified six pairs of meridians whose members resonates each one with the same change phase **wuxing**, five movements: Li-GB wood, H-SI fire, St-Sp earth, Lu-LI metal, and K-B water.

These pairs respond to human influences (**li**) or cosmos ones (**biao**) following the **wuxing** phases, pacing universe and man dynamism. Each movement responds to a coupled **li** meridian and a **biao** meridian. Thus we have two sources of influence, the one from man, and the one from universe: what comes from man resonates on **li** meridians and what comes from the universe does it on **biao** meridians, therefore **biao li** is an interior-exterior notion which expresses the relationships between two coupled meridians and their organs in the *interior of a same element. Su Wen* 25 says that man lives in a body that will never leave **yin yang.**

Biao li is an intra-systemic bond in a close system (the human body) because it functions between the two coupled viscera in each pair. In the organism, **li** represents the internal system (**zang**, organs) and **biao**, the external (**fu,** bowels) and they are distinguished because obverse **biao** subordinates to reverse **li**. **Biao** is the outer lining of the body while **li** is the interior of such lining. In **biao** the idea of manifestation is expressed and in **li** the hidden life one, that which from the interior, from the depth, will show up in the surface going up through the organic layers, and through that same path, what is on the surface will go back to the interior [11].

The obverse-reverse **biao li** binding is different from **nei wai** inside-outside pair. The latter describes an inter-systemic bond: human body is a system and the external environment is a different one, and there are ties between them; **nei wai** [6] ties which evoke those nexus in the internal areas of vitality (**zang fu**) with more external areas, the meridians paths. In turn, **nei wai** and **biao li** are related because the **biao li** interchanges arise from the **nei wai** spatial dynamic so allowing to distinguish visible starting from invisible, to perceive what is active in the latent, to get to the structures through the manifestations as *Suwen* 5 says.

Let's make it clear that **biao li** (obverse-reverse) indicates movements of life whereas **nei wai** (inside-outside) is closer to topographic references.

Among the cosmological roots, we cannot ignore the concept of resonance which is at the innermost core of Chinese cosmology and which appears in various texts from the "Warring States" period and the Empire (III and

II centuries): all things and beings pertaining to analog categories vibrate, resonate in unison, correspond.

"*Surveying Obscurities*", *Huainanzi* [12] chapter 6 deals with the (**ganying**) resonance phenomenon whose existence scholars accept but cannot clearly explain. They describe it as an affinity vibration in the **qi** energy field which goes through the cosmos and it is not just physical resonance but emotional as well as intentional, therefore human actions have clear and predictable effects on the natural world. Hence, observing **Dao** and ruling properly lead to human happiness and celestial harmony. That is to say that not being clear about what **qi** is but its existence confirmed, it claims that each thing is emulated in another one, in that which is analog due to its form or category. Resonances were not and are not abstract, there is always a material substrate for them to happen, and Chinese thinkers attribute field effects (generate energy and drive it) to everything that is alive in nature. This resonance contributes to the visceral functional pairing confirmed by anatomical relationship [13] [14].

These correspondences between macro and micro cosmos, between Heaven and Man realms thanks to *resonance* are not reduced to a simple parallelism, they pose a "vibrational" bond of mutual correspondence whose nature is defined by the **yinyang** relationship and which, according to *Huainanzi* reciprocally activates each other because they share the same breath. **Qi** (vital breath) is a cosmological notion that covers everything and if **yinyang** binomial is vital in its dynamism is because it is ruled by the resonance principle activated by **qi**.

And here we have one of the most endeared themes in the Chinese thought, the numerical game already mentioned by **Lao Zi** 42 [15]

The way generates the one,
The one generates the two,
The two generates the three,
The three generates all beings…

The **yinyang** pairing is met not by two elements but by three because the complementary alternation of two energies generates a third one: the moving force encouraged by duality. **Yinyang** parallelism without the three (emblem of motion) would be self enclosed repeating itself, without functionality: railroads gain sense with the presence of a train. With the three an infinitely transformable "parallelism" opens up. Chinese thought whether of Taoist or Confucian nuance, has always crossed Heaven-Earth influxes, and then crossing is the three conceived to go from duality to the ternary relationship that opens the field of the becoming. Thus the **biao li** pair obtains its dynamism, its "three" from **qi**, the cosmic breath thanks to which all circulations in the body operate.

5. Conclusion

Ever since its first manifestations in divinatory oracles, three millennia previous to our era, the Chinese vision of cosmos-nature facilitates the elaboration of the parallelism concept which evolves towards pairing, a notion that together with resonance phenomenon permeates all Chinese culture since literature—initial form and we believe that it also serves medicine whose practice simply confirms the success of this theoretical approach that this medicine adopts recognizing pairs in a sustained and resonant energetic exchange, in health and in sickness. As an example, the **biao li** binomial represents the use in medical practice of the millenarian Chinese conception of pairing as a form of existential dynamism.

References

[1] Rochat de la Vallée, E. and Larre, P.C. (1993) Su Wen. Les Once Premiers Traités. Maisonneuve, Moulin lès Metz, 123.

[2] Billeter, J.F. (2006) Contre François Jullien. Editions Allia. Paris, 18.

[3] Liu, X. (1995) El corazón de la Literatura y el Cincelado de Dragones. Traducción y notas de Relinque Eleta, A. De Guante Blanco/Comares. Granada.

[4] Chempla, K. (1989) Qu' Apporte la prise en compte du parallelism dans l'etude de textes mathématiques chinois? *Extrême-Orient Extrême-Occident*, **11**, 53-75. http://dx.doi.org/10.3406/oroc.1989.948

[5] Jullien, F. (1989) Une vision du monde fondée sur l'appariement: Enjeux philosophiques textueles (a partir de Wang Fuzhi). *Extrême-Orient Extrême-Occident*, **11**, 45-52. http://dx.doi.org/10.3406/oroc.1989.947

[6] Peluffo, E. (2013) Medicina China. Claves teóricas. Miraguano Ediciones, Madrid.

[7] Gernet, J. (2005) La Raison des Choses: Essai sur la philosophie de Wang Fuzhi 1619-1692. Nrf ëditions Gallimard, Paris.

[8] Cheng, A. (1989) un **Yin**, un **Yang**, telle est la Voie: Les origines cosmologiques du paralelisme dans la pensée chinoise. *Extrême-Orient Extrême-Occident*, **11**, 35-43. http://dx.doi.org/10.3406/oroc.1989.946

[9] Javary, C.J.-D. (2003) Le discourse de la tortue. Découvrir la Pensée Chinoise au Fil du **Yi Jing**. Albin Michel, Paris, 93.

[10] Neal, E. (2012) Introduction to Neijing Classical Acupuncture Part 1: History and Basic Principles. *The Journal of Chinese Medicine*, **100**, 5-14.

[11] Schatz, J., Larre, C. and Rochat de la Vallée, E. (1979) Les seminaires de l'Ecole Europeenne d'Acupuncture. Éditions So-Wen s.a.s., Milan, Épuisé.

[12] Major, J.S., Queen, S.A., Meyer, A.S. and Roth, H.D. (2010) The Huainanzi. Columbia University Press, New York, 207.

[13] Peluffo, E. (2014) Pi Wei Xiang Biao Li and the Trajectory of Zuyangming. *Chinese Medicine*, **5**, 7-15. http://dx.doi.org/10.4236/cm.2014.51002

[14] Peluffo, E. (2011) The Pairing of Heart and Small Intestine Xin Xiao Chang Xiang Biao Li 心小肠相表里. *Chinese Medicine*, **2**, 191-198. http://dx.doi.org/10.4236/cm.2011.24030

[15] Lao Zi (2003) Tao Te King Version Anne-Helène Suarez. Siruela, Madrid.

31

Microsatellite Analysis of *Panax ginseng* Natural Populations in Russia

Galina D. Reunova*, Olga G. Koren, Tamara I. Muzarok, Yury N. Zhuravlev

Department of Biotechnology, Institute of Biology and Soil Science, Far Eastern Branch of the Russian Academy of Sciences, Vladivostok, Russia

Email: *reunova@ibss.dro.ru, academic.secretary@biosoil.ru, muzarok@ibss.dro.ru, zhuravlev@biosoil.ru

Abstract

Panax ginseng **C.A. Meyer is an endangered species in Russia. To restore this species, effective protective measures, including the reintroduction into favorable habitats, must be worked out considering the specificity of genetic structure of ginseng populations. One hundred and thirty-nine *P. ginseng* plants were collected from the forests of nine administrative areas of Primorsky Territory of Russia and transferred to a collection nursery for further investigation. Microsatellite markers were used to study the genetic diversity and the genetic structure of ginseng populations. For populations studied with SSR, the number of observed alleles was ranging from 15 to 25, allelic richness from 1.83 to 3.04, polymorphic loci from 62.5% to 87.7%, observed heterozygosity from 0.410 to 0.512 (an average of 0.453) and expected heterozygosity from 0.304 to 0.479, with an average of 0.393. The values of the inbreeding coefficient within populations (F_{is}) ranged from −0.447 to 0.056, and their average value was −0.296. Genetic differentiation among populations was significant (F_{st} = 0.115) but an isolation-by-distance pattern was not detected. UPGMA and MS-tree confirmed the presence of genetic structure within *P. ginseng* and visualized genetic relationships of populations with similar pattern. STRUCTURE analysis revealed the genetic admixture between different ginseng populations. It was established with SSR markers that *P. ginseng* still preserves substantial genetic resources although all populations are largely exhausted. Because ginseng populations are significantly differentiated all of them should be restored. Considering the admixture of ginseng populations it would be advisable to apply the individual assignment test to verify the content of indigenous populations and to identify the "true" population plants to serve as stock material for reintroduction.**

Keywords

***Panax ginseng*, Genetic Diversity, Genetic Structure, Microsatellites**

---

*Corresponding author.

1. Introduction

The species *Panax ginseng* Meyer (Korean ginseng) belongs to the family Araliaceae and is one of the most important medicinal plants in East Asia. Ginseng represents the herbaceous perennial plant, which prefers to grow in the ripe and dense Korean pine, Korean pine-black-fir-broad-leaved and white beech forests [1] [2]. In nature, ginseng grows singly or in groups ("families"). The lifetime of ginseng plants is approximately 7 - 10 years in plantation and 60 - 100 years in nature. Some authors speculate that ginseng is able to live 400 years. Reproduction of *P. ginseng* occurs exclusively by seeds, which are carried by birds (the hazel grouse, the jay, the cedar bird, etc.) and rodents [1] [2].

In the first half of the 20th century, wild-growing ginseng plants could be found on the large forestlands of China, Korea and the Russian Primorye, but currently, there are almost no wild ginseng plants remaining in China and Korea [2] [3]. Consequently, ginseng is being developed in these countries as a horticultural crop [4]. At the same time, Russia is the only country where *P. ginseng* is still growing in its natural habitat. Because all natural populations of *P. ginseng* are largely exhausted, reintroduction is essential to restore this plant to its former range.

The theoretical aspects of species reintroduction were discussed in the literature [5] [6]. Most researchers agree that for successful reintroduction, a set of rules must be followed to provide the species with the genetic and ecological prosperity inherent in the species' habitat [7]. Genetic variability is critical for a species to adapt to environmental changes and survive in long term [8]. It is important to acknowledge that the genotypic structure of populations is an evolutionary determined characteristic, which, if ignored, would lead to irreparable consequences [9]. Therefore, the assessment of genetic variation and partitioning within and between populations are principal constituents in a species conservation program [9] [10]. The reintroduction strategy must assume the reinstatement of allelic frequencies typical for the population under study [11]. An essential step of reintroduction is the identification of plants intended to be used for the reintroduction in regard of their conformity to ancestral local population. The genetic admixture in local populations of *P. ginseng* might be a consequence; the special care for ginseng among harvesters established a practice of cultivating ginseng on "forest ginseng plantations" where the seeds from wild plants collected in distant populations were used. This practice most likely ensured the sustainable management of ginseng populations; simultaneously, genetic material from different populations was mixed. An immigration rate in the populations of *P. ginseng* could also be provided through effective seed dispersal across the landscape by birds and mammals. Therefore, verifying whether the "indigenous" populations of *P. ginseng* are mixed is necessary.

In recent years, attention has focused mainly on the development of various chemical and molecular techniques for differentiating between samples of *P. ginseng* and authenticating different *Panax* species [12]. However, not much has been reported about genetic variation and the population structure of *P. ginseng* [13]-[16]. In our studies of wild *P. ginseng* populations, a low level of genetic polymorphisms was detected by allozyme and RAPD markers [17] [18], which means effective conservation strategies would be difficult to design using these markers. Fluorescently labeled AFLP markers were highly effective in determining the genetic diversity and genetic structure of *P. ginseng* [19]-[23]. However, because of the dominance of AFLP markers, it was impossible to calculate the allelic frequencies directly to obtain unbiased estimates of population diversity and differentiation. Here, we report the microsatellite analysis of *P. ginseng* populations previously studied with AFLPs [19]-[23].

Among the various molecular markers, microsatellite markers (SSRs) have been successfully used to describe population genetic diversity, because they are codominant and highly polymorphic [24]. Studies using SSR markers in the *Panax* genus have only recently been initiated. Sets of microsatellite markers produced from SSR-enriched libraries [4] [25], bacterial artificial chromosome (BAC) end sequences [26], or expressed sequence tags (EST) [27] were employed to characterize the genetic diversity of ginseng collections.

In this study, our purposes were: 1) to complete previous AFLP study on genetic diversity of *P. ginseng* by estimating the within-population fixation index (F_{is}) with codominant markers; 2) to compare SSR estimates of population diversity and differentiation of *P. ginseng* with those previously obtained in our studies with AFLP markers; and 3) to verify the utility of microsatellites for assigning *P. ginseng* individuals to their population of origin.

2. Materials and Methods

2.1. Sampled Populations

One hundred and thirty-nine (139) *P. ginseng* plants were collected from the forests of nine administrative areas of Primorsky Territory (Russia) and transferred to a collection nursery for further analyses. Geographic locations of sampled populations are shown in **Figure 1** where the populations were coded with the names of the areas. Twenty (20) *P. ginseng* plants were collected from the Chuguevsk area (*Chu*), 22 from the Spassk area (*Spa*), 17 from the Ussuriisk area (*Uss*), 12 from the Dalnerechensk area (*Drech*), 16 from the Dalnegorsk area (*Dgor*), 12 from the Olginsk area (*Olg*), 14 from the Pozharsk area (*Pozh*), 16 from the Partizansk area (*Part*) and 10 from the Yakovlevsk area (*Yak*).

2.2. DNA Extraction and SSR Procedure

Genomic DNA was extracted from fresh leaf tissue according to Zhuravlev *et al.* [20]. Each leaf sample was frozen in liquid nitrogen and then grounded into a fine powder using a mortar and pestle.

Polymerase chain reactions were performed in 12 µL reaction mixtures containing 15 ng of genomic DNA, 0.3 mM dNTP, 5 pM of each primer, 2.8 mM $MgCl_2$, 0.5 unit of *Taq* DNA polymerase and 1× supplied reaction buffer (Fermentas, Canada). The PCR profile using the MyCycler^{TM} (Bio-Rad, Germany) thermocycler program consisted of 1 cycle at 95˚C for 5 min, followed by 34 cycles at 94˚C for 30 s, 56˚ - 60˚ (depending on primer used) for 30 s, and 72˚C for 1 min. PCR concluded with a final extension at 72˚C for 15 min. Eleven SSR polymorphic markers previously developed by Kim *et al.* [25] from *P. ginseng* were analyzed. The primers were synthesized by Syntol (Russia). Forward primers were labeled at the 5'-end with 6-carboxyfluorescein (6-FAM) (Applied Biosystems, USA). The fluorescently labeled PCR products were mixed with the GeneScan-500 LIZ size standard (Applied Biosystems, USA) and separated by capillary electrophoresis using an ABI PRISM 3100 genetic analyzer (Applied Biosystems, USA) for allele detection. Alleles were visualized and sized using the GeneScan 3.7.1 software (Applied Biosystems, USA); alleles were designated by the number of their repeats. All PCRs contained negative and positive controls that were genotyped and analyzed alongside the samples. Genomic DNA was re-extracted for 10% of the individuals and genotyped a second time to check for consistency of allele-calling.

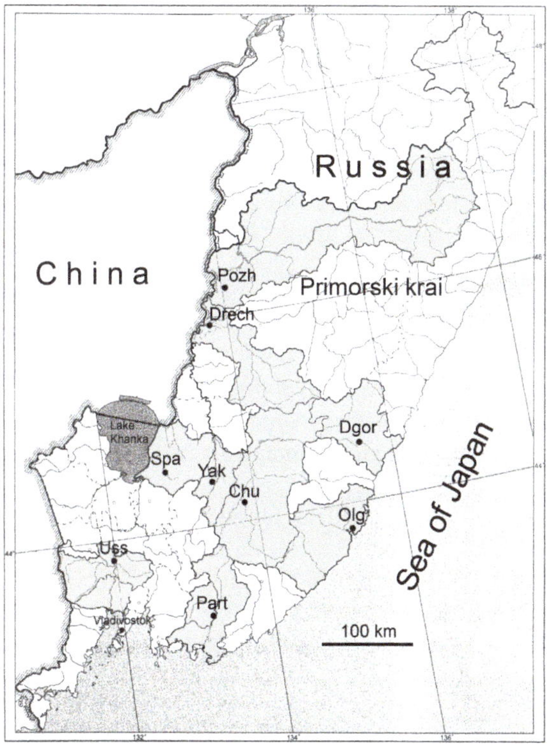

Figure 1. The administrative areas of Primorsky Territory of Russia where *P. ginseng* plants were collected. Names of the areas: Chuguevsk—*Chu*, Spassk—*Spa*, Ussuriisk—*Uss*, Dalnerechensk—*Drech*, Dalnegorsk—*Dgor*, Olginsk—*Olg*, Pozharsk—*Pozh*, Partizansk—*Part*, Yakovlevsk—*Yak*. The administrative centers of the areas are marked with dots.

2.3. Data Analysis

The POPGENE 1.31 [28] software was applied to estimate the frequencies of alleles and to determine the genetic variation parameters, such as the observed number of alleles, percentage of polymorphic loci (*P*), observed heterozygosity (H_O), expected panmictic heterozygosity (H_E), and *F*-statistics of Wright (F_{it}, F_{is}, F_{st}) for loci. The inbreeding coefficient F_{is} [29] for populations was computed using FSTAT 2.9.3 [30]. Allelic richness (A_R) was estimated based on a fixed sample size of 10 plants with FSTAT 2.9.3. GENEPOP [31] online version (http:www.genepop.curtin.edu.au/) and ARLEQUIN 3.1 [32] were used to assess Hardy-Weinberg equilibrium (HWE) and linkage disequilibrium (LD), respectively. An analysis of molecular variance (AMOVA, [33]) was performed with GENALEX 6.0 [34] to estimate the variance components attributable to inter-individual and inter-population differences. Genetic divergence between populations was quantified by estimating pairwise F_{ST} values and calculating their significance by bootstrapping analysis using the ARLEQUIN 3.1 software. To test possible correlations between pairwise genetic and geographic distances, the ARLEQUIN 3.1 software was used to conduct a Mantel test with 5000 permutations by regression analysis $F_{ST}/(1 - F_{ST})$ against the natural logarithm of geographic distance (km) between populations.

Cavalli-Sforza and Edwards' [35] chord distance, D_c, was calculated by the PHYLIP program (online version, http://evolution.gs.washington.edu/phylip/software.html), and tree was constructed among populations with the UPGMA clustering method using NTSYSpc 2.0 [36]. A computer simulation study of various genetic distance measurements found D_c to be the most suitable in obtaining the correct tree topology based on a microsatellite analysis [37]. Using a matrix of Cavalli-Sforza and Edwards' chord distances, the minimum spanning tree (MS-tree) between populations was reconstructed using NTSYSpc 2.0. In addition, the population genetic structure was evaluated by a model-based Bayesian clustering method [38] implemented in STRUCTURE 2.3.2 [39]. To test whether any cluster could be found in studied material, three independent runs with 100-300,000 Markov chain Monte Carlo (MCMC) iterations each and 10-30,000 burn-in periods with *K* between 1 and 10 were performed. In simulations, the admixture model with correlated allele frequencies was used. SSR data were also subjected to individual-based assignment tests by applying the maximum likelihood method with STRUCTURE 2.3.2 [39] to verify the population belonging of every *P. ginseng* individual. Our goal was to detect genetic outliers (*i.e.* migrant genotypes) in the sampled populations.

3. Results

3.1. Genetic Diversity

In this study 139 individual plants were analyzed using 11 SSR primers developed by Kim *et al.* [25] from *P. ginseng* (**Table 1**). One primer pair was monomorphic (PG22) and two primer pairs (PG770 and PG946) did not synthesize fragments. In all populations studied, an aggregate number of 27 alleles across eight SSRs were detected with an average of 3.4 alleles per locus. Approximately 36% of alleles were shared by all *P. ginseng* populations studied. The remaining portion of alleles (64%) was detected in groups consisting of 2 - 8 populations. Every population (except *Yak*) contained some rare alleles (from 1 to 4) occurring with frequencies lower than 0.05. Two private alleles were detected only in *Pozh.* A high proportion of polymorphic loci pairs were found to exhibit LD in *P. ginseng*. Of the examined unique combinations in the nine populations, 53.5% were statistically significant ($p = 0.05$).

In studied populations the number of observed alleles ranging from 15 to 25, allelic richness from 1.83 to 3.04, polymorphic loci from 62.5% to 87.7%, observed heterozygosity from 0.410 to 0.512 (an average of 0.453) and expected heterozygosity from 0.304 to 0.479, with an average of 0.393 (**Table 2**). The values of the inbreeding coefficient within populations (F_{is}) ranged from −0.447 to 0.056, and their average value was −0.296. Generally, deviation from HWE was due to excessive heterozygosity, which was significant in six of the nine populations (**Table 2**).

3.2. Population Structure

The coefficient of population differentiation, F_{st} determined by POPGENE was 0.115. An AMOVA analysis revealed that 9% of the total genetic variation was attributed to the variability among the populations, whereas 91% of the total genetic variation was represented within populations (**Table 3**). The fixation index (F_{ST}) was 0.09 ($p = 0.001$). Moreover, pairwise estimates of F_{ST} ranged from 0.001 to 0.211 (**Table 4**), and only 6 pairs (*Drech*

Table 1. Oligonucleotide primer sequences and annealing temperatures of the 11 microsatellite loci developed by Kim *et al.* [25] from *P. ginseng* and tested in this study.

Locus	Primer sequence, 5'-3'	Annealing temperature, °C
PG22	F: CTGTCTATGCAAGTTGCGGCTG R: ATCAAGTTGGAAATCAGGTGGG	58
PG29	F: AATCAGAAACAAAGAAAGCTAAAAC R: CTCTCTCATCTCTCTCTCTTCC	60
PG281	F: GTAGTAGTAGTAAAAACTTTGCTAACG R: ATTTACAACTCTCTTCTTCCTCTAC	60
PG287	F: GTGGGACTGGTATACAATAAGA R:GTGTTCTTAGTTGCCCATTTG	60
PG668	F: CTGGCATCGAAGTTTCTCCATTC R: TGCATAGCACAGAGAGGAGG	60
PG770	F: CCTCTTTGGGGCAGGGATATTTG R: CCAGCAAACCCAAACCCTCCTC	60
PG946	F: GAATCGAAGTGTTAAGTTGAT R: CTTAAATCGATGATAACACC	56
PG1319	F: GCATGAACGGATACACCTTGAGG R: GGTATGCACCAGAAACGGACTGG	58
PG1419	F: ACTCAAAATTCTACAGCTTCCTC R: GATACCCCAG GCAGTCTGATGAC	56
PG1481	F: GGAGGTGATTGATGTAGTGGAATCC R: GGCTCTCCTATACTCACTATTTCCC	58
PG1663	F: CTACACGCTTTTTCATAGCTTACA R: TGTCTGCATAAAAGAGTTCGAGGC	60

Table 2. Gene diversity statistics in *Panax ginseng* populations estimated based on the analysis of eight polymorphic microsatellite loci.

Population	Number of alleles	A_R	P (%)	H_0	H_e	F_{is}	p (HWE)
Uss	17	2.01	75.35	0.441	0.313	−0.430	0.0001
Spa	17	1.92	87.50	0.457	0.319	−0.447	0.0031
Drech	18	2.16	87.20	0.417	0.342	−0.231	0.1686
Chu	16	1.91	62.50	0.481	0.337	−0.446	0.0001
Dgor	21	2.63	87.70	0.453	0.479	0.056	0.7005
Olg	19	2.30	76.42	0.447	0.352	−0.286	0.0404
Pozh	25	3.04	87.42	0.455	0.424	−0.075	0.7957
Part	15	1.83	62.65	0.410	0.304	−0.366	0.0009
Yak	17	2.12	75.15	0.512	0.359	−0.436	0.0001
Mean	18.33	2.49	77.99	0.453	0.393	−0.296	
Species-level value			100.00				

A_R, allelic richness; P, percent of polymorphic loci; H_0, observed heterozygosity; H_e, expected panmictic heterozygosity; F_{is}, the inbreeding coefficient within population; p (HWE), p value for significance of deviation from Hardy-Weinberg equilibrium.

Table 3. Analysis of molecular variance (AMOVA) for populations of *Panax ginseng*. Level of significance is based on 1023 iterations.

Source of variation	Degree of freedom	Sum of squares	Variance components	Percentage variation
Among populations	8	5644.750	17.747	9.0
Within populations	265	44915.278	169.492	91.0
Total	273	50560.028	187.239	

Fixation index $F_{ST} = 0.09$; p value = 0.001.

Table 4. Pairwise genetic distance matrix based on genetic differentiation (F_{ST}) (lower diagonal) and geographic distance (km, upper diagonal) for populations of *Panax ginseng.*

Population	*Uss*	*Spa*	*Drech*	*Chu*	*Dgor*	*Olg*	*Pozh*	*Part*	*Yak*
Uss	0.000	115	275	165	325	275	325	125	140
Spa	0.178	0.000	170	110	240	220	215	165	60
Drech	0.138	0.005	0.000	210	230	265	50	310	175
Chu	0.127	0.007	0.035	0.000	155	115	245	120	50
Dgor	0.159	0.211	0.171	0.196	0.000	90	245	255	184
Olg	0.135	0.084	0.060	0.069	0.187	0.000	290	190	160
Pozh	0.020	0.126	0.077	0.101	0.065	0.055	0.000	350	220
Part	0.107	0.127	0.063	0.117	0.201	0.032	0.051	0.000	135
Yak	0.063	0.024	0.011	0.014	0.157	0.002	0.024	0.001	0.000

and *Spa*, *Chu* and *Spa*, *Yak* and *Drech*, *Yak* and *Chu*, *Yak* and *Olg*, *Yak* and *Part*) gave nonsignificant results (with $p > 0.05$) after the permutation procedure.

Cavalli-Sforza and Edwards' chord distances among populations ranged from 0.027 to 0.301 (**Table 5**). A UPGMA dendrogram constructed on the basis of the interpopulation chord genetic distances, divided all populations into two main clusters with sub-clusters. One cluster contained *Dgor*, *Pozh* with distant from them *Uss* population and the second cluster contained *Spa*, *Chu*, *Drech*, *Yak* with *Olg* and *Part* being distant from other populations in this cluster (**Figure 2**). The MS-tree similarly divided all populations into two main clusters to visualize the genetic relationships among the *P. ginseng* populations (**Figure 3**). The way the populations tended to cluster using UPGMA (**Figure 2**) and MS-tree (**Figure 3**) appeared to be independent on their geographical origin (**Table 4**). The correlation analysis did not reveal any association between pairwise F_{ST} values and geographical distances among the populations ($r = 0.078$; $p = 0.374$).

The STRUCTURE results revealed that ln(P) is maximized at $K = 4$, suggesting the presence of four genetically distinct groups (**Figure 4**). According to results of STRUCTURE, the group I (red) contained 12 of the 15 *Part*, eight of the 12 *Olg* plants, six of the 10 *Yak* plants, four of the 12 *Drech* plants, and one plant of the other populations, excluding the *Uss*. The STRUCTURE group II (green) included 11 of the 16 *Dgor* plants, six of the 14 *Pozh* plants, and one plant from each of the *Olg* and *Uss* populations. The STRUCTURE group III (blue) contained 17 of the 22 *Spa* plants, 14 of the 20 *Chu* plants, five of the 12 *Drech* plants, three of the 10 *Yak* plants, three of the 12 *Olg* plants, and one plant of the *Part* and *Dgor* populations. The STRUCTURE group IV (yellow) included all of the *Uss* plants (excluding one plant), five of the 14 *Pozh* plants, three of the 16 *Dgor* plants, and five, four, three, two, and one of the *Chu*, *Spa*, *Drech*, *Part* and *Yak* plants, respectively. The individual assignment test with SSR results revealed that only 58 samples out of 139 studied *P. ginseng* samples (42.0%) were assigned to their original populations (results not shown).

4. Discussion

4.1. Genetic Diversity

The populations of *P. ginseng* growing on Primorsky Territory of Russia are characterized by a lower level of allozymes and dominant markers variation than most species with restricted ranges [40]. Our earlier studies demonstrated low levels of genetic variability in *P. ginseng*, as detected by allozymes ($P = 7.6\%$, $H_e = 0.022$), RAPD ($P = 4.0\%$, $H_e = 0.013$) and ISSR ($P = 9.3\%$, $H_e = 0.014$) [17] [19] [21]. These values are consistent with the data from the genetic studies of cultivated ginseng sampled from China and Korea (e.g., [14]). The current study with SSR markers demonstrated a higher genetic diversity in *P. ginseng* comparatively with that obtained with AFLP markers [20] [22] [23]. The polymorphism in *P. ginseng* was 77.99% and 100% at population and species levels, respectively, as estimated by the SSR method. The mean expected heterozygosity (H_e) was 0.393, which is slightly different from those revealed in other studies of *P. ginseng* with SSR markers (0.502, [4];

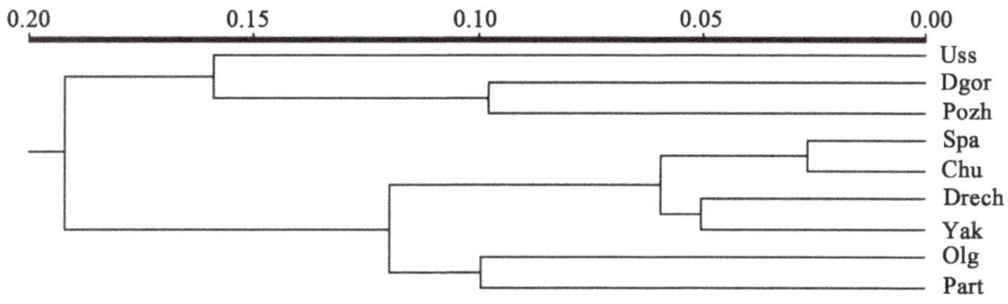

Figure 2. UPGMA dendrogram based on Cavalli_Sforza and Edwards' chord distances among nine *P. ginseng* populations. Population abbreviations are as in "Materials and Methods".

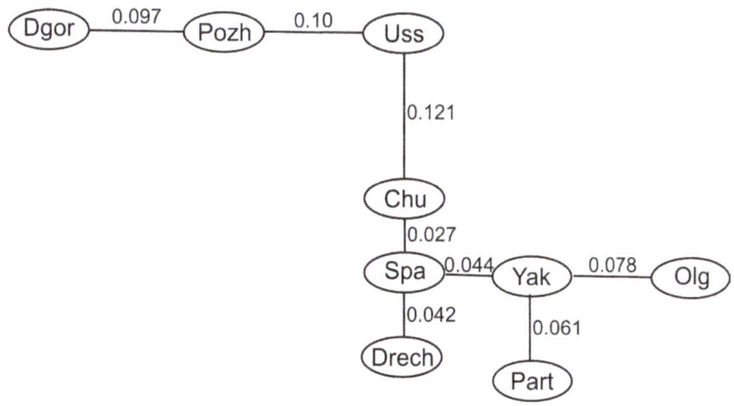

Figure 3. MS-tree representing phylogenetic relationships among nine *P. ginseng* populations. The numbers on lines show Cavalli_Sforza and Edwards' chord distances among populations. Population abbreviations are as in "Materials and Methods".

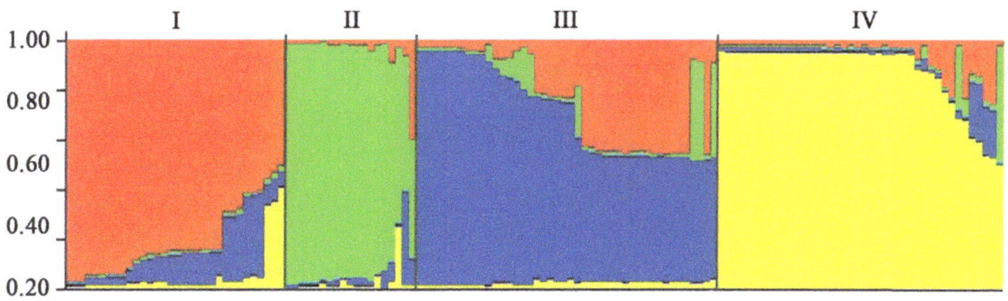

Figure 4. Genetic structure across 139 individuals from nine *P. ginseng* populations using the model-based Bayesian algorithm implemented in the program STRUCTURE. A panel corresponds to K = 4 groups. Fractional membership in each of the clusters (I, II, III, IV) is indicated by *colour*. The populations which created every cluster are described in "Results".

Table 5. Cavalli_Sforza and Edwards' chord distance among populations of *Panax ginseng*.

Population	*Uss*	*Spa*	*Drech*	*Chu*	*Dgor*	*Olg*	*Pozh*	*Part*	*Yak*
Uss	0.000								
Spa	0.172	0.000							
Drech	0.204	0.042	0.000						
Chu	0.121	0.027	0.096	0.000					
Dgor	0.216	0.230	0.205	0.240	0.000				
Olg	0.224	0.142	0.134	0.141	0.246	0.000			
Pozh	0.100	0.163	0.147	0.159	0.098	0.141	0.000		
Part	0.199	0.143	0.105	0.152	0.301	0.099	0.156	0.000	
Yak	0.155	0.044	0.050	0.025	0.251	0.078	0.137	0.061	0.000

0.460, [41]; 0.313, [42]). These differences may be attributed to the source of plant samples, as *P. ginseng* was mainly represented in cultivated forms subjected to artificial breeding and selection. In this study, only wild ginseng was investigated. Furthermore, the populations studied inhabit the northeastern margin of the former range of ginseng, which may be one of the reasons for the observed reduction in the level of genetic variability [40]. Similar values of SSR genetic diversity were observed in two related species, *P. notoginseng* ($H_e = 0.350$, [43]), and *P. vietnamensis* ($H_e = 0.550$, [44]).

Our studies with SSR showed that *P. ginseng* is significantly differentiated ($F_{ST} = 0.09$; $p = 0.001$). The significant differentiation of the ginseng population was also demonstrated in the studies with AFLP markers [20] [22]. The observed genetic differentiation among populations indicates management for the conservation of genetic variability in *P. ginseng* should aim to preserve all investigated populations with the allelic frequencies determined in this study. The populations which exhibited high allelic richness, such as *Pozh* ($A_R = 3.04$), *Dgor* ($A_R = 2.63$), *Olg* ($A_R = 2.30$) and *Drech* ($A_R = 2.16$), should be a priority, as allelic richness was highly recommended as an appropriate measure in the context of genetic conservation [45].

The results obtained indicated an excess of heterozygotes in all populations, except for *Dgor*. The mean observed heterozygosity in populations was 0.453, whereas the mean expected heterozygosity was 0.393. This result is rather unexpected for a species with a restricted and fragmented range. Despite the fact that in the past ginseng was widely distributed in the Far Eastern forests covering present-day territories of northern-east China, Korea and the Russian Primorye, it has been described as a rare plant even in ancient manuscripts [2]. In conditions of low plant density, one would expect a high level of inbreeding within populations, especially considering the peculiarities of the ginseng mating system, such as floral phenology and the inability of insect pollinators (syrphids) to fly long distances [46]. In contrast, the inbreeding coefficient, F_{is}, was negative within almost all populations studied. Additionally, an excess of heterozygotes was shown for *P. ginseng* by Ma *et al.* [4] with SSR markers.

An excess of heterozygotes was found in some long-lived perennial plants with codominant markers, such as those used in the SSR [47] and allozyme analyses [48] [49]. In contrast to well-described reasons causing the deficit of heterozygotes, little is known about the causes of excess of heterozygosity in natural plant populations. Presumably, excess of heterozygosity in populations may be related to overdominance and selection as well as agamospermy [47]. Facultative apomixis was found in *P. ginseng* [50]. However, it has been shown that a type of ginseng agamospermy is similar to diplospory, which can impede inbreeding but not prevent it [19]. Overdominance and selection against homozygotes can play a significant role in the survival of ginseng under severe climate conditions on the northeastern margin of the range. Actually, we observed a high mortality of seedlings during germination experiments. Nevertheless, the existence of the overdominance phenomenon in *P. ginseng* populations requires careful investigation, including an evaluation of the observed heterozygosity and F_{is} indices across different developmental stages (seeds, seedlings and adults).

Another reason for the observed excess of heterozygotes in ginseng populations may be their tetraploid origin. Presumably, *P. ginseng* is allotetraploid, as was demonstrated in comparative studies of the allozyme banding patterns of the two closest species, *P. ginseng* and *P. quinquefolius* [50]. A number of duplicated loci and fixed heterozygotes detected in *P. ginseng* denoted an allotetraploid origin of this species. Allotetraploids usually demonstrate lower levels of allozyme variability than autotetraploids. At the same time, the low variability of allotetraploids is compensated for by the variety of parental genomes that have formed this species. Differences between parental genomes impede free gene recombination during meiosis but increase the species genomic diversity due to fixed heterozygosity, which can be detected with codominant markers. Nevertheless, high levels of observed heterozygosity may be associated with the population structure and reflect the history of its formation under the influences of global climatic and local human-induced impacts.

4.2. Population Structure

To study the genetic structure of *P. ginseng* populations, we used a wide range of analytical methods. The *F*-statistics of Wright (F_{st}) and AMOVA (F_{ST}) revealed genetic structure within *P. ginseng* and showed a moderate population differentiation ($F_{st} = 0.115$; $F_{ST} = 0.09$). The value of F_{ST} was lower than the inter-population variability obtained with AFLP markers ($F_{ST} = 0.36$) [20] [22]. Differentiation is expected to be lower when assessed through microsatellites compared with more slowly evolving markers [51]. This is a consequence of both the higher number of alleles in microsatellites and their higher probability of homoplasy, further decreasing genetic divergence between populations [51].

UPGMA and MS-tree confirmed the presence of genetic structure within *P. ginseng* and visualized genetic relationships of populations with similar pattern. Two main clusters with sub-clusters were obtained (**Figure 2** and **Figure 3**). The Ms-tree **(Figure 3)** did not only confirm the UPGMA data about genetic structure of *P. ginseng* but also allowed discuss the ginseng evolutionary history. The "knot" state of the genetically distant *Uss* and *Chu* populations on Ms-tree (**Figure 3**) testifies that the *P. ginseng* could disperse across the Russian Primorye from south and west. The similar supposition was made in our studies of *P. ginseng* using AFLP markers [20] [22].

The present population relationships inferred from UPGMA and MS-tree were not always consistent with the geographical distribution of the *P. ginseng* populations. For instance, the geographically distant *Uss* and *Pozh* populations were genetically very close but the geographically nearest *Drech* and *Pozh* populations were genetically distant enough (**Table 4**). The population genetic structure of *P. ginseng* derived from SSR analysis was not consistent with a pattern of isolation by distance. Correlation analysis showed that the differences in genetic diversity among the ginseng populations were not related to their geographical distances ($r = 0.078$; $p = 0.374$). This means there was no progressive increase of genetic differentiation with geographic distance, which should be expected if pollen and seed dispersal modes were the main factors influencing the population structure. A negative and nonsignificant ($r = -0.174$; $p = 0.817$) correlation between genetic differentiation and geographic distance was also detected in our study of *P. ginseng* with AFLP markers [22] [23]. The suggestion could be made that, in addition to the effect of species traits, other factors played a very important role in shaping the population genetic structure of *P. ginseng* in Russia.

Tree-based methods that use genetic distances between individuals to discover the species genetic structure are only loosely connected to statistical procedures that allow for the identification of homogeneous clusters of individuals [52]. A Bayesian algorithm implemented in the STRUCTURE program [38] identifies such groups without prior information about number of locations at which the individuals were sampled and also calculates the likelihood of plant belonging to specific group. As detailed in the results, the data obtained by STRUCTURE program are in agree with that obtained using UPGMA (**Figure 2**) and Ms-tree (**Figure 3**). The STRUCTURE analysis defined four homogeneous groups of *P. ginseng* populations (**Figure 4**). The number of STRUCTURE groups was the same as the number of sub-clusters of UPGMA and Ms-tree. The content of "green" and "yellow" STRUCTURE groups corresponded to two sub-clusters of the first main UPGMA and Ms-tree cluster and the plants of "red" and "blue" STRUCTURE groups consisted of plants that could be found in the two sub-clusters of second main cluster of these trees. However, with STRUCTURE the information was revealed that was not evident using UPGMA and Ms-tree. It became clear that none of the studied populations formed a distinct cluster (**Figure 4**). The admixture of ginseng plants belonging to different STRUCTURE clusters was shown. Some individuals showed a stronger genetic resemblance to populations other than their own putative populations. It is unlikely that effective pollen flow could generate such a high genetic resemblance to another population because the male gamete contains only half the genetic load of an individual. Therefore, the outlier genotypes detected by the assignment test in STRUCTURE can be considered the products of successful seed dispersal events, *i.e.*, migrants [53]. The long-distance seed dispersal by birds, animals and also humans could result in the mixing of ginseng plants. Considering the history of controlled and uncontrolled ginseng cultivation in the fields and, more importantly, in the forest farms, we believe that human activity especially influenced on population genetic structure of *P. ginseng* in Russia. The low bootstrap values of the UPGMA dendrogram obtained in this study could be the result of the ginseng plant mixing phenomenon. The high amounts of linkage disequilibrium within *P. ginseng* populations could also be explained by population admixture [54]. The absence of private alleles in most *P. ginseng* populations also testifies to population admixture. At the same time, the genetic similarity of geographically distant ginseng populations may have been due to converging common selection forces in geographically disparate populations [55].

The individual assignment test revealed that only 58 samples out of 139 studied *P. ginseng* samples (42.0%) were assigned to their original populations (*i.e.* having the highest likelihood value of belonging to the populations they came from). The estimated immigration rate in the *P. ginseng* populations, analyzed with AFLP markers was considerably higher and equal 77.7% [22]. Some studied with AFLPs ginseng populations had 100% assignment success [22]. The comparative studies by other authors have also highlighted the higher discriminatory power of AFLP markers over microsatellites in population assignment tests [56]. Thus, in our study, SSR markers demonstrated low efficiency in assigning individuals to their population of origin to be chosen to serve as stock material for *P. ginseng* reintroduction.

5. Conclusion

In the present study using SSR markers, we discovered a high level of genetic diversity and obtained the main genetic characteristics for populations of wild *P. ginseng*. Ginseng in Russia does not require measures such as genetic rescue for species persistence but is in need of recovery measures because natural populations are largely exhausted as a result of the excessive harvesting of ginseng roots. Because ginseng populations are significantly differentiated all of them should be restored with the allelic frequencies determined in this study. Populations with high allelic richness should be granted priority consideration. Due to the mixing of ginseng plants, the *P. ginseng* populations should be checked with individual assignment test to verify the content of indigenous populations and to identify the "true" plants to serve as stock material for reintroduction. Considering the higher discriminatory power of AFLP markers over microsatellites in individual assignment tests, we recommend that the plants which were correctly assigned to their population of origin with AFLP markers should be chosen as material for *P. ginseng* reintroduction.

Competing Interests

The authors declare that they have no competing interests.

Authors' Contributions

YNZ and GDR designed research. GDR and ILK performed the research and analyzed the data. TIM collected the plants. GDR and OGK wrote the manuscript. YNZ helped in writing the manuscript and coordinating the study. All authors read and approved the final version of the manuscript.

Acknowledgements

This study was supported by the Russian Academy of Sciences, research projects No. 12-I-P30-02, No. 12-I-OBN-06 and by RFBR, research project No. 11-04-98515-r_vostok_a. We thank ever so much Irina Kats for participation in this study and mourn over her timeless decease.

References

[1] Grushwitsky, I.V. (1961) Ginseng: The Aspects of Biology. Nauka, Leningrad. (In Russian)

[2] Zhuravlev, Yu.N. and Kolyada, A.S. (1996) Araliaceae: Ginseng and Others. Dalnauka, Vladivostok. (In Russian)

[3] Boehm, C.L., Harrison H.C., Jung, G. and Nienhuis, J. (1999) Organization of American and Asian Ginseng Germplasm Using Randomly Amplified Polymorphic DNA (RAPD) Markers. *Journal of the American Society for Horticultural Science*, **124**, 252-256.

[4] Ma, K.H., Dixit, A., Kim, Y.C., Lee, D.Y., Kim, T.S., Cho, E.G. and Park, Y.J. (2007) Development and Characterization of New Microsatellite Markers for Ginseng (*Panax ginseng* C.A. Meyer). *Conservation Genetics*, **8**, 1507-1509. http://dx.doi.org/10.1007/s10592-007-9284-4

[5] Falk, D.A. and Olwell, M. (1992) Scientific and Policy Considerations in Restoration and Reintroduction of Endangered Species. *Rhodora*, **94**, 287-315.

[6] Falk, D.A., Millar, C.I. and Olwell. M. (1996) Restoring Diversity. Strategies for Reintroduction of Endangered Plants. Island Press, Washington DC.

[7] Schemske, D.W., Husband, B.C., Ruckelshaus, M.H., Goodwillie, C., Parker, I.M. and Bishop, J. (1994) Evaluation Approaches to the Conservation of Rare and Endangered Plants. *Ecology*, **75**, 384-606. http://dx.doi.org/10.2307/1941718

[8] Reed, D.H. and Frankham R. (2003) Population Fitness Is Correlated with Genetic Diversity. *Conservation Biology*, **7**, 230-237. http://dx.doi.org/10.1046/j.1523-1739.2003.01236.x

[9] Altukhov, Yu.P. (2003) Genetic Processes in Populations. Academkniga, Moscow. (In Russian)

[10] Hamrick, J.L. and Godt, M.J.W. (1996) Conservation Genetics of Endemic Plant Species. In: Avise, J.S. and Hamrick J.L., Eds., *Conservation Genetics*: *Case Histories from Nature*, New York, 281-304. http://dx.doi.org/10.1007/978-1-4757-2504-9_9

[11] Zhuravlev, Yu.N., Koren, O.G., Muzarok, T.I., Reunova, G.D., Kozyrenko, M.M., Artyukova, E.V. and Ilushko, M.V. (1999) Molecular Markers for Conservation of Rare Plants of Far East. *Phyziologiya of Rastenii* (*Moscow*), **46**, 953-964.

[12] Hon, C.C., Chow, Y.C., Zeng, F.Y. and Leung, F.C. (2003) Genetic Authentication of Ginseng and Other Traditional Chinese Medicine. *Acta Pharmacologica Sinica*, **24**, 841-846.

[13] Um, J.Y., Chung, H.S., Kim, M.S., Na, H.J., Kwon, H.J., Kim, J.J., Lee, K.M., Lee, S.J., Lim, J.P., Do, K.R., Hwang, W.J., Lyu, Y.S., An, N.H. and Kim, H.M. (2001) Molecular Authentication of *Panax ginseng* Species by RAPD Analysis and PCR-RFLP. *Biological and Pharmaceutical Bulletin*, **24**, 872-875. http://dx.doi.org/10.1248/bpb.24.872

[14] Kim, C. and Choi, H.K. (2003) Genetic Diversity and Relationship in Korean Ginseng (*Panax schinseng*) Based on RAPD Analysis. *Korean Journal of Genetics*, **25**, 181-188.

[15] Seo, S.D., Yuk, J.A., Cha, S.K., Kim, H.H., Seong, B.J., Kim, S.I. and Choi, J.E. (2003) Analysis of Diversity of *Panax ginseng* Collected in Korea by RAPD Technique. *Korean Journal of Medicinal Crop Science*, **11**, 377-384.

[16] Li, S., Li, J., Yang, X.L., Cheng, Z. and Zhang, W.J. (2011) Genetic Diversity and Differentiation of Cultivated Ginseng (*Panax ginseng* C.A. Meyer) Populations in North-East China Revealed by Inter-Simple Sequence Repeat (ISSR) Markers. *Genetic Resources and Crop Evolution*, **58**, 815-824. http://dx.doi.org/10.1007/s10722-010-9618-9

[17] Koren, O.G., Potenko, V.V. and Zhuravlev, Y.N. (2003) Inheritance and Variation of Allozymes in *Panax ginseng* C.A. Meyer (Araliaceae). *International Journal of Plant Sciences*, **164**, 189-195. http://dx.doi.org/10.1086/344758

[18] Zhuravlev, Yu.N., Koren, O.G., Reunova, G.D., Artyukova, E.V., Kozyrenko, M.M., Muzarok, T.I. and Kats, I.L. (2004) Ginseng Conservation Program in Russian Primorye: Genetic Structure of Wild and Cultivated Populations. *Journal of Ginseng Research*, **28**, 60-66. http://dx.doi.org/10.5142/JGR.2004.28.1.060

[19] Zhuravlev, Yu.N., Koren, O.G., Reunova, G.D., Muzarok, T.I., Gorpenchenko, T.Yu., Kats, I.L. and Khrolenko, Yu.A. (2008) *Panax ginseng* Natural Populations: Their Past, Current State and Perspectives. *Acta Pharmacologica Sinica*, **29**, 1127-1136. http://dx.doi.org/10.1111/j.1745-7254.2008.00866.x

[20] Zhuravlev, Yu.N., Reunova, G.D., Kats, I.L., Muzarok, T.I. and Bondar, A.A. (2010) Molecular Variation of Wild *Panax ginseng* C.A. Meyer (Araliaceae) by AFLP Markers. *Chinese Medicine*, **5**, 21.

[21] Reunova, G.D., Kats, I.L., Muzarok, T.I. and Zhuravlev, Yu.N. (2010) Polymorphism of RAPD, ISSR and AFLP Markers of the *Panax ginseng* C.A. Meyer (Araliaceae) Genome. *Russian Journal of Genetics*, **46**, 938-947. http://dx.doi.org/10.1134/S1022795410080053

[22] Zhuravlev, Yu.N., Reunova, G.D., Kats, I.L. and Muzarok, T.I. (2012) New Genetic Provisions for the Reinstatement of the Ginseng Natural Populations. In: Amaya, G. and Jimenez, F., Eds., *Genetic Diversity: New Research*, Nova Science Publishers, Inc., New York, 155-176.

[23] Reunova, G.D., Kats, I.L., Muzarok, T.I., Nguen, C.T.P., Dang, T.T. and Zhuravlev, Yu.N. (2012) Population Genetic Structure of Wild-Growing Ginseng (*Panax ginseng* C.A. Meyer) Assessed Using AFLP Markers. *Russian Journal of Genetics*, **48**, 291-301. http://dx.doi.org/10.1134/S1022795412020135

[24] Kalia, R.K., Rai, M.K., Kalia, S., Singh, R. and Dhawan, A.K. (2011) Microsatellite Markers: An Overview of the Recent Progress in Plants. *Euphytica*, **177**, 309-334. http://dx.doi.org/10.1007/s10681-010-0286-9

[25] Kim, J., Jo, B.H., Lee, K.L., Yoon, E.S., Ryu, G.H. and Chung, K.W. (2007) Identification of New Microsatellite Markers in *Panax ginseng*. *Molecules and Cells*, **24**, 60-68.

[26] Dan, N.V., Ramchiary, N., Choi, S.R., Uhm, T.S., Yang, T.J., Ahn, I.O. and Lim, Y.P. (2010) Development and Characterization of New Microsatellite Markers in *Panax ginseng* (C.A. Meyer) from BAC End Sequences. *Conservation Genetics*, **11**, 1223-1225. http://dx.doi.org/10.1007/s10592-009-9924-y

[27] Choi II, H., Kim, N.H., Kim, J.H., Choi, B.S., Ahn, I.O., Lee, J.S. and Yang, T.J. (2011) Development of Reproducible EST-Derived SSR Markers and Assessment of Genetic Diversity in *Panax ginseng* Cultivars and Related Species. *Journal of Ginseng Research*, **35**, 399-412. http://dx.doi.org/10.5142/jgr.2011.35.4.399

[28] Yeh, F.C. and Boyle, T.J.B. (1997) Population Genetic Analysis of Co-Dominant and Dominant Markers and Quantitative Traits. *Belgian Journal of Botany*, **129**, 157.

[29] Weir, B.C. and Cockerham, C.C. (1984) Estimating F-Statistics for the Analysis of Population-Structure. *Evolution*, **38**, 1358-1370. http://dx.doi.org/10.2307/2408641

[30] Goudet, J. (1995) FSTAT (Version 1.2): A Computer Program to Calculate F-Statistics. *Journal of Heredity*, **86**, 485-486.

[31] Raymond, M. and Rousset, F. (1995) Genepop (Version 1.2): Population-Genetics Software for Exact Tests and Ecumenicism. *Journal of Heredity*, **86**, 248-249.

[32] Schneider, S., Roessli, D. and Excoffier, L. (2000) Arlequin ver. 2.000: A Soft Ware for Population Genetic Data Analysis. Genetics and Biometry Laboratory, University of Geneva, Geneva.

[33] Excoffier, L., Smouse, P.E. and Quattro, J.M. (1992) Analysis of Molecular Variance Inferred from Metric Distances among DNA Haplotypes: Application to Human Mitochondrial DNA Restriction Data. *Genetics*, **131**, 479-491.

[34] Peakall, R. and Smouse, P.E. (2006) GENALEX 6: Genetic Analysis in Excel. Population Genetic Software for

Teaching and Research. *Molecular Ecology Notes*, **6**, 288-295. http://dx.doi.org/10.1111/j.1471-8286.2005.01155.x

[35] Cavalli-Sforza, L.L. and Edwards, A.W.F. (1967) Phylogenetic Analysis Models and Estimation Procedures. *American Journal of Human Genetics*, **19**, 233-257.

[36] Rohlf, F.J. (1993) NTSYS-Pc. Numerical Taxonomy and Multivariate Analysis System, Ver.1.80. Exeter Publishing LTD, New York.

[37] Takezaki, N. and Nei, M. (1996) Genetic Distances and Reconstruction of Phylogenetic Trees from Microsatellite DNA. *Genetics*, **144**, 389-399.

[38] Pritchard, J.K., Stephens, P. and Donnelly, P. (2000) Inference of Population Structure Using Multilocus Genotype Data. *Genetics*, **155**, 945-959.

[39] Pritchard, J.K., Wen, X.Q. and Falush, D. (2007) STRUCTURE ver. 2.2. University of Chicago. http://pritch.bsd.uchicago.edu/software

[40] Artyukova, E.V., Kozyrenko, M.M., Koren, O.G., Kholina, A.B., Nakonechnaya, O.V. and Zhuravlev, Yu.N. (2012) Living on the Edge: Various Modes of Persistence at the Range Margins for Some Far Eastern Species. In: Galiskan, M., Ed., *Genetic Diversity in Plant*, InTech, Rijeka, 349-374. http://dx.doi.org/10.5772/35032

[41] Jo, B.H., Suh, D.S., Cho, E.M., Kim, J., Ryu, G.H. and Chung, K.W. (2009) Characterization of Polymorphic Microsatellite Loci in Cultivated and Wild *Panax ginseng. Genes & Genomics*, **31**, 119-127. http://dx.doi.org/10.1007/BF03191145

[42] Park, S.W., Hyun, Y.S. and Chung, K.W. (2009) Genetic Polymorphism of Microsatellite Markers in *Panax ginseng* C.A. Meyer. *Journal of Ginseng Research*, **33**, 199-205. http://dx.doi.org/10.5142/JGR.2009.33.3.199

[43] Liu, H., Xia, T., Zuo, Y.J., Chen, Z.J. and Zhou, S.L. (2011) Development and Characterization of Microsatellite Markers for *Panax notoginseng* (Araliaceae), a Chinese Traditional Herb. *American Journal of Botany*, **98**, e218-e220. http://dx.doi.org/10.3732/ajb.1100043

[44] Reunova, G.D., Kats, I.L., Muzarok, T.I., Nguyen, T.T.P., Dang, T.T., Brenner, E.V. and Zhuravlev, Yu.N. (2011) Diversity of Microsatellite Loci in the *Panax vietnamensis* Ha et Grushv. (Araliaceae) Population. *Doklady Biological Sciences*, **441**, 408-411. http://dx.doi.org/10.1134/S0012496611060184

[45] Petit, R.J., Mousadik, E.I. and Pons, O. (1998) Identifying Populations for Conservation on the Basis of Genetic Markers. *Conservation Biology*, **12**, 844-855. http://dx.doi.org/10.1046/j.1523-1739.1998.96489.x

[46] Koren, O.G., Krylach, T.Yu., Zaytseva, Yu.A. and Zhuravlev, Yu.N. (1998) Floral Biology and Embryology of *Panax ginseng* C.A. Meyer. *Proceedings of the* 1*st European Ginseng Congress*, Marburg, 6-11 December 1998, 221-231.

[47] Stoeckel, S., Grange, J., Fernandes-Manjarres, J.F., Bilger, I., Frascaria-Lacoste, N. and Mariette, S. (2006) Heterozygote Excess in a Self-Incompatible and Partially Clonal Forest Tree Species-*Prunus avium* L. *Molecular Ecology*, **15**, 2109-2118. http://dx.doi.org/10.1111/j.1365-294X.2006.02926.x

[48] Ford, B.A., McQueen, D.A.R., Naczi, R.F.C. and Reznicek, A. (1998) Allozyme Variation and Genetic Relationships among Species in the *Carex willdenowii* Complex (Cyperaceae). *American Journal of Botany*, **85**, 546-552. http://dx.doi.org/10.2307/2446439

[49] Cabrera-Toledo, D., Gonzalez-Astorga, J. and Vovides, A.P. (2008) Heterozygote Excess in Ancient Populations of the Critically Endangered *Dioon caputoi* (Zamiaceae, Cycadales) from Central Mexico. *Botanical Journal of the Linnean Society*, **158**, 436-447. http://dx.doi.org/10.1111/j.1095-8339.2008.00868.x

[50] Koren, O.G. and Muzarok, T.I. (2010) Nature of Polyploidy in Two *Panax* Species (*Panax ginseng* and *Panax quinquefolius*) Inferred from Allozyme Data. *Proceedings of Cold Spring Harbor Asia Conference from Plant Biology to Crop Biotechnology*, New York, **1**, 58.

[51] Hedrick, P.W. (1999) Perspective: Highly Variable Loci and Their Interpretation in Evolution and Conservation. *Evolution*, **53**, 313-318. http://dx.doi.org/10.2307/2640768

[52] Evanno, G., Regnaut, S. and Goudet, J. (2005) Detecting the Number of Clusters of Individuals Using the Software Structure: A Simulation Study. *Molecular Ecology*, **14**, 2611-2620. http://dx.doi.org/10.1111/j.1365-294X.2005.02553.x

[53] He, T., Krauss, S.L., Lamont, B.B., Miller, B.P. and Enright, N.J. (2004) Long-Distance Seed Dispersal in a Metapopulation of *Banskia hookeriana* Inferred from a Population Allocation Analysis of Amplified Fragment Length Polymorphism Data. *Molecular Ecology*, **13**, 1099-1109. http://dx.doi.org/10.1111/j.1365-294X.2004.02120.x

[54] McVean, G.A.T. (2002) A Genealogical Interpretation of Linkage Disequilibrium. *Genetics*, **162**, 987-991.

[55] Peters, M.D., (Jenny) Xiang, Q.Y., Thomas, D.T., Stucky, J. and Whiteman, N.K. (2009) Genetic Analyses of the Federally Endangered *Echinaceae laevigata* Using Amplified Fragment Length Polymorphisms (AFLP)—Inferences in Population Genetic Structure and Mating System. *Conservation Genetics*, **10**, 1-14.

http://dx.doi.org/10.1007/s10592-008-9509-1

[56] Campbell, D., Duchesne, P. and Bernatchez, L. (2003) AFLP Utility for Population Assignment Studies: Analytical Investigation and Empirical Comparison with Microsatellites. *Molecular Ecology*, **12**, 1979-1991. http://dx.doi.org/10.1046/j.1365-294X.2003.01856.x

Permissions

All chapters in this book were first published in CM, by Scientific Research Publishing; hereby published with permission under the Creative Commons Attribution License or equivalent. Every chapter published in this book has been scrutinized by our experts. Their significance has been extensively debated. The topics covered herein carry significant findings which will fuel the growth of the discipline. They may even be implemented as practical applications or may be referred to as a beginning point for another development.

The contributors of this book come from diverse backgrounds, making this book a truly international effort. This book will bring forth new frontiers with its revolutionizing research information and detailed analysis of the nascent developments around the world.

We would like to thank all the contributing authors for lending their expertise to make the book truly unique. They have played a crucial role in the development of this book. Without their invaluable contributions this book wouldn't have been possible. They have made vital efforts to compile up to date information on the varied aspects of this subject to make this book a valuable addition to the collection of many professionals and students.

This book was conceptualized with the vision of imparting up-to-date information and advanced data in this field. To ensure the same, a matchless editorial board was set up. Every individual on the board went through rigorous rounds of assessment to prove their worth. After which they invested a large part of their time researching and compiling the most relevant data for our readers.

The editorial board has been involved in producing this book since its inception. They have spent rigorous hours researching and exploring the diverse topics which have resulted in the successful publishing of this book. They have passed on their knowledge of decades through this book. To expedite this challenging task, the publisher supported the team at every step. A small team of assistant editors was also appointed to further simplify the editing procedure and attain best results for the readers.

Apart from the editorial board, the designing team has also invested a significant amount of their time in understanding the subject and creating the most relevant covers. They scrutinized every image to scout for the most suitable representation of the subject and create an appropriate cover for the book.

The publishing team has been an ardent support to the editorial, designing and production team. Their endless efforts to recruit the best for this project, has resulted in the accomplishment of this book. They are a veteran in the field of academics and their pool of knowledge is as vast as their experience in printing. Their expertise and guidance has proved useful at every step. Their uncompromising quality standards have made this book an exceptional effort. Their encouragement from time to time has been an inspiration for everyone.

The publisher and the editorial board hope that this book will prove to be a valuable piece of knowledge for researchers, students, practitioners and scholars across the globe.

List of Contributors

Mahsa Hadipour Jahromy
Department of Pharmacology, Tehran Medical Sciences Branch, Islamic Azad University, Tehran, Iran

Shahrzad Khakpour
Department of Physiology, Tehran Medical Sciences Branch, Islamic Azad University, Tehran, Iran

Zhinoos Khorgami
Iranian Tissue Bank and Research Center, Tehran University of Medical Sciences, Tehran, Iran

Sonya K. Sobrian
Department of Pharmacology, Howard University College of Medicine, Washington, USA

Eric Walters
Department of Biochemistry and Molecular Biology, Howard University College of Medicine, Washington, USA

Peishan Xie and Longgang Guo
Guangdong UNION Biotechnology Development Co., Ltd., Guangzhou, China

Yu Zhao
Nikyang Enterprise Co., Ltd., Hong Kong, China

Daniel Bensky
Independent Scholar, Seattle, USA

Erich Stoeger
Plantasia GmbH, Oberndorf, Austria

Azadeh Shariatifar, Mahdieh Riazi, Mona Ebnolelm and Mahsa Hadipour Jahromy
Department of Pharmacology, Medical Sciences Research Center, Tehran Medical Sciences Branch, Islamic Azad University, Tehran, Iran

Zeeshan Ahmed Sheikh, Aqib Zahoor and Saleha Suleman Khan
Department of Research and Development, Herbion Pakistan (Pvt.) Limited, 30/28 Korangi Industrial Area, Karachi, Pakistan

Khan Usmanghani
Department of Research and Development, Herbion Pakistan (Pvt.) Limited, 30/28 Korangi Industrial Area, Karachi, Pakistan
Faculty of Pharmacy, Jinnah University for Women, Karachi, Pakistan

Dalin Song
Department of Geriatric Cardiology, Geriatric Institute, Qingdao Municipal Hospital, Qingdao, China Qingdao University, Qingdao, China

Tongliang Han and Hua Zhang
Department of Geriatric Cardiology, Geriatric Institute, Qingdao Municipal Hospital, Qingdao, China

Tao Tian
Department of Geriatric Cardiology, Linyi People's Hospital, Linyi, China

Mengfen Hu and Yongjun Mao
Qingdao University, Qingdao, China

Li Lei, Ching Wo Tung and Kwai Ching Lo
School of Chinese Medicine, The University of Hong Kong, Hong Kong, China

Oroma B. Nwanodi and Melanie M. Tidman
Department of Interdisciplinary Health Studies, A. T. Still University Arizona School of Health Sciences, Mesa, USA

Yongxing Yan, Lizhen Liang, Yonghui Shen and Yanjing Cao
Department of Neurology, The Third People's Hospital of Hangzhou, Hangzhou, China

Tao Xie
Department of Neurology, University of Chicago Medicine, Chicago, USA

Xiaozhen Fu, Dan Shi, Chao Qu and Guangying Zhong
College of Life Sciences, Liaoning Normal University, Dalian, China

Wei Zou
College of Life Sciences, Liaoning Normal University, Dalian, China
Liaoning Key Laboratories of Biotechnology and Molecular Drug Research and Development, Dalian, China

Jing Liu
The First Affiliated Hospital, Dalian Medical University, Dalian, China

Pou Kuan Leong, Hoi Yan Leung, Hoi Shan Wong, Ji Hang Chen, Wing Man Chan and Kam Ming Ko
Division of Life Science, Hong Kong University of Science and Technology, Hong Kong, China

Chung Wah Ma and Yi Ting Yang
Infinitus (China) Company Ltd., Guangzhou, China

Bo Shuai, Yanping Yang, Lin Shen and Manxiang Wu
Department of Integrated Traditional Chinese and Western Medicine, Union Hospital, Tongji Medical College, Huazhong University of Science and Technology, Wuhan, China

Muhammad Shakil Ahmad Siddiqui
Rafah-e-Aam Dawakhana Ajmali (Clinics) and Rafah-e-Aam Herbal Laboratories, Karachi, Pakistan
Faculty of Eastern Medicine, Hamdard University, Karachi, Pakistan

Khan Usmanghani
Faculty of Eastern Medicine, Hamdard University, Karachi, Pakistan

Khakpour Shahrzad and Mahsa Hadipour Jahromy
Tehran Medical Sciences Branch, Physiology and Pharmacology Research Laboratories of Medical Sciences Research Centre, Islamic Azad University, Tehran, Iran

Najari Mahya, Tokazabani Belasei Fatemeh and Khosravi Maryam
Tehran North Branch, Islamic Azad University, Tehran, Iran

Farhadi Belasei Mohammadreza
Ghazvin Medical Sciences University, Ghazvin, Iran

Xiuming Cui and Jingjing Yang
College of Life Science and Technology, Kunming University of Science and Technology, Kunming, China

Hui Xiao, Yuqin Sun and Yan Zhu
Wenshan Sanqi Research Institute, Wenshan College, Wenshan, China

Tina Dong and Karl Wah-Keung Tsim
Department of Biology and Biotechnology Research Institute, The Hong Kong University of Science and Technology, Hong Kong, China

Electra Peluffo
Faculty of Medicine, Universidad de Valencia, Valencia, Spain

Guohua Lin, Xushan Cha and Qian Li
The First Affiliated Hospital of Guangzhou University of Traditional Chinese Medicine, Guangzhou, China

Yunkuan Yang
Chengdu University of Traditional Chinese Medicine, Chengdu, China

Hongxing Zhang
Wuhan NO.1 Hospital, Wuhan, China

Lixia Li and Chuyun Chen
Guangzhou Hospital of Traditional Chinese Medicine, Guangzhou, China

Yue Liu
The Second Hospital of Traditional Chinese Medicine of Guangdong Province, Guangzhou, China

Pou Kuan Leong, Hoi Yan Leung, Wing Man Chan, Ji Hang Chen, Hoi Shan Wong and Kam Ming Ko
Division of Life Science, The Hong Kong University of Science & Technology, Hong Kong SAR, China

Chung Wah Ma, Shi Yu Zou
Infinitus (China) Company Ltd., Guangzhou, China

Fan Zhao, Xudong Liu, Wenjun Liu, Jiyan Cai, Lingzhi Wang, Huaxin Yu, Lu Wang, Lide Zhang, Deshan Wang and Dehong Shan
Liaoning University of Traditional Chinese Medicine, Shenyang, China

Bo Shuai, Yanping Yang, Lin Shen and Hui Ke
Department of Integrated Traditional Chinese and Western Medicine, Union Hospital, Tongji Medical College, Huazhong University of Science and Technology, Wuhan, China

Bing Yan and Man Guo
School of Life Sciences and Technical, Mudanjiang Normal University, Mudanjiang, China

Liping Zhao
School of Life Sciences, University of Science and Technology of China, Hefei, China

Liang Zhang, Changming Li and Shangju Xie
Research Institute of Orthopedics, Zhejiang Chinese Medical University, Hangzhou, China

Renfu Quan
Department of Orthopedics, Xiaoshan Traditional Chinese Medical Hospital, Hangzhou, China

Pei Yang, Hong Zhou and Hui Yao
Institute of Medicinal Plant Development, Chinese Academy of Medical Sciences and Peking Union Medical

Xiwen Li
Institute of Medicinal Plant Development, Chinese Academy of Medical Sciences and Peking Union Medical College, Beijing, China
Institute of Chinese Materia Medica, China Academy of Chinese Medical Sciences, Beijing, China

Hao Hu and Yitao Wang
State Key Laboratory of Quality Research in Chinese Medicine, Institute of Chinese Medical Sciences, University of Macau, Macau, China

Hui Zhang
Development Center of Traditional Chinese Medicine and Bioengineering, Changchun University of Chinese Medicine, Changchun, China

Wei Sun
Institute of Chinese Materia Medica, China Academy of Chinese Medical Sciences, Beijing, China

Allah Nawaz
Research and Development Department, Herbion Pakistan (Pvt.) Limited, Karachi, Pakistan
First Department of Internal Medicine, Faculty of Medicine, Graduate School of Medical & Pharmaceutical Sciences, University of Toyama, Toyama, Japan

Saira Bano, Zeeshan Ahmed Sheikh and Aqib Zahoor
Research and Development Department, Herbion Pakistan (Pvt.) Limited, Karachi, Pakistan

Khan Usmanghani
Research and Development Department, Herbion Pakistan (Pvt.) Limited, Karachi, Pakistan Jinnah University for Women, Karachi, Pakisntan

Iqbal Ahmad
Baqai Institute of Pharmaceutical Sciences, Baqai Medical University, Karachi, Pakistan

Syed Faisal Zaidi
Department of Basic Medical Sciences, College of Medicine, King Saud bin Abdulaziz University of Health Sciences, Jeddah, KSA

Irshad Ahmad
Department of Pharmacy, The Islamia University of Bahawalpur, Bahawalpur, Pakistan
Clinical Pharmacy and Health Care, Jinnah University for Women, Karachi, Pakistan

Zeli Gao
Department of Gastroenterology, People's Hospital of Pudong New Area, Shanghai, China

Cheng Zhang, Liwen Jin and Wei Yao
Department of Gastroenterology, Zhoupu Hospital, Pudong New Area, Shanghai, China

Longgang Guo, Peishan Xie and Ruiyin Wang
Guangdong UNION Biochemical Development Co. Ltd., Guangzhou, China

Shuai Sun
Guangdong ImVin Pharmaceutical Co. Ltd., Guangzhou, China

He Li
Guangdong UNION Biochemical Development Co. Ltd., Guangzhou, China
Livzon Group Pharmaceutical Factory, Zhuhai, China

Xinjun Xu
School of Pharmaceutical Sciences, Sun Yat-sen University, Guangzhou, China

Sheeraz Siddiqui
Faculty of Eastern Medicine, Hamdard University, Karachi, Pakistan

Khan Usmanghani
Faculty of Eastern Medicine, Hamdard University, Karachi, Pakistan
Research and Development Department, Herbion Pakistan (Pvt.) Limited, Karachi, Pakistan

Aqib Zahoor, Zeeshan Ahmed Sheikh and Saleha Suleman Khan
Research and Development Department, Herbion Pakistan (Pvt.) Limited, Karachi, Pakistan

Daoming Liang, Yi Zhang, Jiayong Chen, Hua Wang and Tao Huang, Xin Xue
Gastrointestinal Surgery Department, Second Affiliated Hospital of Kunming Medical University, Kunming, China

Simao Xu, Weichun Liu and Minhua Li
Department of Physical Education, Guangxi Normal University, Guilin, China

Electra Peluffo
Faculty of Medicine, Universidad de Valencia, Valencia, Spain

Galina D. Reunova, Olga G. Koren, Tamara I. Muzarok and Yury N. Zhuravlev
Department of Biotechnology, Institute of Biology and Soil Science, Far Eastern Branch of the Russian Academy of Sciences, Vladivostok, Russia